# Atlas of
# INFECTIOUS DISEASES

## Volume VIII

## EXTERNAL MANIFESTATIONS OF SYSTEMIC INFECTIONS

Editor-in-Chief

## Gerald L. Mandell, MD

Professor of Medicine
Owen R. Cheatham Professor of the Sciences
Chief, Division of Infectious Diseases
University of Virginia Health Sciences Center
Charlottesville, Virginia

Editor

## Robert Fekety, MD

Professor Emeritus of Internal Medicine
University of Michigan Medical School
Ann Arbor, Michigan

*With 27 contributors*

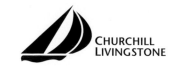

CHURCHILL
LIVINGSTONE

DEVELOPED BY CURRENT MEDICINE, INC.
PHILADELPHIA

## CURRENT MEDICINE
### 400 MARKET STREET, SUITE 700
### PHILADELPHIA, PA 19106

**Library of Congress Cataloging-in-Publication Data**

External manifestations of systemic infections / editor-in-chief, Gerald L. Mandell, editor, Robert Fekety; developed by Current Medicine, Inc.
     p. cm.—(Atlas of infectious diseases; v. 8)
  Includes bibliographical references and index.
  ISBN 0-443-07760-6 (hardcover)
  1. Communicable diseases—Atlases. I. Mandell, Gerald L.
II. Fekety, F. Robert. III. Current Medicine, Inc. IV. Series.
  [DNLM: 1. Communicable Diseases—diagnosis—atlases. WC 17 E93 1997]
RC113.2.E98 1997
616.9—dc20
DNLM/DLC
for Library of Congress
          96-15291
          CIP

| | |
|---|---|
| Development Editors: | Lee Tevebaugh and Michael Bokulich |
| Editorial Assistant: | Elena Coler |
| Art Director: | Paul Fennessy |
| Design and Layout: | Patrick Ward and Lisa Weischedel |
| Illustration Director: | Ann Saydlowski |
| Illustrators: | Elizabeth Carrozza, Beth Starkey, and Gary Welch |
| Production: | David Myers and Lori Holland |
| Managing Editor: | Lori J. Bainbridge |
| Indexer: | Ann Cassar |

Printed in Hong Kong by Paramount Printing Group Limited.

10 9 8 7 6 5 4 3 2 1

# PREFACE

The diagnosis and management of patients with infectious diseases are based in large part on visual clues. Skin and mucous membrane lesions, eye findings, imaging studies, Gram stains, culture plates, insect vectors, preparations of blood, urine, pus, cerebrospinal fluid, and biopsy specimens are studied to establish the proper diagnosis and to choose the most effective therapy. The *Atlas of Infectious Diseases* is a modern, complete collection of these images. Current Medicine, with its capability of superb color reproduction and its state-of-the-art computer imaging facilities, is the ideal publisher for the atlas. Infectious diseases physicians, scientists, microbiologists, and pathologists frequently teach other health-care professionals, and this comprehensive atlas with available slides is an effective teaching tool.

Dr. Robert Fekety is a master teacher, clinician, and investigator with a wealth of experience in all aspects of infectious disease. He and his expert contributors have put together a uniquely useful volume. Systemic and generalized infections may present with overt or subtle external manifestations. This volume presents these manifestations in a format that will be very useful for a broad range of clinicians, educators, and researchers.

**Gerald L. Mandell, MD**
Charlottesville, Virginia

# CONTRIBUTORS

**Donald Armstrong, MD**

*Professor of Medicine*
*Cornell University Medical College*
*Chief, Infectious Diseases Service*
*Department of Medicine*
*Memorial Sloan-Kettering Cancer Center*
*New York, New York*

**Neil Barg, MD**

*Associate Professor of Medicine*
*University of Michigan Medical School*
*Assistant Chief of Infectious Diseases*
*Department of Veterans Affairs Medical Center, Ann Arbor*
*Ann Arbor, Michigan*

**Bruce H. Clements, MD**

*Chief, Clinical Branch*
*Gillis W. Long Hansen's Disease Center*
*Carville, Louisiana*

**Adnan S. Dajani, MD**

*Professor of Pediatrics*
*Wayne State University School of Medicine*
*Director, Infectious Diseases*
*Children's Hospital of Michigan*
*Detroit, Michigan*

**J. Steven Dumler, MD**

*Associate Professor of Pathology, Microbiology, and*
  *Immunology*
*Division of Medical Microbiology*
*The Johns Hopkins University School of Medicine*
*Director, Division of Medical Microbiology*
*The Johns Hopkins Medical Institutions*
*Baltimore, Maryland*

**Janine Evans, MD**

*Assistant Professor of Internal Medicine*
*Yale University School of Medicine*
*New Haven, Connecticut*

**Thomas G. Evans, MD**

*Associate Professor of Internal Medicine*
*Division of Infectious Diseases*
*University of Rochester School of Medicine*
*Rochester, New York*

**Patricia Ferrieri, MD**

*Professor of Laboratory Medicine & Pathology*
  *and Pediatrics*
*University of Minnesota Medical School*
*Director, Clinical Microbiology Laboratory*
*University of Minnesota Hospital*
*Minneapolis, Minnesota*

**Janet R. Gilsdorf, MD**

*Professor of Pediatrics and Communicable Diseases*
*University of Michigan Medical School*
*Director, Pediatric Infectious Diseases*
*University of Michigan Hospital*
*Ann Arbor, Michigan*

**Barney Graham, MD, PhD**

*Associate Professor of Medicine*
*Director of Vaccine Program*
*Vanderbilt University School of Medicine*
*Nashville, Tennessee*

**Clark Gregg, MD**

*Associate Professor of Medicine*
*University of Texas Southwestern*
*Chief of Infectious Diseases*
*Department of Veterans Affairs Medical Center, Dallas*
*Dallas, Texas*

**David Gregory, MD**

*Associate Professor of Medicine*
*Vanderbilt University School of Medicine*
*Chief of Outpatient Services*
*Department of Veterans Affairs Medical Center, Nashville*
*Nashville, Tennessee*

**Carol A. Kauffman, MD**

*Professor of Internal Medicine*
*University of Michigan Medical School*
*Chief, Infectious Diseases Section*
*Veterans Affairs Medical Center*
*Ann Arbor, Michigan*

**Philip E. LeBoit, MD**

*Associate Professor of Clinical Pathology and Dermatology*
*Director of Dermatology Service*
*University of California, San Francisco*
*San Francisco, California*

**Stephen Malawista, MD**

*Professor of Medicine*
*Section of Rheumatology*
*Department of Internal Medicine*
*Yale University School of Medicine*
*New Haven, Connecticut*

**Steven M. Opal, MD**

*Associate Professor of Medicine*
*Department of Internal Medicine*
*Brown University*
*Providence, Rhode Island*
*Staff Physician*
*Memorial Hospital of Rhode Island*
*Pawtucket, Rhode Island*

**Richard D. Pearson, MD**
*Professor of Medicine and Pathology*
*University of Virginia School of Medicine*
*Attending Physician*
*University of Virginia Health Sciences Center*
*Charlottesville, Virginia*

**David H. Persing, MD, PhD**
*Associate Professor of Microbiology and Laboratory Medicine*
*Mayo Medical School*
*Director, Molecular Microbiology Laboratories*
*Director, Legionella and Lyme Serology Laboratories*
*Mayo Clinic*
*Rochester, Minnesota*

**C.J. Peters, MD**
*Chief, Special Pathogens Branch*
*Division of Viral and Rickettsial Diseases*
*Centers for Disease Control and Prevention*
*Atlanta, Georgia*

**D.A. Relman, MD**
*Assistant Professor of Medicine and Microbiology &*
  *Immunology*
*Stanford University School of Medicine*
*Stanford, California*
*Staff Physician*
*Veterans Affairs Palo Alto Health Care System*
*Palo Alto, California*

**P.E. Rollin, MD**
*Chief, Pathogenesis and Immunology Section*
*Special Pathogens Branch*
*Division of Viral and Rickettsial Diseases*
*Centers for Disease Control and Prevention*
*Atlanta, Georgia*

**W. Michael Scheld, MD**
*Professor of Medicine and Neurosurgery*
*Department of Medicine*
*University of Virginia School of Medicine*
*Attending Physician*
*University of Virginia Health Sciences Center*
*Charlottesville, Virginia*

**David M. Scollard, MD, PhD**
*Associate Professor of Pathology*
*Louisiana State University School of Medicine*
*New Orleans, Louisiana*
*Chief of Pathology*
*Gillis W. Long Hansen's Disease Center*
*Carville, Louisiana*

**Thomas Shope, MD**
*Associate Professor of Pediatrics and Communicable*
  *Diseases*
*University of Michigan Medical School*
*Staff Physician*
*University of Michigan Hospitals*
*Ann Arbor, Michigan*

**Anastacio de Q. Sousa, MD**
*Associate Professor of Medicine*
*Universidade Federal de Ceará*
*Núcleo de Medicina Tropical*
*Fortaleza, Ceará*
*Brazil*

**S.R. Zaki, MD, PhD**
*Chief, Molecular Pathology and Ultrastructure Activity*
*Division of Viral and Rickettsial Diseases*
*Centers for Disease Control and Prevention*
*Atlanta, Georgia*

**Stephen H. Zinner, MD**
*Professor and Interim Chairman*
*Director, Division of Infectious Diseases*
*Department of Medicine*
*Brown University School of Medicine*
*Director, Division of Infectious Diseases*
*Roger Williams Medical Center and Rhode Island Hospital*
*Providence, Rhode Island*

# CONTENTS

## Chapter 9
# Leprosy

Bruce H. Clements and David M. Scollard

## Chapter 10
# Viral Hemorrhagic Fevers

C.J. Peters, S.R. Zaki, and
P.E. Rollin

## Chapter 11
# Systemic Fungal Infections

Carol A. Kauffman

## Chapter 12
# Manifestations of Protozoal and Helminthic Diseases in Latin America

Anastacio de Q. Sousa, Thomas G. Evans, and
Richard D. Pearson

## Chapter 13
# Cutaneous Manifestations of Infection in the Immunocompromised Host

Donald Armstrong

# Index

# CHAPTER 1

# Viral Exanthems of Childhood

Janet R. Gilsdorf
Thomas Shope

### Six classic exanthems of childhood

| | |
|---|---|
| First disease | Measles (rubeola) |
| Second disease | Scarlet fever |
| Third disease | German measles (rubella) |
| Fourth disease | Filatov-Dukes |
| Fifth disease | Erythema infectiosum |
| Sixth disease | Exanthem subitum (roseola) |

**FIGURE 1-1** Six classic exanthems of childhood. In the past, six patterns of erythematous rashes in childhood were described, with little understanding of the mechanisms of the rash or cause of the illnesses. Now, we know that most of the classic rash illnesses are viral in origin, although the rashes associated with some of these viral infections (fifth and sixth diseases) reflect immune responses to the virus. Furthermore, the rash of second disease is caused by a bacterial toxin. In recent times, fourth disease is not considered to be a distinct entity.

### Differential diagnosis of viral-type exanthems in children

Viral infections
  Rubella
  Rubeola
  Enterovirus
  Exanthem subitum (roseola)
  Adenovirus
  Infectious mononucleosis
  Dengue
  Erythema infectiosum (parvovirus B16)
Bacterial and parasitic infections
  Toxoplasmosis
  Meningococcemia
  Scarlet fever
  Rickettsia
Noninfectious causes
  Serum sickness
  Kawasaki disease
  Drug rash

**FIGURE 1-2** Differential diagnosis of viral-type exanthems in children. The conditions listed in this figure may present with maculopapular rashes and must be distinguished by their other clinical and laboratory features.

# ERYTHEMA INFECTIOSUM (FIFTH DISEASE)

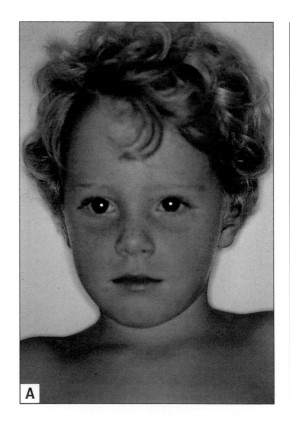

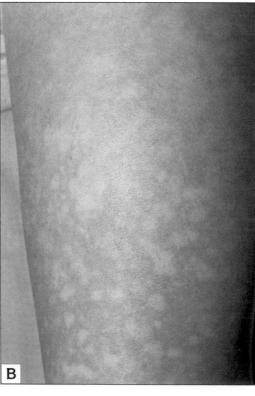

A

B

**FIGURE 1-3** Cutaneous rash of erythema infectiosum. **A,** The initial cutaneous manifestation of erythema infectiosum, which occurs during the recovery phase of the infection and is thought to be immunologically mediated, is a malar flush, giving the characteristic appearance of "slapped cheeks" and circumoral pallor. **B,** The macular erythematous rash then spreads to the arms, trunk, and extremities, where it may fade with a reticulated or lacy pattern.

## Clinical features of erythema infectiosum (fifth disease)

| | |
|---|---|
| Etiology | Parvovirus B19 |
| Incubation period | 4–14 days |
| Epidemiology | Outbreaks in elementary and junior high schools |
| | Household spread common |
| Nature of rash | Symmetric, intensely red, flushed "slapped cheeks" appearance, with caudal spread to arms, trunk, buttocks, and thighs, often in a reticular pattern |
| | Macular erythemic rash may be intermittent, recurring over several months |
| | Rash may fluctuate in intensity depending on environmental conditions, such as temperature, sun exposure, exercise, and stress |
| Other signs and symptoms | Low-grade fever in 15%–30% of patients |
| | Prodrome of mild headache and URI symptoms |
| | Arthritis and arthralgias, more common in adult women |
| | Infection during early pregnancy may result in fetal hydrops and death |
| Laboratory findings | Aplastic crisis in patients with high red cell turnover |
| | Elevated parvovirus-specific IgM antibody during illness |

URI—upper respiratory infection.

**FIGURE 1-4** Clinical features of erythema infectiosum. Erythema infectiosum (fifth disease) is caused by the DNA-containing parvovirus B19, which infects primarily erythroid precursors. Although principally an infection of school-aged children, the virus may cause illness in people of all ages, from fetuses to the elderly.

# ROSEOLA

## Clinical features of roseola infantum

| | |
|---|---|
| Etiology | Human herpesvirus 6 |
| Incubation period | Approximately 9 days |
| Epidemiology | Highest attack rate in children 6–24 mos of age |
| | Rare below age 3 mos and above age 4 yrs |
| | Secondary cases rare |
| | No seasonal pattern |
| Nature of rash | Immediately follows defervescence |
| | Erythematous maculopapular eruption starting on trunk and spreading to face and legs |
| | Rash is temporally associated with appearance of circulating neutralizing antibody |
| Other signs and symptoms | Fever to 42° C for 1–7 days |
| | Seizures in 5%–35% of patients |
| | Adenopathy |
| | Respiratory symptoms |
| | Mild diarrhea |
| | Papular pharyngitis |
| Laboratory findings | Occasional absolute neutropenia and lymphocytosis |

**FIGURE 1-5** Clinical features of roseola infantum. Roseola infantum (sixth disease) is caused by human herpesvirus 6 (HHV-6). Roseola-like illness, however, has been associated with enteroviruses, adenoviruses, and parvovirus B19. The illness typically occurs in infants 6 to 24 months of age and is characterized by sudden onset of fever and irritability lasting 3 to 5 days, followed by rapid return to normal temperature and the appearance of an erythematous maculopapular rash lasting 1 to 2 days.

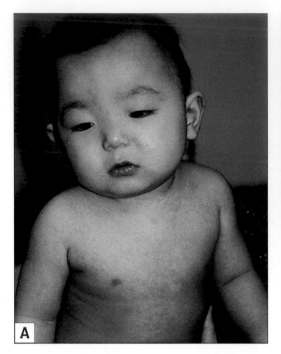
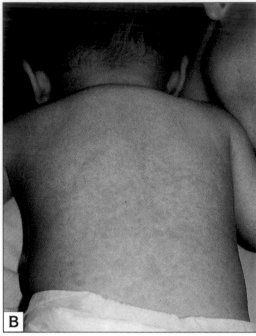

FIGURE 1-6  **A** and **B**, An erythematous maculopapular rash appearing on the face, trunk, and back of a young child. The rash disappears after 1 to 2 days. The child is generally happy and playful during the rash, which results from the host immune response to the virus.

# MEASLES (RUBEOLA)

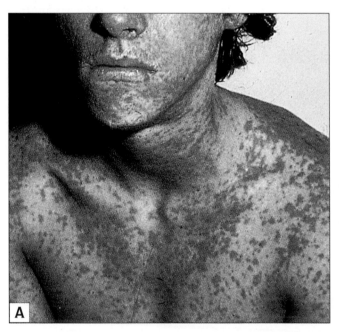
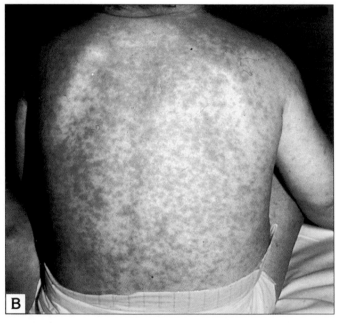

FIGURE 1-7  **A** and **B**, Typical erythematous maculopapular rash of measles. Measles is an acute febrile infection caused by the rubeola virus and characterized by a prodrome of fever and upper respiratory symptoms followed by the characteristic measles exanthem. The rash, which is erythematous and maculopapular, usually begins on the head and spreads downward to involve the trunk and upper and lower extremities.

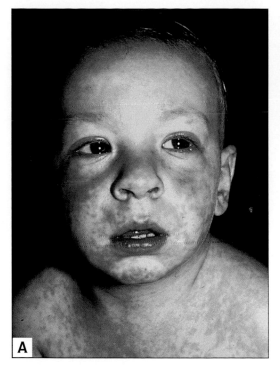

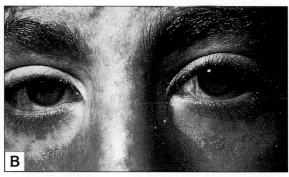

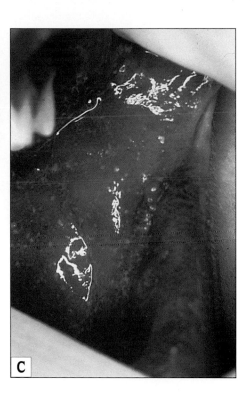

**FIGURE 1-8** Additional clinical manifestations of measles. In addition to the characteristic rash, children with measles experience a variety of other symptoms. **A,** Children appear systemically ill with high fever, malaise, rhinitis, and congestion. **B,** Characteristic features include conjunctivitis with excess lacrimation and eyelid edema. **C,** In some patients, an enanthem, Koplik spots, appears as white specks on the red buccal mucosa near the opening of Stenson's duct. Koplik spots appear 1 or 2 days before the rash and fade as the rash progresses.

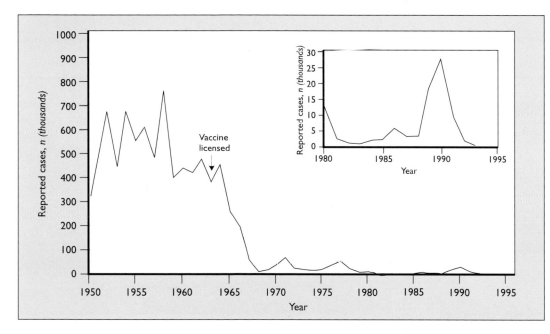

**FIGURE 1-9** Annual incidence of measles in the United States between 1950 and 1993. The introduction of the live, attenuated measles vaccine in 1963 resulted in a dramatic decline in reported measles cases in the United States. The increased incidence of cases in 1989 and 1990 led to the recognition that vaccine-induced immunity wanes over time, especially in a highly vaccinated area where endemic measles does not result in natural boosting, and to the recommendation that a booster immunization be administered either at entry into kindergarten or middle school. (*From* Centers for Disease Control and Prevention [1].)

## Clinical features of measles (rubeola)

| | |
|---|---|
| Etiology | Rubeola virus |
| Incubation period | 8–12 days |
| Epidemiology | Since introduction of the vaccine, measles may be seen in susceptible individuals of all ages |
| | Highly contagious |
| | Transmission via infected respiratory droplets |
| Nature of eruption | Maculopapular rash appears first along hairline, on the neck, and behind the ears; it rapidly spreads over the entire face and proceeds downward, involving the upper arms and chest, trunk, and lower extremities |
| | Occasionally, rash may be urticarial, slightly hemorrhagic, or frankly purpuric |
| Other signs and symptoms | Koplik spots on buccal mucosa before rash erupts |
| | High fever, cough, coryza, conjunctivitis beginning before appearance of rash |
| | Rubeola-specific IgM antibodies detectable days 2–60 after rash appears |
| Laboratory findings | Virus may be isolated from nasopharyngeal secretions, conjunctiva, blood, and urine during acute illness |

**FIGURE 1-10** Clinical features of measles. Measles is a vaccine-preventable acute disease characterized by fever, cough, coryza, conjunctivitis, and an erythematous maculopapular rash.

| Complications of measles |
| --- |
| Otitis media |
| Pneumonia |
| Encephalitis (with residual mental retardation, blindness) |

**FIGURE 1-11** Complications of measles. Before introduction of the measles vaccine, death and serious sequelae from measles were common.

| Prevention of measles |
| --- |
| Active immunization |
|   Rubeola-containing (live virus) vaccine (*ie*, MMR) |
|   Two doses: ages 12–15 mos and prekindergarten or entry into |
|     middle school |
| Passive immunization |
|   Immune serum globulin (0.5 mL/kg intramuscularly) within 5 |
|     days of exposure |

MMR—measles-mumps-rubella.

**FIGURE 1-12** Prevention of measles. Active immunization is recommended for all healthy children, given at 12 to 15 months of age, usually as part of the measles-mumps-rubella multi-vaccine. A booster vaccination is now recommended for children at school entry (age 5–6 years) or entry into junior high school (age 11 years). Passive immunization is recommended for exposed persons who are at high risk to develop severe or fatal measles and who are susceptible, including children with malignant disease, those receiving chemotherapy or radiotherapy, and those with deficits in cell-mediated immunity.

# ATYPICAL MEASLES

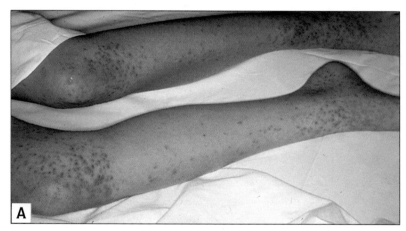

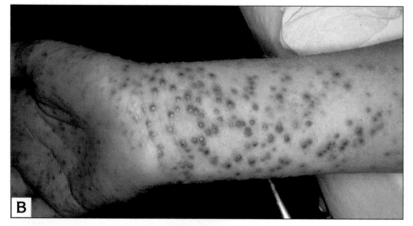

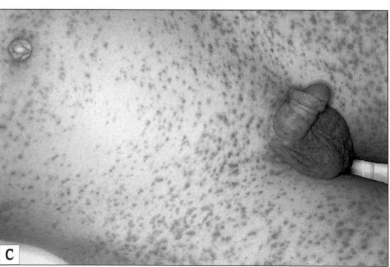

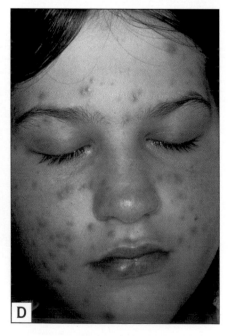

**FIGURE 1-13** Clinical appearance of atypical measles. Atypical measles occurs in individuals who have been vaccinated with the killed measles vaccine and then exposed to natural measles. Two to 3 days after the onset of high fever and headache, the rash begins. It resembles that of typical rubeola and is erythematous and maculopapular, but it is more discrete and appears initially in the distal extremities. **A** and **B**, The rash is predominant on the ankles and wrists. **C**, The rash extends cephalad, often to involve the trunk. **D**, Unlike typical measles, it only sparsely involves the face.

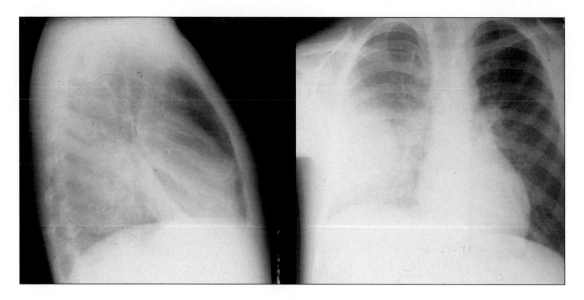

**FIGURE 1-14** Chest radiograph showing pulmonary involvement in atypical measles. Pulmonary involvement, with hilar adenopathy and segmental pneumonia, is present in the vast majority of patients with atypical measles. It is the most frequent cause of death.

**FIGURE 1-15** Clinical features of atypical measles. The clinical features of atypical measles are not unique and overlap with those of other clinical entities, making the diagnosis sometimes difficult. With the passage of time since the killed measles vaccine has been used, and with the low level of endemic measles in the United States, atypical measles is now extremely rare.

## Clinical features of atypical measles

| | |
|---|---|
| Etiology | Rubeola |
| Incubation period | 7–14 days |
| Epidemiology | Occurs in individuals vaccinated with killed measles vaccine and then exposed to natural measles |
| | Extremely rare |
| Nature of eruption | Erythematous maculopapular rash (may also be urticarial, hemorrhagic, or vesicular) |
| | Begins peripherally and progresses cephalad |
| | Pathogenesis appears to be hypersensitivity to measles virus in a partially immune host |
| Other signs and symptoms | High fever (up to 40.6° C) |
| | Headache |
| | Abdominal pain |
| | Dry, nonproductive cough |
| | Pleuritic chest pain |
| | Dyspnea and rales |
| Laboratory findings | Extremely high rubeola antibody titer |
| | Hilar adenopathy, pleural effusion, and focal pulmonary infiltrates on chest radiograph |

# RUBELLA (GERMAN MEASLES)

**FIGURE 1-16**
Typical nonspecific rash of rubella on the extremities.
**A** and **B**, Rubella (German measles, third disease) is generally a mild infection (one third of cases are completely asymptomatic) characterized by a faint, discrete, erythematous, maculopapular, nonconfluent rash that begins on the face and spreads downward to the trunk, arms, and

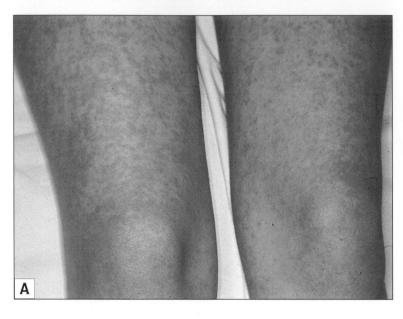

legs. The rash itself is not easily distinguished from the rashes of many other viruses, bacterial toxins, and drug reactions, but an association with lymphadenopathy helps narrow the differential. Adolescents and adults may also experience transient polyarthralgia and polyarthritis, particularly involving the wrist, hand, and knees, a finding especially common among women and girls.

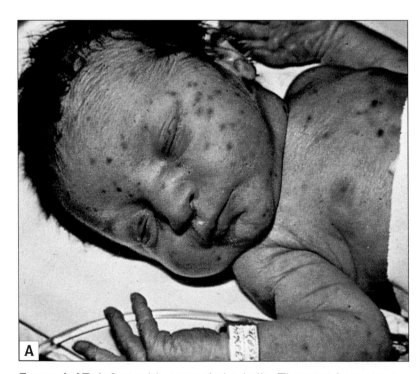

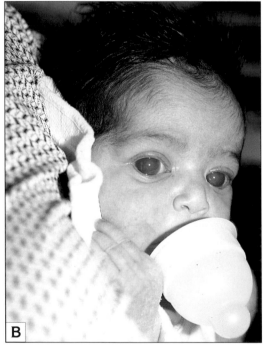

**FIGURE 1-17** Infant with congenital rubella. The most important clinical sequela of rubella occurs in infants exposed to the virus in utero. **A**, Although the extent of fetal involvement may be variable, babies with severe congenital infection display multiple discrete purpuric skin lesions on a background of yellow skin, known as *blueberry muffin spots*, secondary to dermal erythropoiesis and underlying jaundice. **B**, Another infant demonstrates congenital cataracts and corneal cloudiness due to congenital glaucoma, which result from congenital rubella infection. (Panel 17B *courtesy of* D. Stevens, MD.)

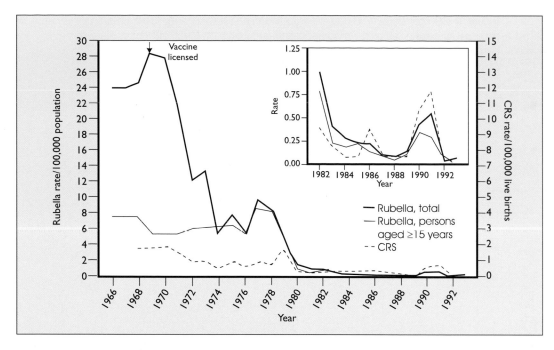

**FIGURE 1-18** Annual incidence for rubella and congenital rubella syndrome in the United States between 1966 and 1993. Introduction of live, attenuated rubella vaccine in 1969 resulted in dramatic decreases in both rubella and congenital rubella syndrome (CRS). However, there have been resurgences, as focal outbreaks continue to occur, especially in poorly immunized populations, such as urban, medically underserved children and members of religious communities who traditionally refuse vaccination. Recent focal outbreaks also have occurred among persons in prisons, colleges, and work settings. (*From* Centers for Disease Control and Prevention [2].)

## Clinical features of postnatal rubella

| | |
|---|---|
| Etiology | Rubella virus (Togaviridae) |
| Incubation period | Usually 16–18 days, may range to 14–21 days |
| Epidemiology | Peak incidence in late winter and early spring, with epidemics occurring in 6–9-yr cycles |
| | Affected children < 10 yrs of age, with occasional cases in young, susceptible adults |
| Nature of eruption | Maculopapular, nonconfluent, erythematous eruption evolves over 12–24 hours and lasts 3–5 days |
| | Rash begins on face and progresses down the body |
| Other signs and symptoms | Adenopathy involving postauricular, suboccipital, and posterior cervical chains, may remain enlarged for several weeks |
| | Fever, if present, is low-grade and lasts 1 day |
| Laboratory findings | Rubella-specific IgM antibody in single serum specimen, or better, ≥ 4-fold rise in antibody titer in two specimens |
| | Virus culture from throat secretions and urine (usually not done) |

**FIGURE 1-19** Clinical features of postnatal rubella. Rubella is caused by the rubella virus, which is an RNA virus in the Togaviridae family. The disease is generally mild and was considered of minor importance until the recognition, in 1941, of the link to congenital rubella syndrome. Since, its occurrence has been markedly altered by vaccine use, and in the postvaccine era, cases are seen in young, unvaccinated adults during outbreaks in colleges and occupational settings.

## A. Early manifestations of congenital rubella

| | |
|---|---|
| Growth retardation, low birthweight* | Hemolytic anemia* |
| Eye defects | Cerebral defects |
|   Cataracts |   Psychomotor retardation |
|   Glaucoma |   Microcephaly |
|   Retinopathy |   Encephalitis |
|   Microphthalmia |   Spastic quadriparesis |
| Cardiac defects |   Cerebrospinal fluid pleocytosis* |
|   Patent ductus arteriosus | Hepatomegaly* (rarely hepatitis, jaundice) |
|   Ventricular septal defect | Splenomegaly* |
|   Pulmonic stenosis and coarctation | Bone lesions* |
|   Myocardial abnormalities | Large anterior fontanelle* |
| Hearing loss | Cryptorchidism |
| Thrombocytopenic purpura* | Inguinal hernia |

*Transient.

**FIGURE 1-20** Congenital effects of intrauterine rubella infection. In general, the extent and severity of clinical manifestations depend on the time during gestation that infection occurs. Damage is most severe when infection occurs in the first and early second trimesters. Damage that occurs in the third trimester is more subtle, for instance, resulting in learning disabilities. **A,** Early manifestations. These changes are present at birth or shortly thereafter. A variety of manifestations are transient because they are not associated with tissue damage and therefore are not associated with long-term structural abnormalities. (*continued*)

**B. Late manifestations of congenital rubella**

Infancy
  Chronic rubelliform rash
  Interstitial pneumonitis
  Recurrent pulmonary infection
  Chronic diarrhea
  Hypogammaglobulinemia
Childhood
  Sensorineural deafness
  Central auditory imperception
  Speech defects
  Diabetes mellitus
  Growth hormone deficiency
  Thyroid disorders
  Progressive panencephalitis
  Behavioral disorders
  Central language disorders

**FIGURE 1-20** (*continued*) **B,** Late manifestations. These changes, which are not necessarily evident at birth, may appear weeks to years later, yet they relate to damage caused by initial or continued viral replication.

**Immunization against rubella**

| Age | Rationale |
|---|---|
| 12–18 mos | Immunization of infants to protect childbearing-age women from exposure and to provide lifelong protection to the vaccine immune cohort |
| 11–12 yrs, unless required for school entry | Reimmunization to protect those who previously received vaccine, but whose immunity may be incomplete because of poor response or failure of initial vaccine |
| Adulthood | Immunization of susceptible adult women of childbearing age (usually just after birth of a child) |

**FIGURE 1-21** Immunization against rubella. Live attenuated rubella vaccine was licensed in 1969 and is routinely provided as part of the measles-mumps-rubella multi-vaccine. The rationale for its use is primarily to prevent congenital rubella by controlling postnatal rubella. The vaccine, when properly administered, produces seroconversion in approximately 95% of persons.

# VARICELLA (CHICKENPOX)

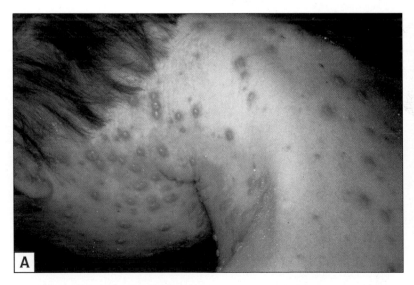

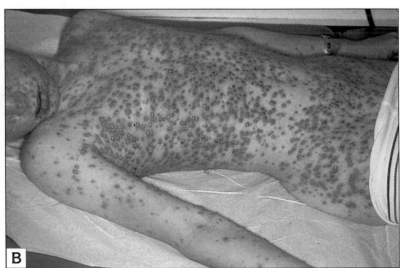

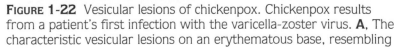

**FIGURE 1-22** Vesicular lesions of chickenpox. Chickenpox results from a patient's first infection with the varicella-zoster virus. **A,** The characteristic vesicular lesions on an erythematous base, resembling a dew drop on a rose petal, develop around the hair line and on the face. **B,** Over the next several days, the lesions become more widespread, with marked variability in their density. (*continued*)

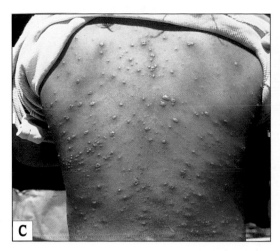

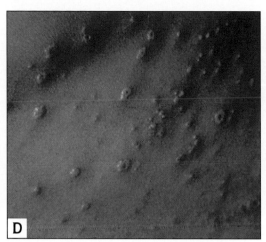

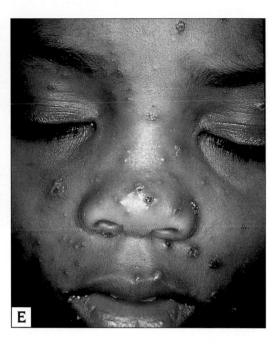

**FIGURE 1-22** (*continued*) **C,** Over several days, the vesicles mature into pustular-appearing lesions that then develop central umbilication. **D** and **E,** Finally, with healing, the lesions become crusted. New lesions may appear for only a few days, but they occasionally will continue to appear for 7 to 10 days before evolving to the pustular, then crusted lesions.

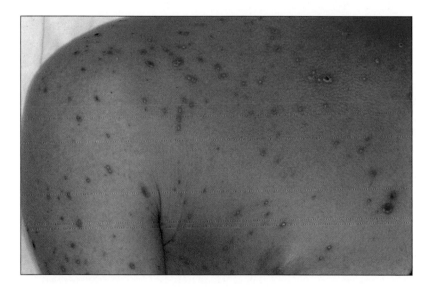

**FIGURE 1-23** Bacterial superinfection of varicella lesions. Because the lesions are ulcerative and pruritic, occasionally they become superinfected with skin flora, primarily staphylococci and strepto-cocci. A resultant cellulitis, as seen here, or even bacteremia, with seeding of distant foci, may develop.

| Clinical features of chickenpox | |
|---|---|
| Etiology | VZV (Herpesviridae) |
| Incubation period | Usually 14–15 days from exposure to appearance of vesicles (range, 10–20 days) |
| Epidemiology | Annual epidemics occur from fall to spring |
| | Preschool and school-aged children most often infected |
| | Transmission by close contact |
| Nature of eruption | Vesicular lesions on erythematous base, progressing to pustular, then crusting over at 3–5 days |
| Other signs and symptoms | Enanthem on palate and nasopharynx of most children during the first days of rash |
| | Mild fever in early phase of illness |
| | Malaise, pruritus, anorexia, listlessness |
| Laboratory findings | Culture of vesicular fluid yields virus |
| | VZV-specific IgM antibody in single serum specimen or ≥ 4-fold rise in antibody titer on two serum specimens |
| | Direct fluorescent antibody staining of scrapings from vesicular lesions |

VZV—varicella-zoster virus.

**FIGURE 1-24** Clinical features of chicken-pox. The varicella-zoster virus is a DNA virus belonging to the Herpesviridae family. The illness is contagious over several days preceding the rash, so the actual moment of exposure is seldom known. Chickenpox occurs in annual epidemics, often beginning in the fall and extending through to the next spring. Preschool and school-aged children are usually infected, with 3 to 4 million cases occurring each year. Infection is associated with close contact, with exposure over 20 to 30 minutes being most efficient. Secondary attack rates within classrooms approximate 20%, but within households it is 70% to 90%. With the introduction of vaccine, the epidemiology will change, but illness will continue to affect those who remain susceptible.

### Complications of varicella

Central nervous system
  Acute cerebellar ataxia
  Encephalitis
  Reye syndrome
Pneumonitis
Disseminated disease (especially severe in perinates
  and immunocompromised persons)
Herpes zoster (late recurrence)

**FIGURE 1-25** Complications of varicella. The most common extra-cutaneous site of involvement is the central nervous system. Acute cerebellar ataxia occurs in one of 4000 cases with recovery in 2 to 4 weeks. Encephalitis is a rare life-threatening complication often associated with sequelae in survivors. Though some degree of pneumonitis occurs in many individuals with chickenpox, clinically remarkable pneumonitis (varicella pneumonia), associated with tachypnea, cough, dyspnea, and fever, can be life threatening, especially when occurring late in pregnancy or in immunocompromised persons. Dissemination to involve visceral organs, seen in neonates and in immunocompromised persons, is a cause of significant morbidity and mortality.

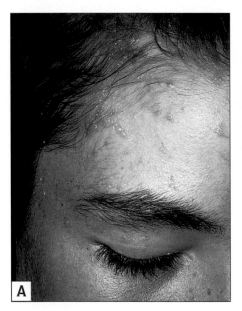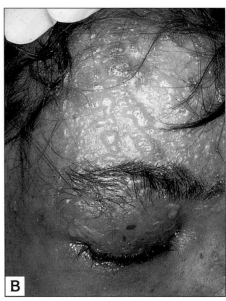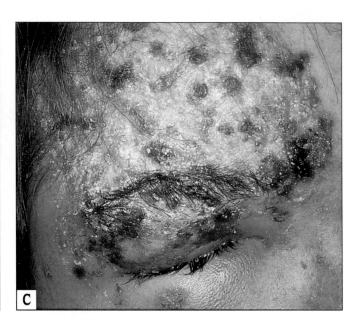

**FIGURE 1-26** Outbreak and progression of herpes zoster on the forehead of a boy aged 12 years. Though not a complication of primary infection, herpes zoster (shingles) occurs, usually years later, among approximately 20% of individuals who had chickenpox. Zoster is a manifestation of recrudescent replication of the virus that caused the chickenpox, which then remained latent in dorsal root ganglion neurons. Herpes zoster is not commonly seen among children, but under certain circumstances the condition can occur. **A,** Usually ushered in by hours to days of pain localized to a dermatome, the rash begins as an erythematous patch, with small vesicles filled with clear fluid, as seen here at day 2. **B,** By day 5, there is coalescence of vesicles. **C,** Eventually, vesicles crust over, as seen in this patient on day 8. Early, the vesicular fluid contains infectious virus. Although rare in children, pain may continue long beyond healing.

### Therapy and prevention of varicella

| | |
|---|---|
| Acyclovir | Approved for use in management of chickenpox and herpes zoster in normal and immunocompromised patients |
| Varicella-zoster immune globulin | May prevent or alleviate chickenpox in exposed susceptible person if given within 72 hours of exposure |
| Varicella vaccine | Recommended for routine use in all healthy children who are susceptible and who are > 1 year of age |
| | Infants and children < 13 years of age require a single dose; those ≥ 13 require two doses separated by at least 1 month |

**FIGURE 1-27** Therapy and prevention of varicella. Acyclovir, a guanine derivative, is activated through phosphorylation by the virus-specified thymidine kinase and selectively inhibits the viral DNA polymerase. Varicella zoster immune globulin (VZIG) is derived from individuals recovering from zoster. Candidates for VZIG include certain susceptible immunocompromised individuals under age 15 years, susceptible women in pregnancy, and neonates exposed within 5 days before delivery or 48 hours postpartum. Varicella vaccine, licensed in March 1995, is now recommended as routine for all healthy children who are susceptible to chickenpox and who are past their first birthday.

# HERPES SIMPLEX

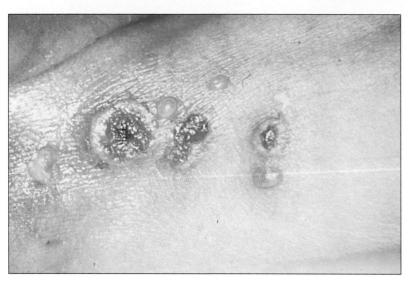

**FIGURE 1-28** Cluster of herpes simplex vesicles showing phases of maturation. Neonatal herpes simplex infection is a systemic disease in which skin manifestations are characterized by clusters of vesicles located anywhere on the body representative of the varied portals of entry for the virus. Infection is generally acquired during birth. Characteristically, lesions appear at points where skin integrity was interrupted, such as at insertion sites for fetal monitors and near abrasions caused by instrumentation. Lesions also appear after hematogenous dissemination of the virus. In this photograph, a cluster of lesions is seen demonstrating the phased progression of lesions from early, clear, fluid-filled vesicles, to more mature, umbilicated vesicles, to healing lesions that are beginning to crust.

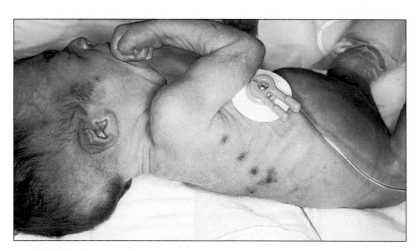

**FIGURE 1-29** Widespread lesions in neonatal herpes simplex. Lesions occurred in a linear arrangement along the infant's chest. The patch of vesicles anterior the ear developed at a site of forceps application during delivery. Neonatal infection may be widespread, involving the brain and other viscera, such as the liver and lungs. This child's "fisting" is a manifestation of brain involvement secondary to central nervous system destruction by viral replication in the brain.

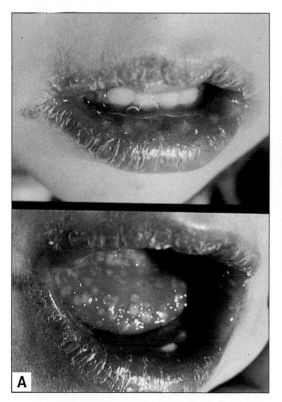

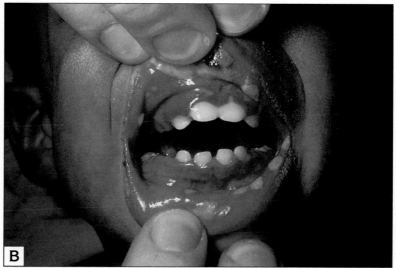

**FIGURE 1-30** Herpes simplex gingivostomatitis. **A** and **B**, Herpes simplex infection in children and infants beyond the newborn period presents most commonly as gingivostomatitis and pharyngitis. Although beginning as small mucosal vesicles, shallow ulcers rapidly evolve as vesicles rupture. Involved areas include the soft palate, buccal mucosa, tongue, floor of the mouth, and lips. Pain may be extreme; some children become dehydrated because of refusal to eat or drink. (Panel 30B *courtesy of* A.M. Margileth, MD.)

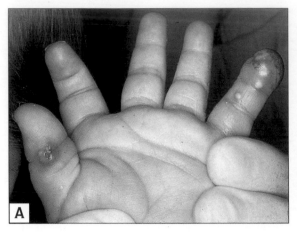
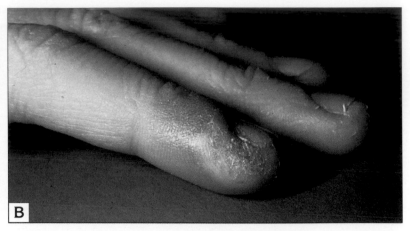

**FIGURE 1-31** Herpetic whitlow. Not uncommonly, infants and children with primary gingivostomatitis transfer infection to other parts of their bodies. **A,** Herpes simplex involves the thumb and little finger, the favorite fingers that this child sucked for comfort. **B,** An older child with stomatitis transferred infection to her index finger around the nailbed when she trimmed her nails with her teeth.

## Clinical features of childhood herpes simplex

| | |
|---|---|
| Etiology | HSV (Herpesviridae) types 1 and 2 |
| Epidemiology | Childhood, usually HSV-1 with oropharyngeal entry |
| | Adolescence and early adulthood: usually HSV-2 with sexual transmission |
| | Neonatal infection: usually acquired during delivery, predominantly HSV-2 |
| Nature of eruption | Clear fluid-filled vesicles, with a narrow base of erythema, appear in clusters |
| | Vesicles progress to cloudy, then umbilicated, then crusted lesions |
| | Lasts 7–10 days |
| Other signs and symptoms | Vary widely, may show visceral involvement |
| Laboratory findings | Vesicular fluid and nasopharangeal secretions yield virus on culture |
| | Viral antigens demonstrated by direct fluorescent antibody staining of vesicle scrapings or enzyme immunoassay detection in vesicular fluid |

HSV—herpes simplex virus.

**FIGURE 1-32** Clinical features of childhood herpes simplex. Herpes simplex virus (HSV) is a DNA virus belonging to the Herpesviridae family. HSV type 1 is the most frequent cause of infection during childhood, usually by way of an oropharyngeal portal of entry. Type 2 is the most frequent cause of infection during adolescence and early adulthood, usually by way of anal/genital contact. Neonatal infection is most frequently acquired during delivery and therefore predominantly HSV type 2, although type 1 causes 10% to 20% of the infections. Illness may begin within hours of birth but generally appears 5 to 10 days after birth. Early symptoms are variable and include respiratory distress syndrome, sepsis syndrome, and convulsions. Only two thirds of neonatal herpes infections involve the skin, and only one third present with skin lesions as the initial indication of infection.

## Clinical variants of neonatal herpes simplex

| | |
|---|---|
| Generalized, systemic | May be fulminant, disseminated illness involving the liver, lungs, and brain (encephalitis) |
| | Associated with high mortality (80%), even with treatment (30%), and neurologic sequelae |
| Localized central nervous system | Spares extracranial viscera but may cause extensive brain damage |
| | Neurologic sequelae include seizures, paralysis, deafness, mental retardation |
| Localized SEM disease | Mildest form with best prognosis |
| | Skin lesions may recur at 3–4-week intervals throughout childhood but recrudescent episodes are not associated with continued damage or risk of dissemination |

SEM—skin, eyes, mouth.

**FIGURE 1-33** Clinical variants of neonatal herpes simplex. If untreated, > 70% of neonates will develop disseminated or central nervous system infection; the mortality rate is 65% to 85%, with neurologic and developmental sequelae in > 90% of survivors. Antiviral therapy has reduced the mortality to 25%. Skin, eyes, and mouth disease is associated with virtually no deaths but involves frequent recurrences.

| Therapy for neonatal herpes simplex | |
| --- | --- |
| Acyclovir | 30 mg/kg/day intravenously |
| Vidarabine | 30 mg/kg/day intravenously |

**FIGURE 1-34** Therapy for neonatal herpes simplex. Acyclovir and vidarabine are both effective for treatment of neonatal herpes simplex infections. Outcomes are best for disease limited to the skin, eyes, and mouth (SEM disease); are intermediate for disease limited to the brain; and are least effective for disseminated disease. Because acyclovir is less toxic and easier to use than vidarabine, it has become the agent of choice in management of neonatal herpes simplex.

# CYTOMEGALOVIRUS INFECTIONS

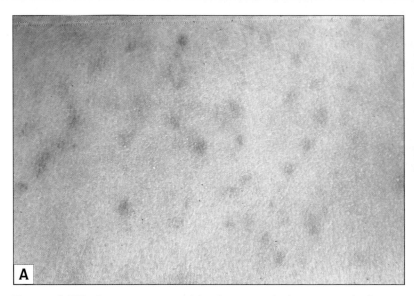

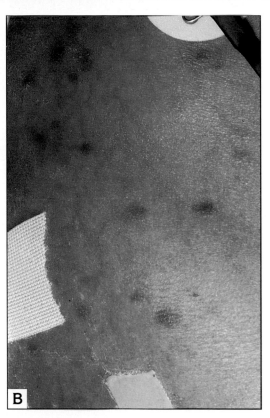

**FIGURE 1-35** Cutaneous petechiae in congenital cytomegalovirus (CMV) infection. Manifestations of intrauterine CMV infection range from no abnormalities to extensive illness. The classic illness is congenital cytomegalic inclusion disease and is characterized by jaundice, hepatosplenomegaly, and multiple organ involvement. **A** and **B**, Cutaneous manifestations involve multiple scattered flat petechiae or purpura resulting from thrombocytopenia. (Panel 35B *courtesy of* J. Neff, MD.)

| Clinical features of congenital cytomegalovirus infection | |
| --- | --- |
| Etiology | Cytomegalovirus (Herpesviridae) |
| Incubation period | 3–5 wks after exposure, depending on dose, route of exposure, and host immune responsiveness |
| Epidemiology | Ubiquitous, found in 80% of adult population |
| | Virus is generally latent but periodically replicates without symptoms |
| | Spread by person-to-person contact through exchange of body fluids, including nasopharyngeal secretions, human milk, uterine cervical secretions, semen, urine, blood |
| | Also spread in human donor organs and bone marrow at transplantation |
| Nature of eruption | Rash not an integral part of infection |
| | Petechiae and purpura result from a complication such as thrombocytopenia and subsequent microvascular bleeding into skin |
| Other signs and symptoms | Multiple organ involvement (hepatomegaly with jaundice, splenomegaly with thrombocytopenia, neuronal damage with microcephaly, intracranial calcifications, chorioretinitis, deafness, mental retardation) |
| | Intrauterine or perinatal infection is usually asymptomatic |
| Laboratory findings | Culture of body fluids |
| | Cytomegalovirus-specific IgM antibody |

**FIGURE 1-36** Clinical features of congenital cytomegalovirus (CMV) infection. CMV is a DNA virus of the Herpesviridae family. Like other herpesviruses, CMV can remain latent and reappear later as recrudescent disease, usually under conditions of change in effectiveness of host defense. There is some suggestion that reinfection also occurs, but there seems to be only one strain of virus. Congenital infection can cause extensive damage, including multiple organ involvement, but most frequently, intrauterine or perinatal infection is asymptomatic, resulting in an immune response for life. Techniques for rapid identification of viral replication have been developed. As with other perinatal infections, serology needs to differentiate between maternal, transplacentally transferred antibody, and the baby's own antibody production. CMV-specific IgM antibody, when present, will substantiate infection of the infant.

| Clinical variants of cytomegalovirus infection in infants and children | |
| --- | --- |
| Congenital | Potential for serious illness with chronic sequelae, including isolated microcephaly with mental retardation and other learning impairment |
| Perinatal | Often benign illness, occasionally with subtle long-term sequelae |
| | Potential for recrudescent illness |
| Acquired | |
| Normal host | Often benign illness, may present as mononucleosis syndrome, but most cases are asymptomatic |
| | Potential for serious illness with chronic active disease |
| Immunocompromised host | Particularly problematic in HIV-infected, transplant, and cancer chemotherapy populations |
| Recrudescent illness | Replication and illness occurs with change in host immune responsiveness |

**FIGURE 1-37** Clinical variants of cytomegalovirus infection in infants and children. Infection in normal individuals is followed by recovery, but the virus remains sequestered in latent form. Occasionally, especially when the individual's immune response is compromised, the latent genomes reactivate, virus replicates, and new episodes of illness (recrudescence) occur. This illness may take the form of interstitial pneumonitis, hepatitis, chronic gastroenteritis, retinitis, or central nervous system disease.

# ENTEROVIRUS INFECTIONS

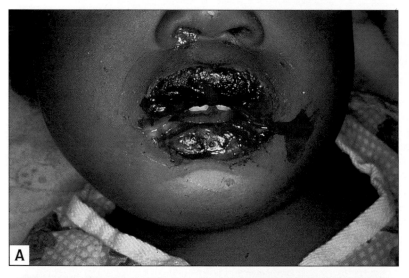

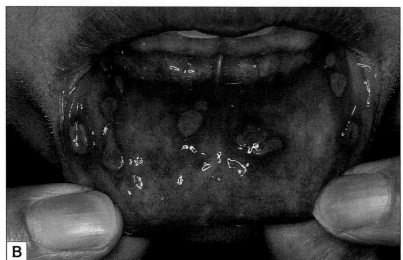

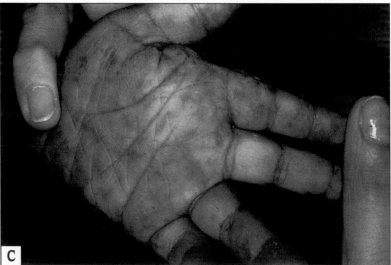

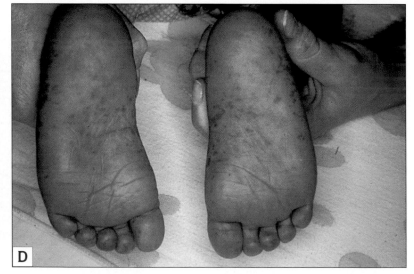

**FIGURE 1-38** Hand, foot, and mouth disease. Enterovirus infection in children manifests as a variety of cutaneous lesions. The only sufficiently distinctive rash to permit definitive diagnosis on clinical grounds is hand, foot, and mouth disease, which most commonly is associated with coxsackievirus A16. **A** and **B**, Vesicular and ulcerative lesions of the mouth or lips. **C** and **D**, Erythematous, sometimes painful, vesicular lesions occur on the palmar and plantar surfaces of the hands and feet, respectively. (Panel 38B *courtesy of* R. Holderman, DDS.)

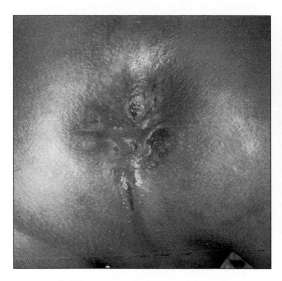

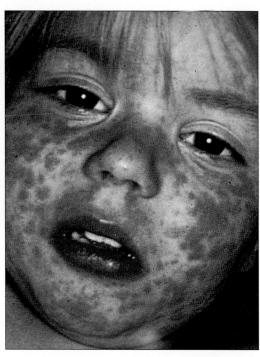

**FIGURE 1-39** Hand, foot, and mouth disease presenting in perianal area. Rarely, other mucous membranes, such as the perirectal area, may be involved.

**FIGURE 1-40** Vibrant maculapapular rash associated with echovirus 9 infection. Maculopapular, erythematous exanthems, ranging from brightly distinctive (as pictured) to only faintly apparent, are the most common cutaneous manifestation of infection with enteroviruses. Exanthems are especially common in echo 9 and 16, but are also common with a variety of coxsackie A and B viruses and other echoviruses. Exanthems are usually accompanied by fever, pharyngitis, and malaise, but patients may also experience headache or other central nervous system disturbance, cough and other pulmonary symptoms, and a variety of gastrointestinal, cardiac, and musculoskeletal complaints. Newborn infants may have fulminant illness and even fatal outcome.

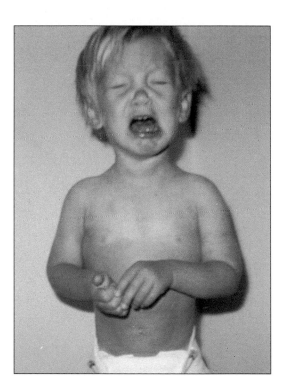

**FIGURE 1-41** Urticarial rash in an angry child with coxsackie A9 infection. Just as with virtually all other infectious organisms, urticaria may accompany infection with enteroviruses.

| Enteroviruses associated with exanthems | |
|---|---|
| Hand, foot, and mouth Exanthem | Coxsackievirus A (5, 7, 9, 10, 16) |
| | Coxsackievirus A (2, 4, 5, 9, 16) |
| | Coxsackievirus B (1, 3, 4, 5) |
| | Echovirus (especially 9 and 16, but also 1–8, 11, 14, 18, 19, 25, 30, 32, 33) |

**FIGURE 1-42** Enteroviruses associated with exanthems. Aside from hand, foot, and mouth disease, the rashes due to the coxsackieviruses and echoviruses are not distinctive enough to permit diagnosis on clinical appearance. The rashes may be rubelliform or morbilliform, roseoliform, vesicular (herpetic-like), or petechial and are included in these differential diagnoses.

### Clinical spectrum of infection with coxsackieviruses and echoviruses*

| | Coxsackievirus group A | Coxsackievirus group B | Echovirus |
|---|---|---|---|
| **Illness associated with many enteroviruses** | | | |
| Asymptomatic infection | + | + | + |
| Febrile illness with or without respiratory symptoms | + | + | + |
| Aseptic meningitis | 1–11, 14, 16–18, 22, 24 | 1–6 | All except 24, 26, 29, 32 |
| Encephalitis | 2, 5, 6, 7, 9 | 1–3, 5, 6 | 2–4, 6, 7, 9, 11, 14, 17–19, 25 |
| Paralysis | 4, 6, 7, 9, 11, 14, 21 | 1–6 | 1–4, 6, 7, 9, 11, 14, 16, 18, 19, 30 |
| **Illness more characteristic of particular groups or serotypes** | | | |
| Herpangina | 2–6, 8, 10, 22 | | |
| Exanthem | 2, 4, 5, 9, 16 | 1, 3–5 | Especially 9, 16; also 1–8, 11, 14, 18, 19, 25, 30, 32, 33 |
| Hand, foot, mouth syndrome | 5, 7, 9, 10, 16 | | |
| Pleurodynia | | 1–5 | |
| Lymphonodular pharyngitis | 10 | | |
| Pericarditis | | 1–5 | |
| Myocarditis | | 1–5 | |
| Generalized disease of newborns | | 1–5 | 4, 6, 7, 9, 11, 12, 14, 19, 21, 51 |
| Epidemic conjunctivitis | 24 | | |
| Neonatal diarrhea | | | 11, 14, 18 |
| Chronic meningoencephalitis (in agammaglobulinemics) | | | 2, 3, 5, 9, 11, 19, 24, 25, 30, 33 |
| **Etiologic role undefined** | | | |
| Diarrhea | + | + | + |
| Hemolytic-uremic syndrome | 4 | 2, 4 | 22 |
| Myositis | 9 | 2, 6 | 9, 11 |
| Guillain-Barré syndrome | 2, 5, 9 | | 6, 22 |
| Reye syndrome | + | + | |
| Mononucleosis-like syndrome | 5, 6 | 5 | + |
| Infectious lymphocytosis | + | | 25 |
| Diabetes mellitus | | + | |

*Implicated serotypes are listed.

+—serotype not specified.

**FIGURE 1-43** Clinical spectrum of infection with coxsackieviruses and echoviruses. The enteroviruses are capable of causing a vast array of clinically different illnesses. This figure lists the viruses more commonly associated with specific enteroviral infections. (*Adapted from* Modlin [3].)

# EPSTEIN-BARR VIRUS INFECTIONS

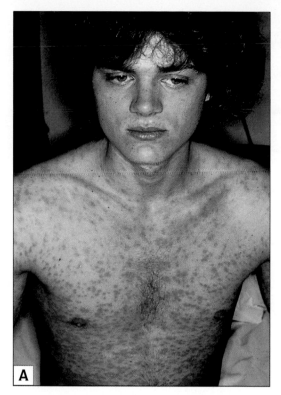

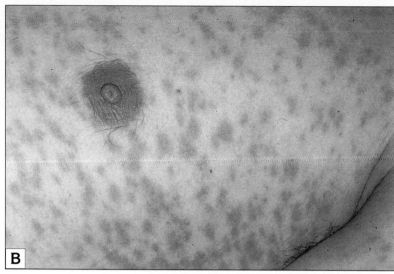

**FIGURE 1-44** Epstein-Barr virus infection is classically associated with signs and symptoms of lymphoproliferative disease (fever, sore throat with tonsillar hypertrophy, lymphadenopathy, splenomegaly, and sometimes hepatomegaly); the illness is called *infectious mononucleosis*. **A** and **B**, Occasionally (5%–10% incidence), a rash—usually faint, widely scattered, erythematous, and maculopapular—appears in the early days of infectious mononucleosis. Patients given ampicillin/amoxicillin are highly prone to develop the rash, as seen in this patient.

| Clinical features of infectious mononucleosis syndrome | |
|---|---|
| Etiology | Heterophile-positive: EBV |
| | Heterophile-negative: EBV (especially in young children); also cytomegalovirus, toxoplasmosis, viral hepatitis, rubella, streptococcal pharyngitis, HIV-1 |
| Incubation period | 4–5 wks for EBV-induced illness |
| Epidemiology | EBV infection occurs in ~50% of individuals by age 5 years, with a second wave during adolescence and early adulthood |
| | Peak incidence of infectious mononucleosis is in people 15–24 year of age |
| Nature of eruption | Eruption in absence of ampicillin is rare |
| | Rash usually appears on all parts of body within 24 hrs after antibiotic, disappears over subsequent days when drug is stopped |
| Other signs and symptoms | None |
| Laboratory findings | None |

EBV—Epstein-Barr virus.

**FIGURE 1-45** Clinical features of infectious mononucleosis syndrome. The eruption rarely occurs in the absence of ampicillin, and the usual onset occurs in association with administration of the antibiotic, usually within the initial 24 hours but occasionally delayed (even sometimes after antibiotic has been stopped). The rash is thought to be secondary to breakdown of ampicillin to toxic subproducts. There are no associated signs and symptoms that accompany the rash, and erythema recedes over a short time.

# REFERENCES

1.  Centers for Disease Control and Prevention: Summary of notifiable diseases, United States, 1993. *MMWR* 1993, 42(53):38.

2.  Centers for Disease Control and Prevention: Rubella and congenital rubella syndrome, United States, January 1, 1991–May 7, 1994. *MMWR* 1994, 43:391.

3.  Modlin JF: Coxsackieviruses, echoviruses, and newer enteroviruses. *In* Mandell GL, Bennett JE, Dolin R (eds.): *Principles and Practice of Infectious Diseases*, 4th ed. New York: Churchill Livingstone; 1995:1620–1636.

# SELECTED BIBLIOGRAPHY

Cherry JD: Contemporary infectious exanthems. *Clin Infect Dis* 1993, 16:199–207.

Farrar WD, Wood MJ, Innes JA, Tubbs H (eds.): *Infectious Diseases Text and Color Atlas*, 2nd ed. London: Gower Medical Publishing; 1992.

Feigin RD, Cherry JD (eds.): *Textbook of Pediatric Infectious Diseases*, 3rd ed. Philadelphia: W.B. Saunders; 1992.

Mandell GL, Bennett JE, Dolin R (eds.): *Principles and Practice of Infectious Diseases*, 4th ed. New York: Churchill Livingstone; 1995.

Remington JS, Klein JO (eds.): *Infectious Diseases of the Fetus and Newborn Infant*, 4th ed. Philadelphia: W.B. Saunders; 1995.

# CHAPTER 2

# Infective Endocarditis

W. Michael Scheld

## Controversial issues related to infective endocarditis in the 1990s

1. Clinical diagnosis of endocarditis in at-risk patients with no classic stigmata
2. Diagnosis of endocarditis in patients with *Staphylococcus aureus* bacteremia
3. Optimal treatment for *S. aureus* endocarditis
4. Use of ceftriaxone for treatment of endocarditis due to viridans streptococci
5. Role of endocardiography in diagnosis and management of endocarditis
6. Administration of chemoprophylaxis for endocarditis
7. Optimal therapy for prosthetic valve endocarditis due to coagulase-negative staphylococci
8. Management of extracardiac complications, especially cerebrovascular mycotic aneurysms

**Figure 2-1** Controversial issues related to infective endocarditis in the 1990s. Many controversial issues need to be considered in the approach to patients with suspected endocarditis in the 1990s. (*Adapted from* Bayer [1]).

# EPIDEMIOLOGY

## Epidemiology of infective endocarditis

~0.3–3.0 cases/1000 hospital admissions
3.8 cases/$10^5$ person-years, 1950–1981
Age peak: 45–65 yrs
Male:female = 1.7:1.0
Nosocomial endocarditis = 14%–28%
Valves involved: mitral > aortic > tricuspid > pulmonic

**Figure 2-2** Epidemiology of infective endocarditis. Although increasing in frequency, infective endocarditis is a relatively rare infection, accounting for 0.3 to 3 cases per 1000 hospital admissions. For the years 1950 to 1981, 3.8 cases occurred per 100,000 population per year in one hospital-based survey. The peak age of affected individuals has increased over the past several decades and is now in the 45 to 65-year-old range. Men predominate slightly over women, and nosocomial endocarditis accounts for 14% to 28% of cases in recent reports. The valves involved, in order of frequency, are the mitral, aortic, tricuspid, and pulmonic.

## Predisposing factors in infective endocarditis

Rheumatic heart disease ~25%–30%
Congenital heart disease
  Bicuspid aortic valve
  Marfan's syndrome
  Ventricular septal defect
  Mitral valve prolapse (~30%)
Prosthetic valves, pacemakers
Asymmetric septal hypertrophy
Intravenous drug use
"Degenerative" heart disease (> 50% over age 60 yrs)

**Figure 2-3** Predisposing factors in infective endocarditis. In recent decades, the proportion of infective endocarditis cases secondary to rheumatic heart disease has declined to the range of 25% to 30% overall. Various forms of congenital heart disease, including a bicuspid aortic valve, Marfan's syndrome, ventricular septal defect, and especially mitral valve prolapse (occurs as an antecedent event in approximately 30% of infective endocarditis cases overall), remain important. Insertion of prosthetic valves and intravenous drug use continue as causes of infective endocarditis. Asymmetric septal hypertrophy or idiopathic hypertrophic subaortic stenosis is rarely implicated. Conversely, so-called degenerative heart disease has accounted for an increasing proportion of cases and is involved in 50% of cases of infective endocarditis in patients over age 60 years.

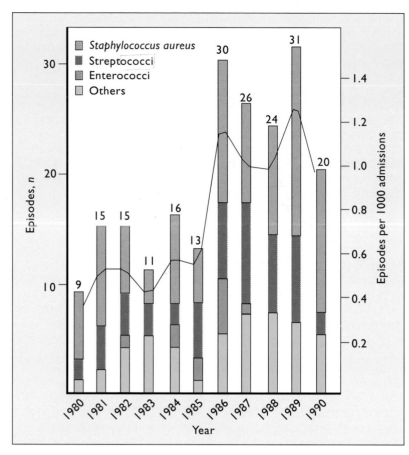

**FIGURE 2-4** Increasing frequency of infective endocarditis between 1980 and 1990. A survey of a decade's experience at one large community teaching hospital reveals the changing trends in infective endocarditis. Through the 1980s, a total of 210 episodes of infective endocarditis occurred in 204 patients. The frequency of this infection increased steadily over the decade. The proportion of cases due to *Staphylococcus aureus* also increased. The median patient age was > 60 years. Twenty-nine cases involved prosthetic valves, and 33 cases involved intravenous drug abuse (*Adapted from* Watanakunakorn and Burkert [2].)

## Changing epidemiology of infective endocarditis: Duke University Medical Center, 1992

| 148 episodes in 136 patients | |
|---|---|
| Male:female | 74:74 |
| Mean age | 47 yrs |
| Previous heart disease | 70% |
| Injected drug user | 29% |
| Mitral valve disease | 16% |
| Prosthetic valve endocarditis | 15% |
| HIV infection | 5% |
| Valve replaced | 37% |

**FIGURE 2-5** Changing epidemiology of infective endocarditis at Duke University Medical Center in 1992. During the year 1992, 148 episodes of infective endocarditis were documented in 136 patients, with an equal male:female distribution. The mean age was 47 years, and previous heart disease was documented in 70% of patients. Nearly 30% had injected drugs previous to their episode of infective endocarditis, and mitral valve disease particularly was an important antecedent heart lesion. Prosthetic valve endocarditis accounted for 15% of the total, and 5% of the cases occurred in patients with HIV infection. The need for valve replacement during the initial episode was documented in more than one third of cases. (*Courtesy of* D. Durack, MD.)

# PATHOGENESIS

## Pathogenetic factors in infective endocarditis

1. NBTE
2. Hemodynamic factors
3. Bacteremia
4. Microorganism–NBTE interaction
5. Immunopathologic factors

NBTE—nonbacterial thrombotic endocarditis.

**FIGURE 2-6** Pathogenetic factors in infective endocarditis. The pathogenesis of infective endocarditis involves five major factors. Nonbacterial thrombotic endocarditis (NBTE), consisting of fibrin-platelet deposits on valvular endothelium, serves as a common predisposing factor. Hemodynamic factors may determine localization of vegetations within the heart. Bacteremia, occasionally occurring after invasive procedures, may seed the NBTE lesion, resulting in initial colonization followed by a microorganism–NBTE interaction that produces a mature vegetation. Various immunopathologic factors also may contribute to the clinical course.

## Nonbacterial thrombotic endocarditis

1. Fibrin-platelet composition
2. Nidus for colonization; involves free edge valve leaflet
3. Found at autopsy: cancer, renal failure, rheumatic heart disease, congenital heart disease, systemic lupus erythematus, Swan-Ganz, acute illness, etc.
4. Induced experimentally; stress, valve trauma, cold, high altitude, high cardiac output, hypersensitivity, lymphatic obstruction, hormonal manipulations, etc.

**FIGURE 2-7** Nonbacterial thrombotic endocarditis (NBTE) consists of fibrin-platelet deposits and may serve as a nidus for colonization. NBTE usually involves the free edge of the valve leaflet and is seen frequently at autopsy in patients with rheumatic heart disease, congenital heart disease, renal failure, debilitating conditions such as cancer, systemic lupus erythematosus, following Swan-Ganz catheterization, and with various acute illnesses. Experimentally, NBTE can be induced by virtually any stress, including valve trauma, cold exposure, simulated high altitude, high cardiac output states, hypersensitivity reactions, lymphatic obstruction, and various hormonal manipulations. In one large series of 3404 autopsies performed in Japan, NBTE was found in 2.4%, especially in elderly individuals with chronic wasting diseases [3].

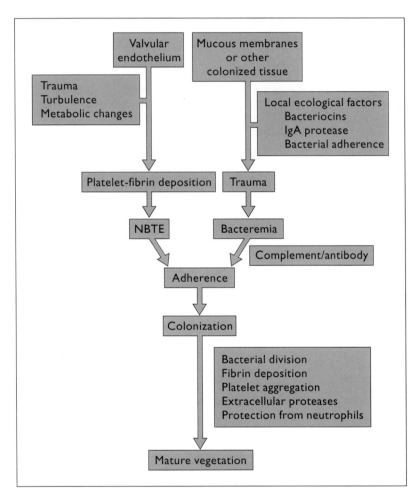

**FIGURE 2-8** Proposed scheme for the pathogenesis of infective endocarditis. As noted, valvular endothelium subjected to trauma, turbulence such as in rheumatic or congenital heart disease, or metabolic changes may induce platelet-fibrin deposition (nonbacterial thrombotic endocarditis [NBTE]). Mucous membranes or other colonized tissue subjected to trauma may induce bacteremia that, if the organisms can escape host complement–antibody-mediated clearance mechanisms, may adhere to NBTE. Various surface constituents, such as dextran, may facilitate adherence of oral streptococci to NBTE. Following adherence, further bacterial division, fibrin deposition, platelet aggregation, the production of extracellular proteases and partial protection from neutrophils may facilitate development of a mature vegetation. (*Adapted from* Scheld and Sande [4]).

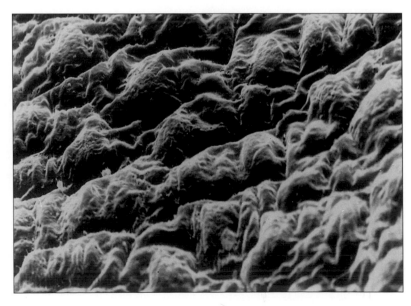

**FIGURE 2-9** Scanning electron micrograph of normal endothelial surface of the aortic valve from a New Zealand white rabbit. Despite its ruffled appearance, this intact endothelium is remarkably resistant to colonization during bacteremia.

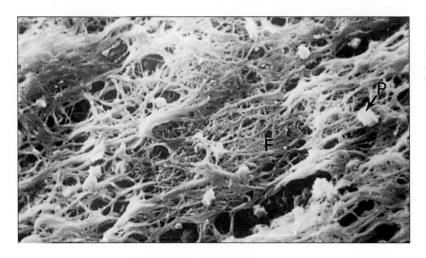

**FIGURE 2-10** Experimental nonbacterial thrombotic endocarditis. Following 1 hour of catheter-induced aortic valve trauma, fibrin-platelet deposits are readily evident on the endothelium of the aortic valve from this New Zealand white rabbit prior to inoculation of bacteria to induce experimental endocarditis.

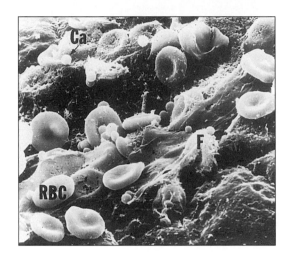

**FIGURE 2-11** Scanning electron micrograph of the surface of an aortic valve subjected to catheter-induced trauma. In a New Zealand white rabbit, fibrin (*F*) deposits are evident as well as scattered red blood cells (*RBC*). This animal was inoculated with *Candida albicans* (*Ca*), which is readily apparent adherent to areas of fibrin-platelet deposits on the traumatized endothelial surface.

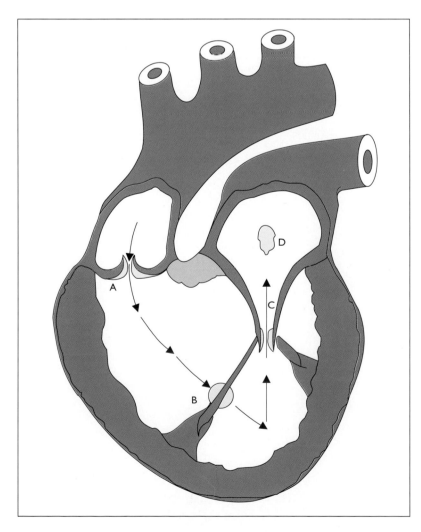

**FIGURE 2-12** Characteristic sites of vegetations within the heart. In the presence of aortic insufficiency, vegetations characteristically occur on the ventricular surface of the aortic valve (*A*) or on the chordae tendinae or papillary muscles (*B*). In mitral regurgitation, the vegetations characteristically are located on the atrial surface of the mitral valve (*C*) or at sites of jet lesions (*D*) on the atrial wall.

| Incidence of transient bacteremia after various procedures | |
| --- | --- |
| Procedure/manipulation | Positive blood cultures, % |
| Dental | |
| Dental extraction | 18–85 |
| Periodontal surgery | 32–88 |
| Chewing candy or paraffin | 17–51 |
| Tooth brushing | 0–26 |
| Oral irrigation device | 27–50 |
| Upper airway | |
| Bronchoscopy (rigid scope) | 15 |
| Tonsillectomy | 28–38 |
| Nasotracheal suctioning/intubation | 16 |
| Gastrointestinal | |
| Upper gastrointestinal endoscopy | 8–12 |
| Sigmoidoscopy/colonoscopy | 0–9.5 |
| Barium enema | 11 |
| Percutaneous needle biopsy of liver | 3–13 |
| Urologic | |
| Urethral dilatation | 18–33 |
| Urethral catheterization | 8 |
| Cystoscopy | 0–17 |
| Transurethral prostatic resection | 12–46 |
| Obstetric/gynecologic | |
| Normal vaginal delivery | 0–11 |
| Punch biopsy of cervix | 0 |
| Removal/insertion of intrauterine device | 0 |

**FIGURE 2-13** Incidence of transient bacteremia after various procedures. Several procedures may induce a transient bacteremia. In general, the bacteremia is characterized by the presence of gram-positive cocci and other oral microbial flora, in low numbers ( ≤ 10 cfu/mL) and with a transient course (~ 15–30 min). Extraction of teeth is associated with bacteremia in most cases, as is the performance of periodontal surgery. Urologic surgery, especially in the presence of infected urine, is commonly associated with a transient bacteremia. Bacteremia in the setting of a normal vaginal delivery is extremely rare. Various diagnostic procedures, such as endoscopy, bronchoscopy, barium enema, and sclerosis of esophageal varices, are infrequently associated with bacteremia. Although the occurrence of transient bacteremia is important in the initiation of infective endocarditis, its presence after various procedures also is relevant to the prophylaxis of this condition.

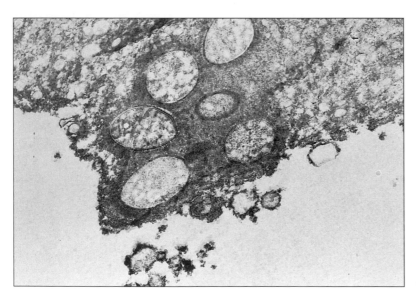

**FIGURE 2-14** Transmission electron micrograph demonstrating *Streptococcus sanguis* adherent to fibrin-platelet deposits (nonbacterial thrombotic endocarditis [NBTE]) following injection of a New Zealand white rabbit. The coarse material surrounding the streptococci is dextran, potentially important in facilitating adhesion of this organism to NBTE and in initiating the infection.

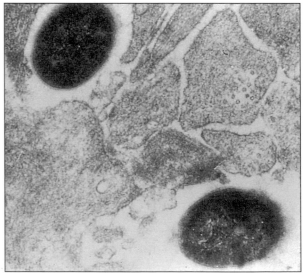

**FIGURE 2-15** Transmission electron micrograph demonstrating two streptococci (*Streptococcus mutans*) in and on the surface of a vegetation in a patient with endocarditis. The amorphous nature of the vegetation between the streptococci consists of fibrin and platelets.

**Immunopathologic factors in the pathogenesis of infective endocarditis**

1. Stimulates humoral immunity
   Hypergammaglobulinemia, rheumatoid factor, antinuclear antibodies, cryoglobulins
   Circulating immune complexes occur with hypocomplementemia, nephritis
2. Role of preformed antibody
3. Stimulates cell-mediated immunity: splenomegaly, macrophages in peripheral blood

**FIGURE 2-16** Immunopathologic factors in the pathogenesis of infective endocarditis. Humoral immunity is stimulated during infective endocarditis, resulting in hypergammaglobulinemia, and the presence of rheumatoid factor, antinuclear antibodies, or cryoglobulins in the circulation. Circulating immune complexes may rise to high levels with the development of hypocomplementemia and, occasionally, immune complex-mediated glomerulonephritis. Preformed antibody is probably protective and does not facilitate the infection in experimental animals. Stimulation of cell-mediated immunity also occurs, with the consequences of splenomegaly and occasionally the presence of macrophages in the peripheral blood.

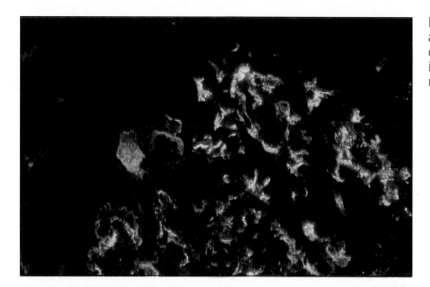

**FIGURE 2-17** Immunofluorescent staining of the glomerulus from a patient with immune complex-mediated nephritis. The figure documents the presence of immune complexes consisting of IgM in a "lumpy-bumpy" pattern throughout the glomerulus. (Original magnification, $\times$ 25.)

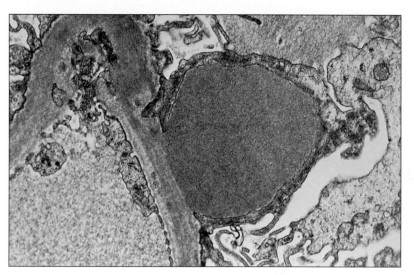

**FIGURE 2-18** Transmission electron micrograph depicting a subepithelial deposit resulting from immune complex-mediated deposition within the glomerulus. This patient had streptococcal endocarditis and glomerulonephritis.

# PATHOLOGY

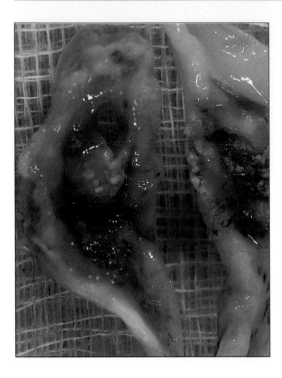

**FIGURE 2-19** Gross specimen from a patient with *Staphylococcus aureus* endocarditis. The patient, a man aged 63 years, developed an acute syndrome characterized by fever, rigors, myalgias, and the rapid onset of shortness of breath. *S. aureus* was isolated from multiple blood cultures, and pulmonary edema was evident on the chest radiograph. At surgery, a bicuspid aortic valve was resected with multiple vegetations. Perforation of this bicuspid valve also is evident, resulting in severe and acute congestive heart failure.

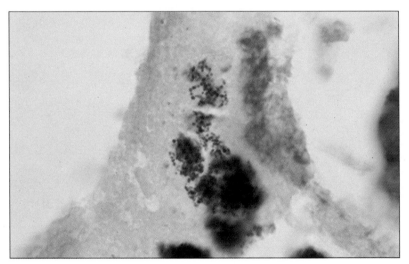

**FIGURE 2-20** Histopathologic examination of infective endocarditis showing microcolonies of streptococci within a mature vegetation. This mitral valve specimen has been stained with the Brown and Hoppes stain.

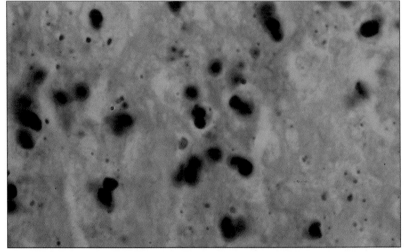

**FIGURE 2-21** Histopathologic examination of aortic valve from a patient with streptococcal endocarditis. Again, the Brown and Hoppes stain reveals microcolonies of *Streptococcus mutans* within the mature vegetation.

**FIGURE 2-22** Intraoperative specimen demonstrating multiple vegetations along the free edge of a trileaflet aortic valve.

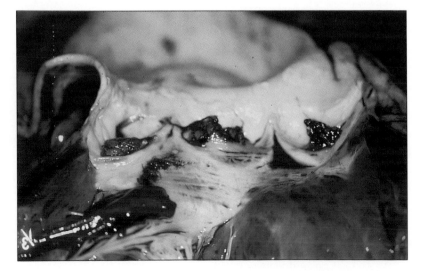

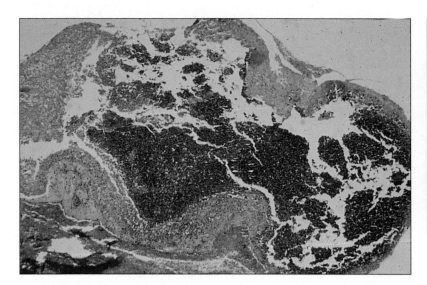

**FIGURE 2-23** Histopathologic findings in experimental endocarditis. This large vegetation attached to the aortic valve leaflet is nearly full of a dense mat of *Streptococcus sanguis*. The specimen was resected from the valve leaflet 3 days following inoculation with *S. sanguis*.

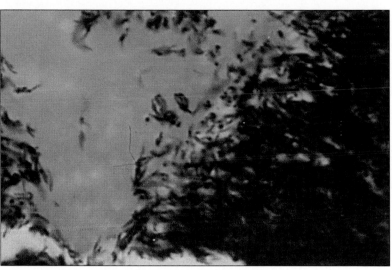

**FIGURE 2-24** Histopathologic findings in fungal endocarditis. This specimen demonstrates thick, matted mycelia of *Aspergillus fumigatus* attached to and invading the mature vegetation.

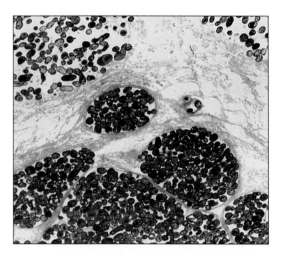

**FIGURE 2-25** Transmission electron micrograph of a mature vegetation from experimental endocarditis.

# ETIOLOGY

### Etiologic agents in infective endocarditis

|  | Cases, % |
|---|---|
| Streptococci | 60–80 |
| Viridans streptococci | 30–40 |
| Enterococci | 5–18 |
| Other streptococci | 15–25 |
| Staphylococci | 20–35 |
| Coagulase-positive | 10–27 |
| Coagulase-negative | 1–3 |
| Gram-negative aerobic bacilli | 1.5–13 |
| Fungi | 2–4 |
| Miscellaneous bacteria | < 5 |
| Mixed infections | 1–2 |
| "Culture negative" | < 5–24 |

**FIGURE 2-26** Etiologic agents in infective endocarditis. Gram-positive cocci are the major etiologic agents isolated from cases of infective endocarditis. Streptococci account for 60% to 80% of cases in multiple series. Viridans streptococci remain important. Enterococci, including *E. faecalis* and *E. faecium*, are responsible for 5% to 18% of cases. *Staphylococcus aureus* accounts for 10% to 27% of infective endocarditis on native valves and is a major cause in intravenous drug users. *Staphylococcus epidermidis* is the major cause of prosthetic valve endocarditis but is isolated rarely in native valve disease. A wide variety of gram-negative aerobic bacilli have been isolated. Members of the HACEK group have been recognized with increasing frequency and include organisms belonging to the genera *Haemophilus*, *Actinobacillus*, *Cardiobacterium*, *Eikenella*, and *Kingella*. Miscellaneous bacteria, rarely implicated in endocarditis in the present era, include gram-negative cocci, gram-positive bacilli, anaerobic organisms, and multiple other agents. Fungal endocarditis usually is seen in narcotic addicts, patients after reconstructive cardiovascular surgery, and after prolonged intravenous and/or antibiotic therapy and is usually due to species of *Candida* or *Aspergillus*. Other fungi have been implicated rarely. Mixed infections are unusual, and culture-negative endocarditis occurs with variable frequency in published series. (*From* Scheld and Sande [4].)

## Major streptococci causing infective endocarditis

| Viridans group | S. bovis |
|---|---|
|   S. sanguis | Enterococcus spp |
|   S. mutans | S. pneumoniae |
|   S. mitis (mitior) | S. agalactiae |
|   S. intermedius | S. suis |
|   S. constellatus | S. anginosus |
|   S. milleri | Gemella haemolysans |
|   S. salivarius | |
|   S. defectivus | |
|   S. adjacens | |

**FIGURE 2-27** Major streptococci causing infective endocarditis. Streptococci account for the majority of cases of infective endocarditis in multiple series. The viridans streptococci are a heterogeneous group that consists of multiple organisms, including *S. mitis*, *S. sanguis*, *S. mutans*, *S. salivarius*, the nutritionally variant streptococci (such as *S. adjacens*, *S. defectivus*), and some isolates of the *S. intermedius* group, among others. Isolation of *S. bovis* from blood cultures should prompt a search for lesions of the gastrointestinal tract.

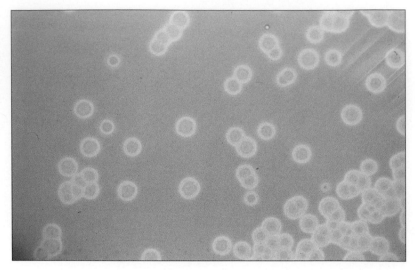

**FIGURE 2-28** Blood agar plate showing colonies of *Streptococcus sanguis* from a patient with infective endocarditis. A green zone surrounds each colony, documenting α-hemolysis.

## Important properties of nutritionally deficient streptococci

1. Usually *Streptococcus mitior*
2. Require vitamin $B_6$ or cysteine
3. Stain gram-positive with negative subculture
4. Relatively common (5% of infective endocarditis)
5. Slow response to therapy

**FIGURE 2-29** Important properties of nutritionally deficient streptococci. Most strains classified as nutritionally deficient are *Streptococcus mitior* and require vitamin $B_6$ or cysteine in subculture for growth. Laboratories recognize these strains as gram positive from the original blood culture with negative subcultures, unless supplemented with the above constituents. Nutritionally deficient streptococci are a relatively common cause of infective endocarditis, accounting for approximately 5% of cases, and they are characteristically slow to respond to therapy.

## Fastidious, slow-growing gram-negative bacteria causing endocarditis (HACEK group)

1. *Haemophilus aprophilus, H. parainfluenzae, H. paraaphrophilus*
2. *Actinobacillus actinomycetemcomitans*
3. *Cardiobacterium hominis*
4. *Eikenella corrodens*
5. *Kingella kingae*

**FIGURE 2-30** Fastidious, slow-growing, gram-negative bacteria causing endocarditis (HACEK group). The HACEK group, defined as organisms belonging to *Haemophilus*, *Actinobacillus*, *Cardiobacterium*, *Eikenella*, and *Kingella* species, are important causes of infective endocarditis. Commonly labeled "culture-negative" initially, these fastidious organisms may require up to 3 weeks of culture for demonstrable growth. Cases of infective endocarditis due to the HACEK group are characterized by large vegetations with frequent embolization, congestive heart failure, and the need for surgery when compared with viridans streptococcal disease. Nevertheless, mortality remains low with appropriate therapy.

**Causes of "culture-negative" infective endocarditis**

HACEK organisms
*Bartonella* spp
*Coxiella burnetii*
*Legionella* spp
*Chlamydia* spp
*Brucella* spp
*Spirillum minor*

**FIGURE 2-31** Causes of "culture-negative" infective endocarditis. Culture-negative endocarditis occurs with variable frequency in published series of infective endocarditis. Occasional "culture-negative" cases are due to unusual organisms, such as *Coxiella burnettii*, *Brucella*, *Spirillum minor*, or *Chlamydia*. Two other causes for culture negativity are recent antimicrobial therapy and failure to incubate blood cultures for 3 weeks.

# CLINICAL MANIFESTATIONS

**Factors influencing the pathogenesis and clinical course of infective endocarditis**

Constant bacteremia
Local invasion
Embolization
Circulating immune complexes

**FIGURE 2-32** Factors influencing the pathogenesis and clinical course of infective endocarditis. Four major factors contribute to the clinical manifestations of infective endocarditis. Constant bacteremia contributes to the fever, chills, rigors, sweats, myalgias, malaise, fatigability, and other constitutional symptoms. Local invasion of the valve may lead to fulminant pulmonary edema, heart block, myocardial abscess, coronary artery emboli, pericarditis, and other complications. Embolization can occur to virtually any organ in the body and result in bland or septic infarcts, mycotic aneurysm formation, and abscess formation. Emboli most commonly involve the skin, central nervous system, kidney, spleen, and lung (in the presence of right-sided infective endocarditis). Circulating immune complexes may contribute to various manifestations, including skin lesions, retinal deposits, and kidney involvement.

**A. Clinical manifestations of infective endocarditis: Symptoms**

| | % |
|---|---|
| Fever | 80 |
| Chills | 40 |
| Weakness | 40 |
| Dyspnea | 40 |
| Sweats | 25 |
| Anorexia | 25 |
| Weight loss | 25 |
| Malaise | 25 |
| Cough | 25 |
| Skin lesions | 20 |
| Stroke | 20 |
| Nausea/vomiting | 20 |
| Headache | 20 |
| Myalgia/arthralgia | 15 |
| Edema | 15 |
| Chest pain | 15 |
| Abdominal pain | 15 |
| Delirium/coma | 10–15 |
| Hemoptysis | 10 |
| Back pain | 10 |

**B. Clinical manifestations of infective endocarditis: Signs**

| | % |
|---|---|
| Fever | 90 |
| Heart murmur | 85 |
| Changing murmur | 5–10 |
| New murmur | 3–5 |
| Embolic phenomenon | > 50 |
| Skin manifestations | 18–50 |
| Osler nodes | 10–23 |
| Splinter hemorrhages | 15 |
| Petechiae | 20–40 |
| Janeway lesion | < 10 |
| Splenomegaly | 20–57 |
| Septic complications (pneumonia, meningitis, etc.) | 20 |
| Mycotic aneurysms | 20 |
| Clubbing | 12–52 |
| Retinal lesion | 2–10 |
| Signs of renal failure | 10–15 |

**FIGURE 2-33** Clinical manifestations of infective endocarditis. **A**, Symptoms. Constitutional findings such as fever, chills, weakness, dyspnea, sweats, anorexia, weight loss, malaise, and others are relatively frequent in patients with infective endocarditis. Rheumatic manifestations, including arthralgias, arthritis, and back pain, are not infrequent presenting features. Unfortunately, patients may present with prominent central nervous system manifestations. **B**, Signs. The physical findings relate to fever, heart murmur, and the consequences of emboli or immunopathologic manifestations. Infective endocarditis should be considered in any patient with a fever and heart murmur. Changing murmurs are unusual but of particular importance in the evaluation of a patient with known cardiac risk factors. Older designations of infective endocarditis as "acute or subacute" should be abandoned in favor of classification schemes dependent on isolation of the etiologic agent. (*From* Scheld and Sande [4]).

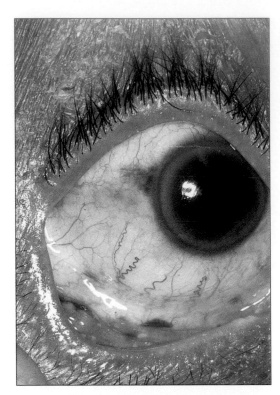

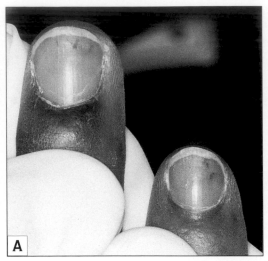

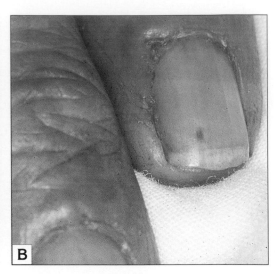

**FIGURE 2-35** **A** and **B**, Splinter hemorrhages in the nailbed of patients with endocarditis. Although nonspecific, splinter hemorrhages in the distal nailbed of a "fresh" nature (red as opposed to brown) may be more indicative of infective endocarditis.

**FIGURE 2-34** Conjunctival hemorrhages in a patient with *Staphylococcus aureus* endocarditis.

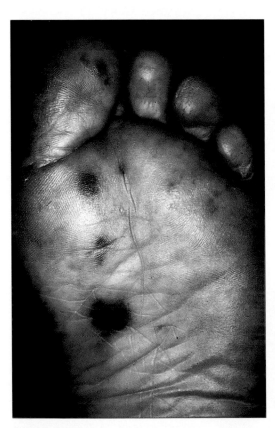

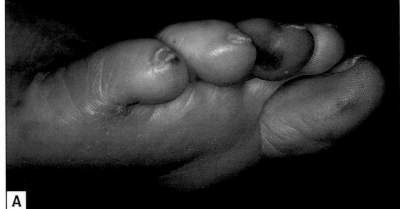

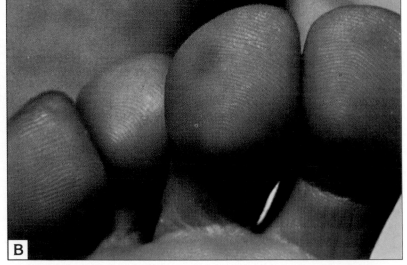

**FIGURE 2-36** Janeway lesions in a patient with *Staphylococcus aureus* endocarditis. Janeway lesions are generally painless, flat, and occasionally hemorrhagic, as in this case. Embolic in origin with microabscess formation in the dermis, they are almost pathognomonic of *S. aureus* endocarditis. (*From* Sande and Strausbaugh [5]; with permission).

**FIGURE 2-37** **A** and **B**, Osler's nodes in patients with infective endocarditis. These lesions usually occur in the tufts of the fingers or toes and are painful and evanescent. They likely are mediated by immunopathologic factors.

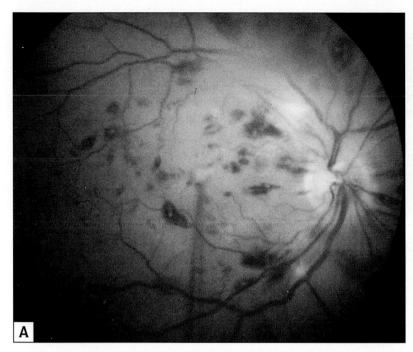

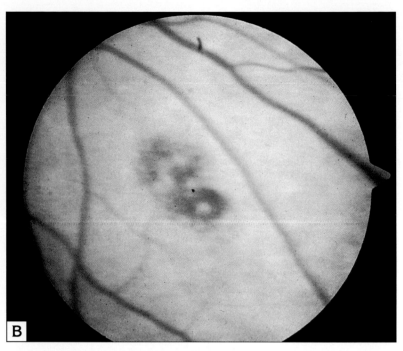

**FIGURE 2-38 A** and **B**, Roth spots in infective endocarditis. Of uncertain pathogenesis, these lesions usually are characterized by a central clear area surrounded by hemorrhage. Multiple lesions may be present in the retina, as seen in *panel 38A*.

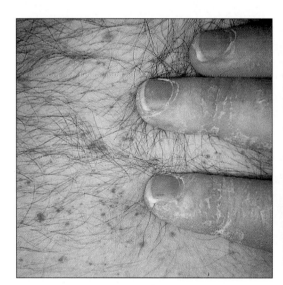

**FIGURE 2-39** Diffuse petechial rash in a patient with *Staphylococcus aureus* endocarditis. Occasionally, a fulminant case of *S. aureus* endocarditis may mimic meningococcemia. Careful inspection of the petechiae may reveal some lesions with a pustular center, which almost always test positive on Gram stain.

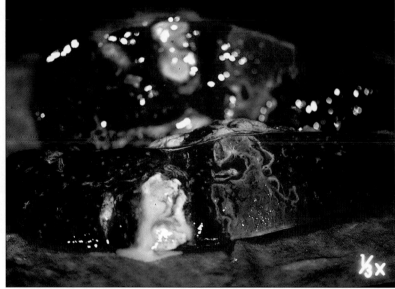

**FIGURE 2-40** Gross specimen of spleen resected from a patient with *Staphylococcus aureus* endocarditis. The patient developed acute left upper quadrant pain and tenderness, and a computed tomography scan documented multiple filling defects within the spleen. This gross specimen demonstrates both bland infarct and abscess formation, with visible pus following emboli to the organ.

**FIGURE 2-41** Small hemorrhagic infarct in the toe of a patient with infective endocarditis. *Streptococcus mutans* was isolated from the lesion as well as from multiple blood cultures.

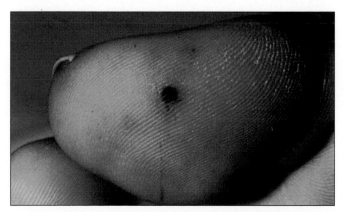

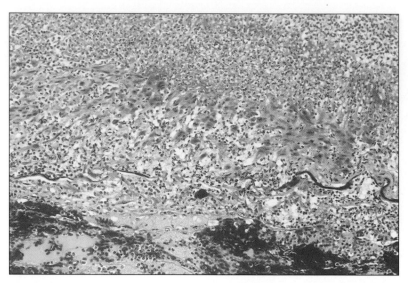

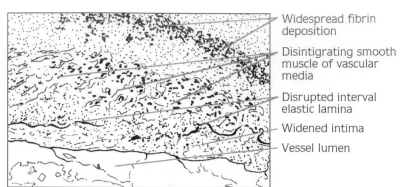

Widespread fibrin deposition

Disintigrating smooth muscle of vascular media

Disrupted interval elastic lamina

Widened intima

Vessel lumen

**FIGURE 2-42** Histologic findings of cerebrovascular mycotic arteritis. Vegetations associated with *Staphylococcus aureus* infective

endocarditis tend to embolize. Once the infected vegetations enter the cerebrovascular circulation, they may occlude a vessel, leading to an infarct. Or, if the embolus is infected, the organisms may cause acute inflammation in, and destruction of, the vessel walls. In this photomicrograph, disruption of the internal elastic lamina and disintegration of the vascular media are apparent. (Hematoxylin, phloxine, and saffron; × 38.) (*Courtesy of* D.A. Ramsay, MB, and G.B. Young, MD.)

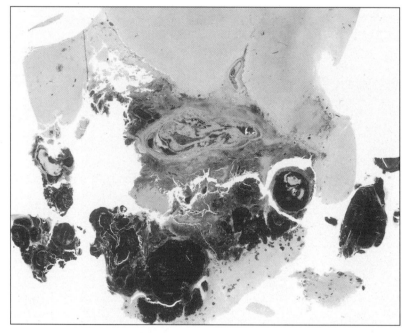

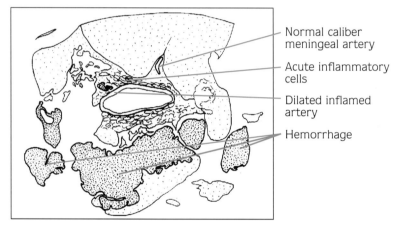

Normal caliber meningeal artery

Acute inflammatory cells

Dilated inflamed artery

Hemorrhage

**FIGURE 2-43** Histologic section demonstrating cerebrovascular mycotic aneurysm formation and rupture in septic arteritis. The

mycotic arteritis weakens the blood vessel wall, which then dilates and eventually ruptures. In this figure, a greatly dilated blood vessel is surrounded by a haze of acute inflammatory cells, and a hemorrhage is obvious. (A vessel of normal caliber is identified for comparison.) Hemorrhage in most cases of *Staphylococcus aureus* endocarditis may be due to septic arteritis, whereas a closer link between streptococcal endocarditis and mycotic aneurysm rupture has been suggested [6]. (Hematoxylin, phloxine, and saffron; × 1.) (*Courtesy of* D.A. Ramsay, MB, and G.B. Young, MD.)

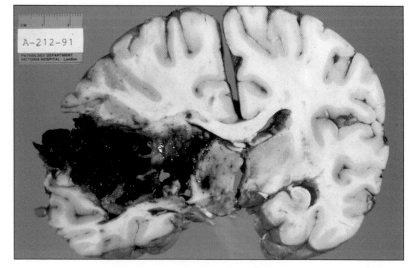

**FIGURE 2-44** Gross specimen showing endocarditic intracerebral hemorrhage. In the case shown in Figure 2-43, the septic arteritis caused a fatal massive left temporal intracerebral hemorrhage. Intracerebral hemorrhage occurs in approximately 5% of patients with native-valve bacterial endocarditis, and in some cases it can be predicted by radiologic identification of "mycotic" aneurysms. Most of the cerebrovascular complications of bacterial endocarditis occur early, and the risk of these complications diminishes rapidly as the infection is controlled. (*Courtesy of* D.A. Ramsay, MB, and G.B. Young, MD.)

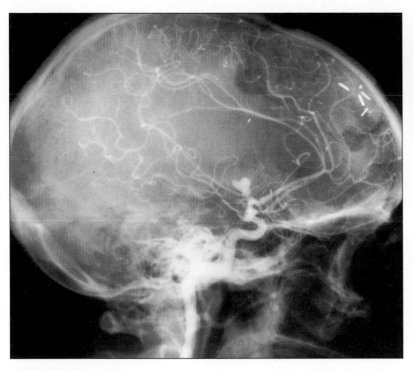

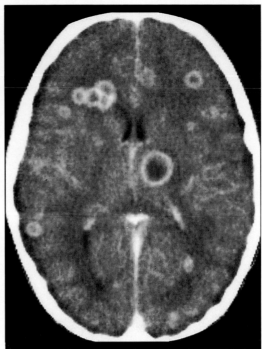

**FIGURE 2-46** Contrast-enhanced cranial computed tomography scan showing multiple brain abscesses. These scans are from a boy aged 10 years who developed headaches, fever, altered mental status, and frontal lobe signs. The ring-enhancing abscesses are similar to those found in bacterial endocarditis, although the cause was not found in this patient. The symptoms and radiologic signs of abscesses resolved with antibiotic therapy. (*From* lagarashi [7]; with permission.)

**FIGURE 2-45** Angiogram showing intracerebral mycotic aneurysms. Mycotic aneurysms typically involve the branch points of small, secondary arteries (the site of the clip on the angiogram). Since the clipping, a larger, multilobulated aneurysm has developed at the bifurcation of the internal carotid artery.

# DIAGNOSIS

## Proposed new criteria for diagnosis of infective endocarditis

**Definite infective endocarditis**
 Pathologic criteria
  Microorganisms: demonstrated by culture *or* histology in vegetation, or in vegetation
   that has embolized, or in intracardiac abscess; *or*
  Pathologic lesions: vegetation or intracardiac abscess present, confirmed by histol-
   ogy showing active IE
 Clinical criteria (*see* definitions in Fig. 2-48)
  Two major criteria, *or*
  One major and three minor criteria, *or*
  Five minor criteria
**Possible infective endocarditis**
 Findings consistent with IE that fall short of *definitive* but not *rejected*
**Rejected**
 Firm alternative diagnosis explaining evidence of IE, *or*
 Resolution of endocarditis syndrome with antibiotic therapy for ≤ 4 days, *or*
 No pathologic evidence of IE at surgery or autopsy, after antibiotic therapy for ≤ 4 days

IE—infective endocarditis.

**FIGURE 2-47** Proposed new criteria for the diagnosis of infective endocarditis. New criteria for the diagnosis of infective endocarditis have been proposed by Durack *et al.* that are based largely on the presence of typical microorganisms for endocarditis from blood cultures and characteristic findings on echocardiography. These new criteria have been validated by several other groups in recent years. (*Adapted from* Durack *et al.* [8].)

## A. Terminology used in the proposed new criteria for infective endocarditis: Major criteria

Positive blood culture for IE
  Typical microorganisms for IE from two separate blood cultures
    Viridans streptococci, *Streptococcus bovis*, HACEK group, *or*
    Community-acquired *Staphylococcus aureus* or enterococci, in the absence of a primary focus, *or*
  Persistently positive blood culture, defined as microorganism consistent with IE from:
    Blood cultures drawn > 12 hours apart, *or*
    All of three or majority of four or more separate blood cultures, with first and last drawn at least 1 hour apart
Evidence of endocardial involvement
  Positive echocardiogram for IE
    Oscillating intracardiac mass on valve or supporting structures, or in path of regurgitant jets, or on iatrogenic devices, in the absence of alternative anatomic explanation, *or*
    Abscess, *or*
    New partial dehiscence of prosthetic valve, *or*
  New valvular regurgitation (increase or change in preexisting murmur *not* sufficient)

IE—infective endocarditis.

**FIGURE 2-48** Terminology used in the proposed new criteria for infective endocarditis. **A**, Major criteria. The major criteria reflect positive blood cultures with typical or atypical microorganisms under appropriate clinical conditions, evidence of endocarditis involvement on an echocardiogram, or new valvular regurgitation.

## B. Terminology used in the proposed new criteria for infectious endocarditis: Minor criteria

Predisposition: predisposing heart condition *or* intravenous drug use
Fever: ≥ 38.3° C (100.4° F)
Vascular phenomena: arterial embolism, septic pulmonary infarcts, mycotic aneurysm, intracranial hemorrhage, Janeway lesions
Immunologic phenomena: glomerulonephritis, Osler nodes, Roth spots, rheumatoid factor
Echocardiogram: consistent with infective endocarditis but not meeting major criterion
Microbiologic evidence: positive blood culture but not meeting major criterion, *or* serologic evidence of active infection with organism consistent with infective endocarditis

**B**, Minor criteria. Multiple minor criteria also are included. Various combinations of the major and minor criteria are proposed for the diagnosis of infective endocarditis. (*Adapted from* Durack *et al.* [8].)

## Principles of blood cultures in the evaluation of suspected endocarditis

Obtain three sets before antibiotics
Obtain blood cultures from referring hospital
Talk to the microbiologist
Aerobic (5%–10% $CO_2$) and anaerobic
Hold ≥ 3 wks
Blind subcultures
Look for granular growth
Value of hypertonic media, antibiotic-removal resins, and arterial or bone marrow cultures unproven
Fungal cultures if intravenous drug abuse, prosthetic valve endocarditis

**FIGURE 2-49** Principles of blood cultures in the evaluation of suspected infective endocarditis. Blood cultures are the most important test performed in the initial evaluation of patients with suspected infective endocarditis. Ideally, three sets of blood cultures should be collected before the institution of antimicrobial therapy. The timing of these blood cultures depends on the clinical scenario and should be rapid in cases with a fulminant or acute onset. If the patient is referred from an outside hospital, obtain the blood cultures from that institution for further evaluation in the laboratory. Proper communication with the microbiology laboratory is essential. Blood cultures should be incubated aerobically in 5% to 10% $CO_2$ and anaerobically and held for at least 3 weeks to detect fastidious microorganisms. Blind subcultures are useful, especially in the detection of nutritionally variant streptococci and other fastidious organisms. Granular growth may be a clue to their early diagnosis. The use of hypertonic media, antibiotic-removal resins, arterial cultures, and cultures of bone marrow are of unproven benefit. In intravenous drug users and suspected prosthetic valve endocarditis, blood cultures for fungi are absolutely essential.

| Transesophageal echocardiography for infectious endocarditis |
|---|
| Sensitivity: ~95% for TEE vs ~60% for TTE |
| Superior to TTE for detecting valve ring abscess, local complications |
| Not a screening tool; expensive |

TEE—transesophageal echocardiography;
TTE—transthoracic echocardiography.

**FIGURE 2-50** Transesophageal echocardiography (TEE) for the diagnosis of infective endocarditis. TEE is a relatively new technique that has altered the diagnostic approach to some patients with suspected infective endocarditis. It utilizes a 5-MHz phase-array transducer with Doppler and color flow–encoding capabilities mounted on the tip of a flexible endoscope. Biplane imaging is improved over that possible with transthoracic echocardiography (TTE) because of better spatial resolution, lack of acoustic interference, and proximity to posterior structures (such as the mitral valve, left atrium, interatrial septum, and descending aorta). The sensitivity of TEE for the detection of vegetations is approximately 95%, compared with approximately 60% for conventional TTE. TEE is clearly superior to TTE in detecting local invasive phenomena, such as valve ring abscess, and other local complications. TEE is not a screening tool, however, and is expensive. TEE is also much more sensitive in the diagnosis of prosthetic valve endocarditis than are transthoracic techniques. TEE should be performed, unless contraindicated, in all infective endocarditis patients with a complicated course when perivalvular extension is suspected. Magnetic resonance imaging also appears promising for the detection of these complications.

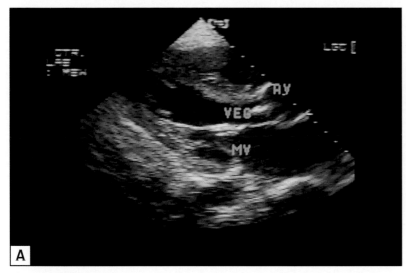

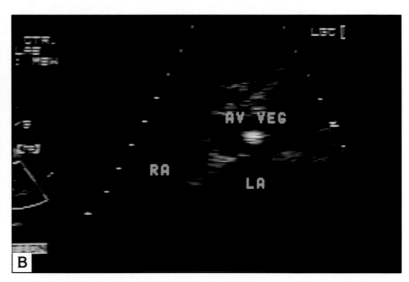

**FIGURE 2-51** Transthoracic echocardiographic views of aortic valve endocarditis. **A,** Parasternal long-axis view shows an aortic valve vegetation prolapsing into the left ventricular outflow tract. **B,** Short axis view of the aortic valve shows a prominent vegetation in the same patient.

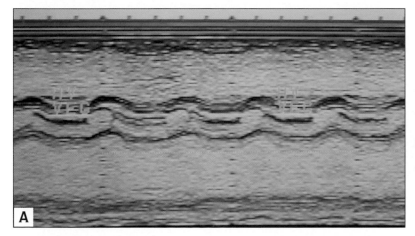

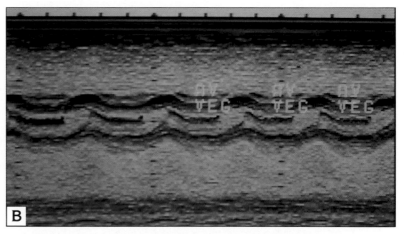

**FIGURE 2-52** M-mode transthoracic echocardiographic (TTE) views of aortic valve endocarditis. **A,** TTE M-mode examination of the same patient shown in Figure 2-51 depicts the aortic valve with a vegetation during valve closure. **B,** TTE M-mode examination documents high-frequency reverberations of the vegetation during diastole.

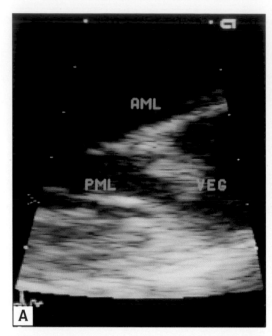

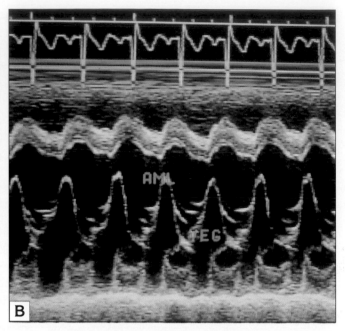

**FIGURE 2-53** Transthoracic echocardiographic (TTE) views of mitral valve endocarditis.
**A**, TTE shows a large vegetation on the anterior mitral valve leaflet prolapsing into the left atrium.
**B**, M-mode TTE shows mitral valve vegetation prolapsing into the left atrium during systole.

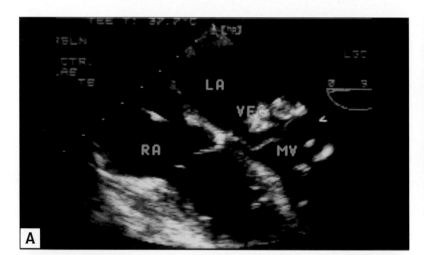

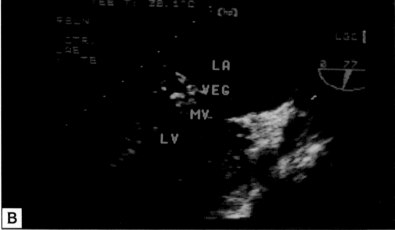

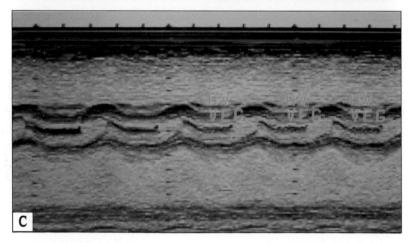

**FIGURE 2-54** Transesophageal echocardiographic (TEE) examination in mitral valve endocarditis. **A**, A TEE four-chamber view shows a large mitral valve vegetation prolapsing into the left atrium in systole. **B**, In the same patient, a long-axis view by TEE shows the same findings. **C**, TEE documents high-frequency reverberations of the vegetations.

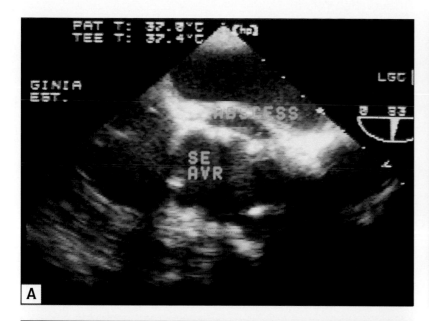

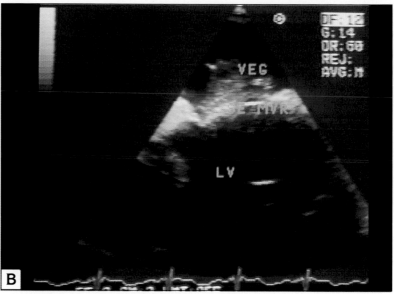

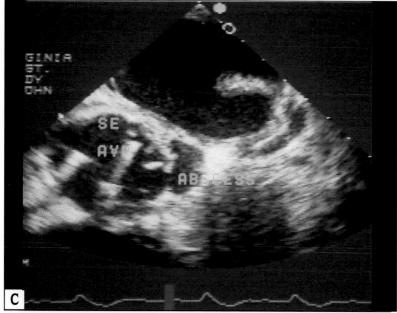

FIGURE 2-55 Transesophageal echocardiographic (TEE) evaluation of prosthetic valve endocarditis. **A**, TEE short-axis view of a Starr-Edwards aortic valve and a ring abscess pocket that bulges toward the left atrium during systole. **B**, TEE four-chamber view shows a huge vegetation on a Starr-Edwards mitral valve prosthesis. **C**, Short-axis TEE view of a Starr-Edwards aortic valve showing a ring abscess pocket.

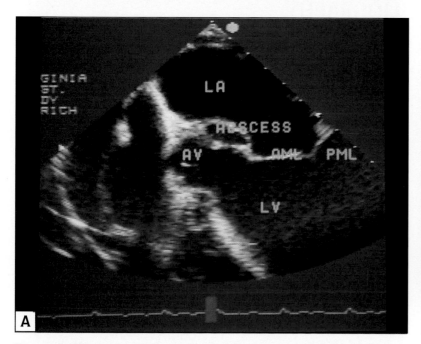

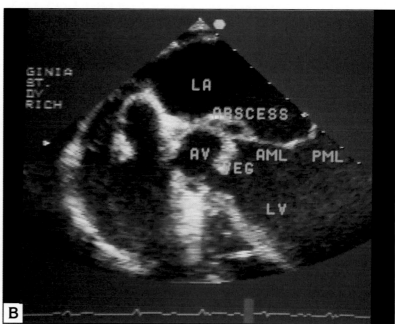

FIGURE 2-56 Transesophageal echocardiographic (TEE) view of native aortic valve endocarditis. **A**, TEE four-chamber view shows a native aortic valve ring abscess involving the anterior mitral leaflet. **B**, In the same patient, a TEE study shows the aortic vegetation with a valve ring abscess extending into the anterior mitral valve leaflet.

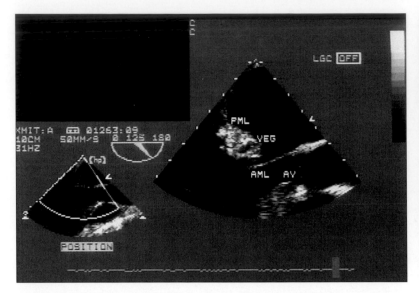

**Figure 2-57** Transesophageal echocardiogram depicting a large posterior mitral valve leaflet vegetation prolapsing into the left atrium during systole.

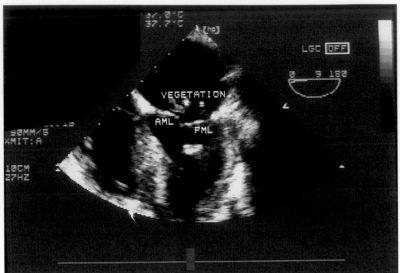

**Figure 2-58** Transesophageal echocardiogram showing a large vegetation involving both the anterior and posterior mitral valve leaflets.

# REFERENCES

1. Bayer AS: Infective endocarditis. *Clin Infect Dis* 1993, 17:313–320.

2. Watanakunakorn C, Burkert T: Infective endocarditis at a large community teaching hospital, 1980–1990: A review of 210 episodes. *Medicine* 1993, 72:90–102.

3. Chino F, Kodama A, Otake M, *et al.*: Nonbacterial thrombotic endocarditis in a Japanese autopsy sample: A review of 80 cases. *Am Heart J* 1975, 90:190.

4. Scheld WM, Sande MA: Endocarditis and intravascular infections. *In* Mandell GL, Bennett JE, Dolin R (eds.): *Principles and Practice of Infectious Diseases*, 4th ed. New York: Churchill Livingstone; 1995:740–783.

5. Sande MA, Strausbaugh LJ: Infective endocarditis. *In* Hook EW, Mandell GL, Gwaltney JM Jr, *et al.* (eds.): *Current Concepts in Infectious Diseases*. New York: Wiley; 1977.

6. Hart RG, Foster JW, Luther MF, Kanter MC: Stroke in infective endocarditis. *Stroke* 1990, 21:695–700.

7. Igarashi M: Multiple brain abscesses. *N Engl J Med* 1993, 329:1083.

8. Durack DT, Lukes AS, Bright DK, *et al.*: New criteria for diagnosis of infective endocarditis. *Am J Med* 1995, 96:200–209.

# SELECTED BIBLIOGRAPHY

Kaye D (ed.): *Infective Endocarditis*, 2nd ed. New York: Raven Press; 1992.

Scheld WM, Sande MA: Endocarditis and intravascular infections. *In* Mandell GL, Bennett JE, Dolin R (eds.): *Principles and Practice of Infectious Diseases*, 4th ed. New York: Churchill Livingstone; 1995:740–783.

Wilson WR, Steckelberg JM (eds.): Infective endocarditis. *Infect Dis Clin North Am* 1995, 7:1–170.

# CHAPTER 3

## Sepsis and Bacteremia

Steven M. Opal
Stephen H. Zinner

# EPIDEMIOLOGY AND PREDISPOSING FACTORS

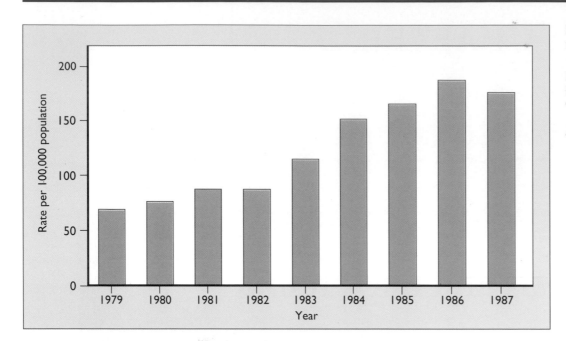

**FIGURE 3-1** Increasing incidence of bacterial sepsis in the United States between 1979 and 1987. There has been a steady progression of bacterial sepsis over the past two decades despite the development of more potent broad-spectrum antibiotics. (*Adapted from* Centers for Disease Control and Prevention [1].)

**Potential explanations for the increasing incidence of sepsis**

Aging patient population
Increased use of immunosuppressive therapies
Innovations in surgery (implantable devices)
Invasive monitoring (intravascular and urinary catheters)
Increase in bacterial sepsis from HIV infection
Prevalence of multidrug-resistant bacteria

**FIGURE 3-2** Potential explanations for the increasing incidence of sepsis. The presence of more elderly persons and more premature infants, as well as the wider use of more potent immunosuppressive conditions to treat malignancies and allow organ transplantation, certainly has rendered the population more susceptible to infections in general. The use of implantable devices and invasive monitoring of body systems in hospitals has also increased the access of sepsis-causing pathogens in the patient population. The incursion of HIV infection has certainly affected the rates of bacterial infection, and patients with AIDS are at risk of bacterial sepsis. In the past 10 years, the increased frequency and spectrum of bacteria resistant to many antibiotics surely has affected the incidence of bacterial sepsis, and this trend is likely to continue until new antibiotics are available and more attention is paid to prevention of bacterial infection.

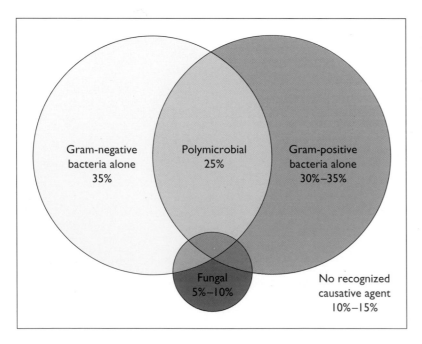

**FIGURE 3-3** Distribution of pathogens causing septic shock. In recent clinical series, the distribution of microorganisms responsible for sepsis emphasizes the fact that gram-negative bacteria are not the sole causes of this clinical syndrome. Although gram-negative and gram-positive bacteria each account for about one third of cases, fungal and mixed infections certainly may cause a clinical picture of sepsis. A minority of patients with sepsis do not have a causative agent identified. (*Adapted from* Bone [2].)

## Predisposing factors and associated pathogens in bacteremic patients

| Predisposing factor | Associated organisms |
| --- | --- |
| HIV infection | Encapsulated gram-positive bacteria |
| | *Salmonella* |
| | *Haemophilus influenzae* |
| Neutropenia | Gram-negative enteric organisms |
| | *Pseudomonas* spp |
| | *Candida* |
| | *Staphylococcus aureus* |
| Soft-tissue injury | Group A streptococci |
| | Clostridia |
| | *Vibrio* spp |
| Intravascular catheters | Coagulase-negative staphylococci |
| | *Staphylococcus aureus* |
| | Candida |
| Asplenia | Pneumococci |
| | Meningococci |
| | *Haemophilus* spp |
| Humoral immune deficiencies | Encapsulated gram-positive organisms |
| | Meningococci |
| | Haemophilus spp |

**FIGURE 3-4** Predisposing factors and associated pathogens in bacteremic patients. This figure associates the common infecting organisms and the host factors that predispose to bacteremia or fungemia. HIV infection results in defective antibody responses to new antigens, and these patients are often infected with encapsulated bacteria, such as pneumococci, *Haemophilus influenzae*, and *Salmonella* species. Neutropenic patients classically are at risk of severe sepsis due to gram-negative enteric rods, and these infections have the highest mortality rate. Recently, an increase in gram-positive infections with streptococcal species has been noted in these patients. Patients who suffer burns or other soft-tissue injuries are at particular risk of streptococcal infections, and patients with long-term intravascular catheters are at risk of bacteremia with coagulase-negative staphylococci. Patients with functional or anatomic asplenia are at risk of serious infections with encapsulated organisms, as are those with humoral immune deficiencies or complement defects.

# PATHOPHYSIOLOGY

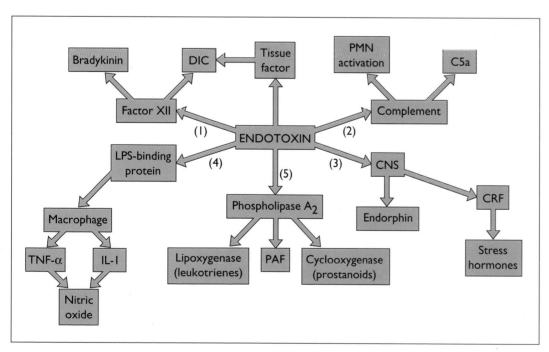

**FIGURE 3-5** Systemic effects of endotoxin. Bacterial endotoxin (such as lipopolysaccharide [LPS] in gram-negative bacteria) activates a cascade of inflammatory mediators from various systems, including the coagulation and fibrinolytic systems (*1*), complement system (*2*), neuroendocrine system (*3*), and eicosanoid pathway (*4*). LPS also activates the monocyte/macrophage cell line (*5*) to release interleukin-1 (IL-1) and tumor necrosis factor-α (TNF-α) via a carrier protein, a LPS-binding protein. *1*, Factor XII in concert with circulating high-molecular-weight (tissue) kininogen converts prekallikrein to kallikrein, which catalyzes kininogen breakdown to the vasoactive peptide bradykinin. Activated factor XII and tissue factor (factor III) further activate the entire coagulation cascade and fibrolytic system, ultimately resulting in disseminated intravascular coagulation (DIC). *2*, Complement activation leads to the release of anaphylatoxins, such as C3a and C5a, which contribute to vasomotor instability in sepsis. *3*, Endotoxin also activates the stress hormone response and β-endorphins, which centrally mediate hypotension. *4*, The eicosanoids are a family of vasoactive cyclic endoperoxides that contribute to the systemic inflammatory response. *5*, The monocyte-macrophage components are the principal elaborators of the inflammatory cytokines, IL-1, IL-6, IL-8, IL-12, and TNF. Shock or hypotension itself is directly produced by cytokine-induced nitric oxide synthesis and release, platelet-activating factor (PAF), bradykinin, complement components, and perhaps other host-derived mediators [2,3]. (CNS—central nervous system; CRF—corticotropin-releasing factor; PMN—polymorphonuclear leukocytes.)

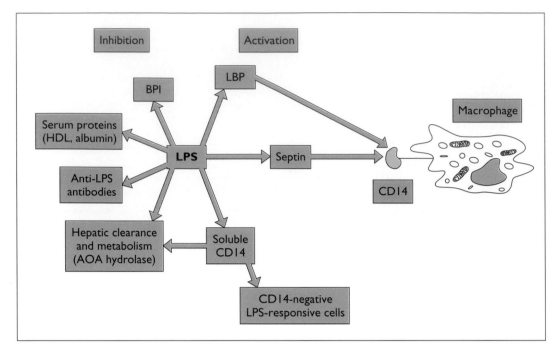

**FIGURE 3-6** Potential host responses to endotoxin. The potential host responses to endotoxin (lipopolysaccharide [LPS]) are in a state of dynamic balance between inhibitory and activating effects. Endotoxin activity may be inhibited by several endogenous host-defense mechanisms, including bactericidal/permeability-inducting protein (BPI), a neutrophil-derived protein that neutralizes endotoxin; serum proteins, such as high-density lipoproteins (HDL) and albumin, which bind to help clear LPS; preformed anti-LPS antibodies, which also bind LPS; and hepatic clearance and metabolic activity, including acyl-oxy-acyl (AOA) hydrolase. LPS effects may be activated by a series of endogenous proteins, including: LPS-binding protein (LBP) and septin (a series of proteolytic enzymes that may activate macrophages), both of which facilitate the delivery of endotoxin to membrane-bound CD14 receptor on the macrophage. The binding of endotoxin to this receptor, in turn, results in activation of a separate signal transduction mechanism with the ultimate release of cytokines. Soluble CD14 may play a dual role in either the activation or clearance of LPS from the circulation [4].

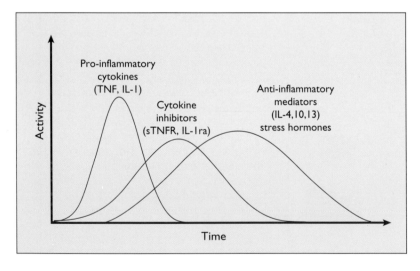

**FIGURE 3-7** Sequence of cytokine responses to infection over time. The initial response to an infectious stimulus is the generation of the proinflammatory cytokines tumor necrosis factor-$\alpha$ (TNF-$\alpha$) and interleukin (IL)-1. Other cytokines, such as IL-6, IL-8, and IL-12, may also participate. Soon, specific cytokine inhibitors are released, such as soluble TNF receptor (sTNFR) and IL-1 receptor antagonist (IL-1ra), which downregulate cytokine activity. Subsequently, anti-inflammatory cytokines, such as IL-4, IL-10, and IL-13, and stress hormones (epinephrine, glucocorticoids) further modulate the response [5].

# CLINICAL MANIFESTATIONS

## Clinical signs and symptoms of sepsis

Fever, chills, hypotension
Hypothermia
Hyperventilation
Alteration in mental status
Bleeding or oozing from wounds or puncture sites
Evidence of infection in lung, urinary tract
Ecthyma gangrenosum, petechiae, bullae
Evidence for organ failure: jaundice, cyanosis, oliguria/anuria,
  heart failure

**FIGURE 3-8** Common clinical signs and symptoms associated with bacterial sepsis. Some patients may present with very subtle signs early in their course. For example, hyperventilation or altered mental status may be the only manifestation in some patients. Others, notably neutropenic patients, may present with only fever. Eventually, there is evidence of infection at some body site or in association with specific evidence for organ failure.

## Laboratory abnormalities in sepsis

Leukopenia or leukocytosis
Anemia, thrombocytopenia
Evidence of disseminated intravascular coagulation, fibrin split products
Elevated serum creatinine, lactic acidosis
Hyperbilirubinemia
Diffuse pulmonary infiltrates, hypoxia, normal left ventricular end-diastolic pressure
  (consistent with acute respiratory distress syndrome)
High cardiac index, low systemic vascular resistance

**FIGURE 3-9** Clinical laboratory findings associated with bacterial sepsis. Abnormalities involve white blood cells, red cells, and platelets. Renal failure may occur, as may altered bilirubin metabolism. The cardiovascular effects of sepsis often contribute significantly to the clinical presentation.

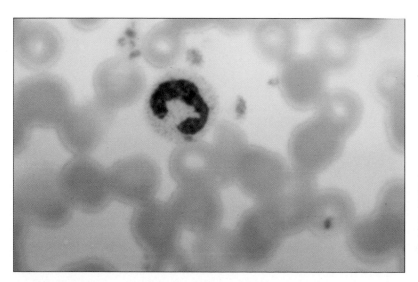

**FIGURE 3-10** Döhle inclusion body. A cytoplasmic inclusion is seen in this Wright-stained neutrophil from the peripheral blood of a septic patient. Döhle bodies are believed to be precipitated components of the endoplasmic reticulum. These cells may reflect the presence of bacterial sepsis, although they may also be found in other acute inflammatory states.

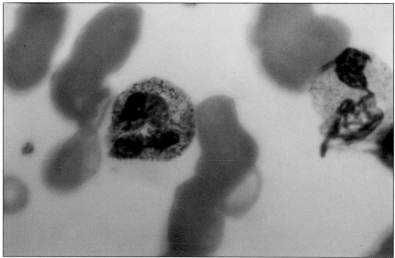

**FIGURE 3-11** Toxic granules within polymorphonuclear leukocytes in a Wright-stained smear of peripheral blood from a bacteremic patient. These granules are believed to be prominent lysosomal granules and usually indicate serious bacterial infection.

# Streptococcal Sepsis

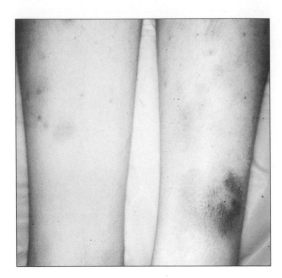

**FIGURE 3-12** Erythema nodosum in a patient with severe streptococcal pharyngitis, peritonsillar abscess, and bacteremia. This painful skin lesion may often be found accompanying several clinical situations, including severe infections caused by *Streptococcus pyogenes*, fungi, and *Mycobacterium* species. Erythema nodosum also may be seen as an adverse effect of some antibiotics (*eg*, penicillins, sulfonamides).

# Staphylococcal Bacteremia

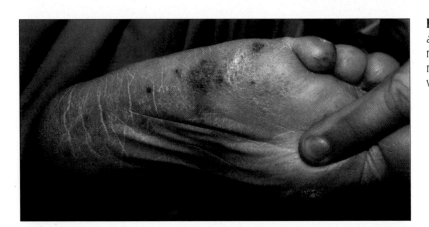

**FIGURE 3-13** Septic emboli in a patient with *Staphylococcus aureus* bacteremia. The emboli originated from an abdominal mycotic aneurysm. This lesion is usually painful and ultimately results in cutaneous necrosis. Similar lesions may occur in patients with bacterial endocarditis.

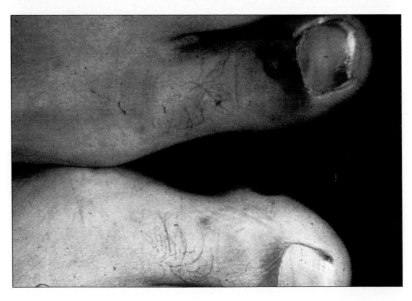

**FIGURE 3-14** Peripheral septic embolus to the skin in a patient with *Staphylococcus aureus* bacteremia without endocarditis. This patient had severe untreated dermatophytosis (tinea pedis), which may have served as an entry for staphylococci. In this case, the patient had no other underlying diseases and responded promptly to antistaphylococcal antibiotics and supportive therapy. The dermatophytosis also responded to vigorous antifungal therapy.

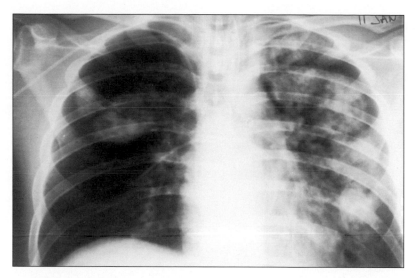

**FIGURE 3-15** Chest radiograph showing multiple septic pulmonary emboli in a patient with suppurative phlebitis at the site of an intravascular catheter insertion. *Staphylococcus aureus* was cultured from the blood and the removed catheter tip. Right-sided bacterial endocarditis should be considered in patients with similar presentations. (*Courtesy of* S. Lowry, MD.)

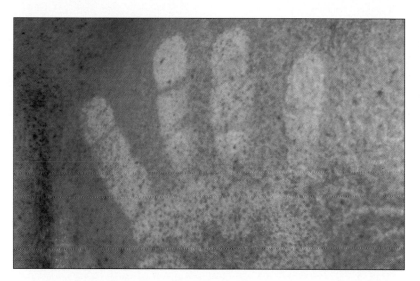

**FIGURE 3-16** Typical erythroderma associated with early staphylococcal toxic shock syndrome. A characteristic blanching of the skin can be seen in the early stage of this syndrome. This condition is caused by a toxin-producing strain of *Staphylococcus aureus* that is usually producing infection at some distant site. Supportive therapy is critical to successful outcome, and treatment with antistaphylococcal antibiotics is associated with lower recurrence rates. (*Courtesy of* C. Fisher, MD.)

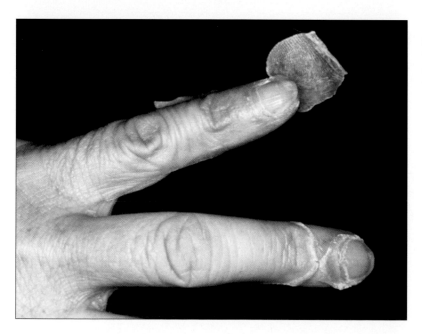

**FIGURE 3-17** Desquamation of the epidermis in late toxic shock syndrome. Similar manifestations can be seen with serious streptococcal infections, including scarlet fever and the "toxic streptococcal syndrome." In several cases the nail is sloughed as well as the superficial epidermis. (*Courtesy of* C. Fisher, MD.)

## Clostridial Sepsis

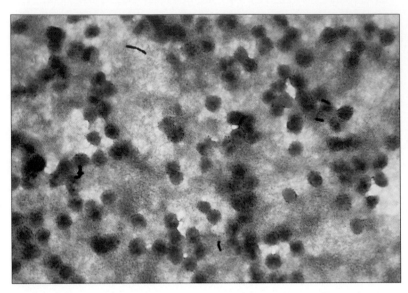

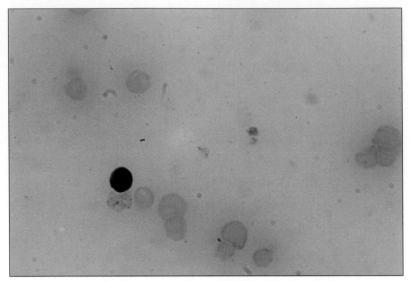

**FIGURE 3-18** Gram-positive bacilli in a peripheral blood buffy coat in clostridial sepsis. Peripheral blood smears of the buffy coat from this patient with clostridial bacteremia and sepsis revealed stainable bacteria and red blood cell ghosts. This patient had clostridial sepsis secondary to a widely metastatic uterine carcinoma with colonic fistula formation. She also experienced hemoglobinuria and acute renal failure and died from refractory septic shock. High-grade bacteremia with *Clostridium perfringens* or other gram-positive bacteria may be detected occasionally in buffy coat smears.

**FIGURE 3-19** Wright-stained smear of peripheral blood in clostridial sepsis. Peripheral blood smear from the same patient as in Figure 3-18 shows a paucity of intact erythrocytes and platelets indicative of massive intravascular hemolysis. This hemolysis is due to the generation of clostridial alpha-toxin, which has phospholipase activity that destroys cell membranes. Exchange transfusions have been used with some success to control intravascular hemolysis in these patients.

## Meningococcemia

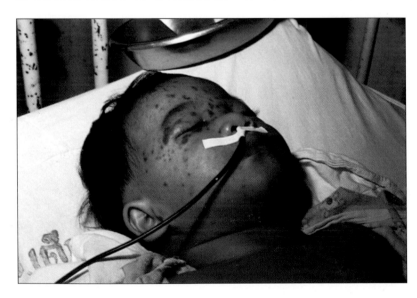

**FIGURE 3-20** Petechial and purpuric lesions of early acute meningococcemia. This child aged 3 years with meningitis has disseminated intravascular coagulation, as noted by the hemorrhagic return in the nasogastric tube. Fulminant meningococcemia is frequently fatal despite the institution of antibiotics, fluids, and cardiovascular support.

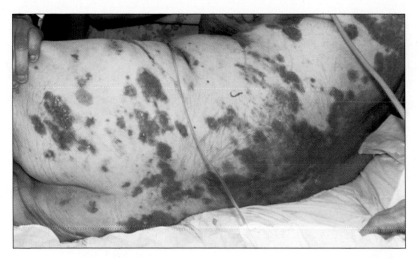

**FIGURE 3-21** Erythematous sedulations in early meningococcemia. Approximately 5 days into the course of meningococcemia, an adult with meningitis caused by *Neisseria meningitidis* shows the characteristic cutaneous necrosis. These lesions are the result of intravascular coagulation induced by direct activation of the coagulation and thrombolytic pathways. The lesions may heal over several weeks, but terminal digits may necrose completely and slough. (*Courtesy of* H. Levy, MD.)

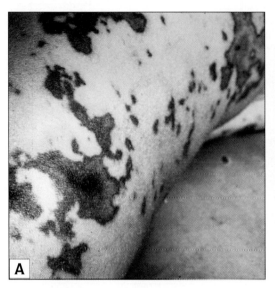

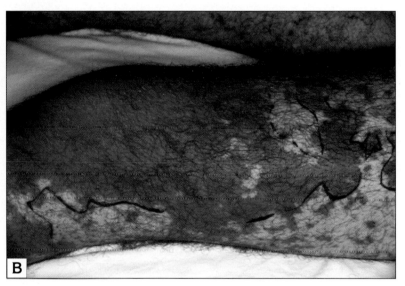

**FIGURE 3-22** Late skin lesions in fulminant meningococcemia. **A,** As meningococcemia progresses, petechial skin lesions, seen here on the thigh, coalesce into large areas of cutaneous necrosis (sedulations). Meningococcemia may present subtly with or without meningeal involvement. If treated promptly with appropriate antibiotics, these cutaneous consequences may be prevented. **B,** Extensive cutaneous involvement and coalesced necrotic lesions are seen in a patient with fulminant meningococcemia.

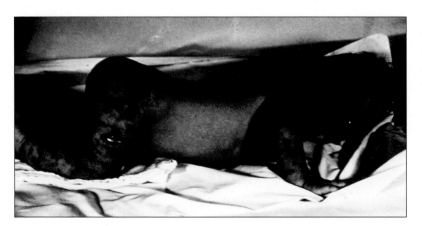

**FIGURE 3-23** Extensive extremity sedulations in a child aged 2 years with meningococcal meningitis and bacteremia. As a manifestation of disseminated intravascular coagulation in severe bacteremia, similar lesions may occur in the kidney, bone, and central nervous system. The patient survived following an extensive course of antibiotics and supportive therapy.

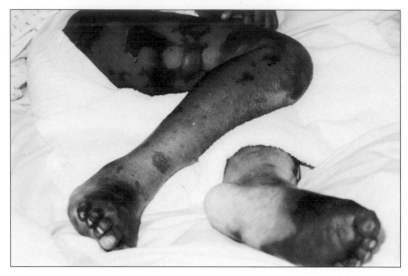

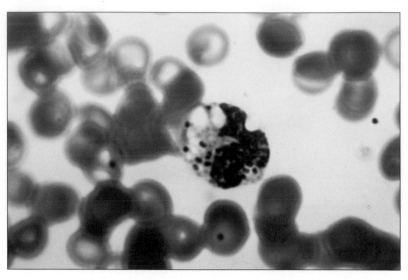

**FIGURE 3-24** Extensive cutaneous, soft-tissue, and bone necrosis following meningococcal sepsis. These lesions are the result of extensive microthrombi in the skin and supporting tissues that result from endotoxin activation of the clotting cascade. Inflammatory cytokines, such as interleukin (IL)-1, IL-6, and tumor necrosis factor, play a prominent role in the development of these lesions. (*Courtesy of* G. Slotman, MD.)

**FIGURE 3-25** Wright-stained smear of peripheral blood in fulminant *Neisseria meningitidis* bacteremia. Note the presence of extracellular and intracellular gram-negative diplococci. Direct visualization of meningococci on unspun peripheral blood is quite unusual. However, similar smears can be obtained by direct aspiration of necrotic skin lesions.

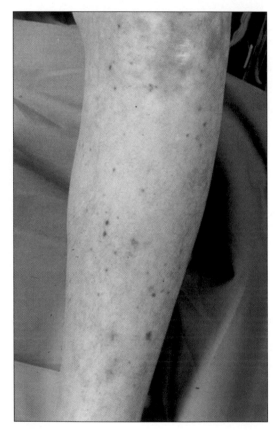

**FIGURE 3-26** Discrete petechial skin lesions in chronic meningococcemia. Chronic meningococcemia is a subacute illness with subtle presentations, such as low-grade fever, malaise, and septic arthritis. Recurrent meningococcemia may be a clue to the presence of late complement component deficiencies, as in this patient who has an inherited C6 deficiency.

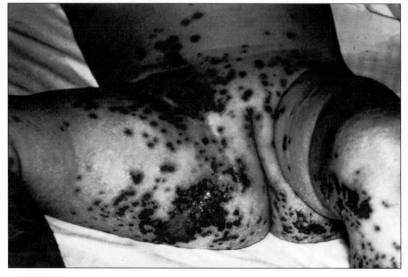

**FIGURE 3-27** Eczema vaccinatum in an infant. This lesion may develop in severely immunocompromised patients who receive smallpox vaccine. Although these lesions may resemble necrotic skin lesions of acute meningococcemia, the individual lesions in eczema vaccinatum are smaller and become encrusted like those of other poxvirus infections. These patients usually recover uneventfully with no specific therapy.

# Cutaneous Manifestations of Sepsis

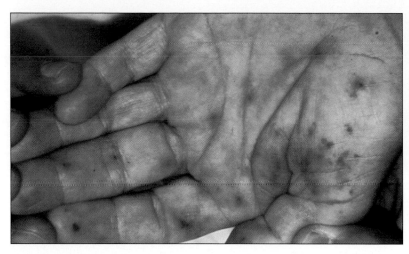

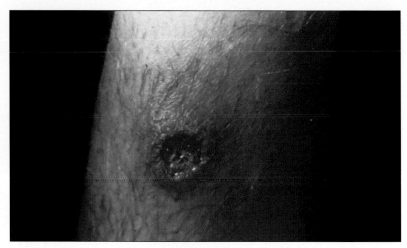

**FIGURE 3-28** Janeway lesions in bacteremia and sepsis. Typical Janeway lesions, punctate painless embolic manifestations of endovascular infection, are seen on a patient's palm. These lesions are typical for subacute bacterial endocarditis caused by viridans streptococci but can also be seen in patients who do not have endocarditis. This patient had bacteremia and sepsis due to an abdominal aortic graft infected by *Acinetobacter calcoaceticus*. This patient died, and no evidence of endocarditis was found at postmortem examination.

**FIGURE 3-29** Early lesion of ecthyma gangrenosum. This granulocytopenic patient had bacteremia due to *Pseudomonas aeruginosa*. Note the raised hemorrhagic border with a prominent central depression. These lesions occur as a poor prognostic sign in severely immunocompromised, bacteremic patients and are usually seen in patients with acute leukemia in blast crisis. Although most commonly seen with *P. aeruginosa* bacteremic, they may occur in association with other gram-negative infections [6]. (*Courtesy of* A. Cross, MD.)

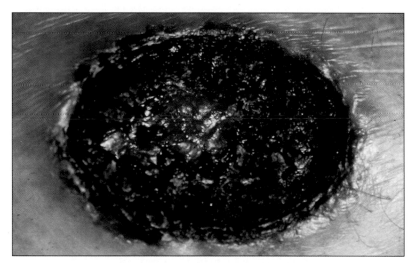

**FIGURE 3-30** Late manifestations of ecthyma gangrenosum. In an immunocompromised patient with *Pseudomonas aeruginosa* bacteremia, a late lesion of ecthyma shows discrete borders and a necrotic center. It is unusual to find more than 6 to 10 such lesions widely scattered over the body. Aspiration of the necrotic center usually reveals necrotic debris, bacteria, and a notable absence of granulocytes. (*Courtesy of* A. Cross, MD.)

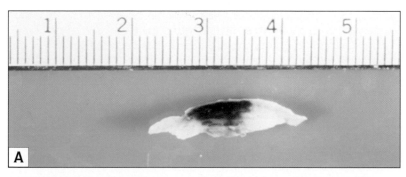

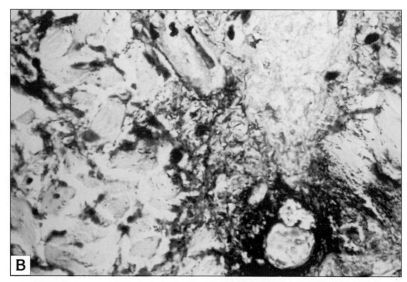

**FIGURE 3-31** Skin biopsy of an ecthyma gangrenosum lesion. This severely burned patient was bacteremic with *Pseudomonas aeruginosa*. **A,** Gross examination of the biopsy specimen shows a discrete area of hemorrhagic necrosis extending into the subcutaneous tissues. **B,** On Gram-staining, there is an absence of polymorphonuclear leukocytes and the presence of gram-negative bacilli in and around the vessel adventitia and media. (*Courtesy of* C.W. Goodwin, MD.)

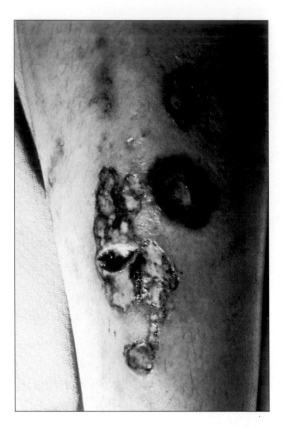

**FIGURE 3-32**
Two lesions of ecthyma gangrenosum adjacent to an area of burn wound sepsis due to *Pseudomonas aeruginosa*. Note the violaceous ecchymotic areas around the central necrosis. This patient was not neutropenic. (*Courtesy of* C.W. Goodwin, MD.)

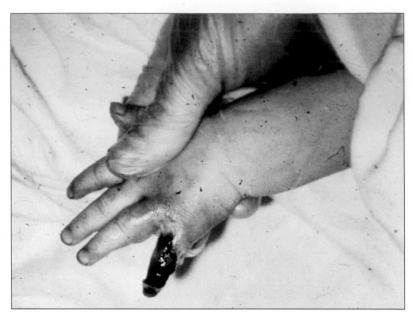

**FIGURE 3-33** Digital necrosis and sloughing in a child with *Pseudomonas aeruginosa* bacteremia. The bacteremia developed following rupture of a gangrenous appendix. This is an unusual manifestation of sepsis given the current antibiotics active against gram-negative bacteria. This patient presented before the availability of specific antipseudomonal antibiotics and did not survive.

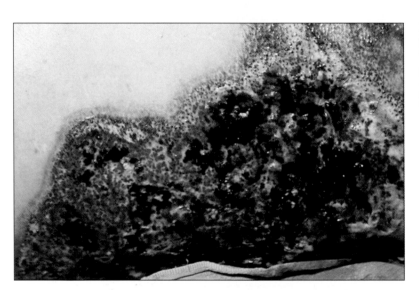

**FIGURE 3-34** Burn wound sepsis and *Pseudomonas aeruginosa* infection. There are extensive areas of necrosis above the wound. Tissue necrosis at various sites is often seen with severe pseudomonal infections, probably due in part to the elaboration of pseudomonal exotoxins such as exotoxin A, elastase, and phospholipases. (*Courtesy of* C.W. Goodwin, MD.)

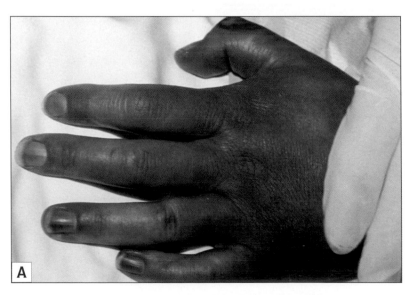

**A**

**FIGURE 3-35** Catecholamine-associated digital cyanosis and necrosis in bacteremia. **A**, Digits from a patient with dopamine-induced cyanosis. This patient had refractory septic shock due to *Escherichia coli* bacteremia. Vasoactive amines, such as catecholamines, may precipitate this process in patients with unresponsive sepsis. (*continued*)

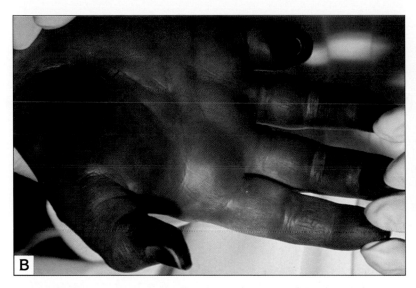

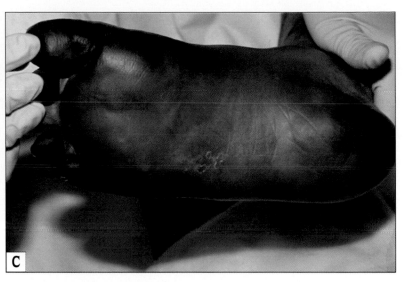

**Figure 3-35** (*continued*) **B**, The ventral aspect of the hand shows acral necrosis. **C**, The plantar view of the foot shows extensive cyanosis and necrosis. Note the absence of discrete demarcated borders as seen in meningococcemia. (*Courtesy of* H. Levy, MD.)

# MANAGEMENT AND PREVENTION

**Patient evaluation in suspected sepsis**

Complete history and physical examination (determine predisposing factors and likely source of infection)
Blood cultures (*before* antibiotic therapy)
Cultures of urine, secretions, wounds, abscess aspirates, etc.
Stool examination for fecal leukocytes and culture, if indicated
Complete blood count, platelet count, coagulation profiles, lactate levels, hepatic and renal function tests
Lumbar puncture with cerebrospinal fluid culture if headache or mental status change (and no increased intracranial pressure)

**FIGURE 3-36** Evaluation of patients with suspected sepsis. A careful history and physical examination will reveal the presence of risk factors for and the early clinical signs of sepsis. Blood cultures *before* the addition of antibiotic therapy remain the critical diagnostic step to determine the causative organism, and this identification is crucial to the correct use of antibiotics. If any neurologic symptoms are present, lumbar puncture with cerebrospinal fluid examination is important (although lumbar puncture is not indicated in the presence of increased intracranial pressure).

**Treatment of bacterial sepsis**

Maintain airway and venous access
Intravenous antibiotics directed to likely pathogens
Monitor systemic arterial pressure, pulmonary wedge pressures, oxygenation, respiratory status
Fluid and electrolyte replacement to maintain tissue perfusion
Surgical drainage of purulent collections

**FIGURE 3-37** General approach to the treatment of septic patients. As with other emergency conditions, it is critical to establish a patent airway and intravenous access. Antibiotics directed against the likely pathogens must be started promptly after diagnostic blood cultures are obtained. Because many of the complications of sepsis involve organ failure, it is crucial to maintain tissue perfusion with pressure monitoring and fluid and electrolyte management. Prompt surgical drainage is indicated for any suspected purulent collections.

## Experimental therapies for sepsis

| | |
|---|---|
| Organism-specific | Polyvalent antibody (*eg*, O-side chains of gram-negative bacteria, exotoxin of *Staphylococcus aureus* and *Streptococcus*, cell wall antigens of *Enterococcus* and *Staphylococcus*) |
| Endotoxin-specific | Monoclonal antibody lipid A antibodies; polymyxin; bacterial permeability-increasing protein; CAP 18 (cationic protein in human neutrophils); endotoxin-binding membranes; lipid A analogs and antagonists |
| Endogenous mediator-specific | Anticytokines against tumor necrosis factor and IL-1; anti-inflammatory cytokines (IL-10); therapies against platelet activating factor, nitric oxide, bradykinin, white cell integrins, eicosanoids |

IL—interleukin.

**Figure 3-38** Experimental therapies for sepsis. There has been an explosion of research into the prevention and treatment of bacterial sepsis. However, no new modalities have yet been successfully introduced to the clinical armamentarium for sepsis management. Potential treatments undergoing critical evaluation include attempts to block or modify bacterial endotoxin or other bacterial antigens and products, to block proinflammatory cytokines, or to stimulate anti-inflammatory cytokines or their function.

## Prognostic factors in sepsis and bacteremia

Severity of underlying disease*
Level of immunosuppression
Presence of shock
Polymicrobial bacteremia
Hypothermia, multiorgan failure
High APACHE score or other acute physiologic indicators
*Pseudomonas* bacteremia, *Candida* infection

*Most important predictor.

**Figure 3-39** Prognostic factors in sepsis and bacteremia. Several factors affect the outcome of episodes of bacterial sepsis. The most important predictive factor is the severity of the underlying disease. Patients with rapidly fatal underlying conditions (such as acute leukemia in blast crisis) are at serious risk of death from associated bacterial sepsis. The degree of patient immunocompromise also affects the outcome from sepsis, with more intense immunocompromise conferring a poorer prognosis with sepsis. Other poor prognostic indicators include polymicrobial bacteremia, multiorgan failure, hypothermia, and high APACHE scores. Pseudomonal and candidal infections are listed as poor prognostic indicators, but these infections often occur in the most immunocompromised patients who are otherwise at risk.

## Prevention of bacteremia and sepsis

Bacterial vaccines—in asplenic patients, elderly, immunocompromised
Judicious use and meticulous maintenance of catheter devices
Limit degree of immunosuppressive therapy (if possible)
Protect integument and mucosal barriers, nutritional support, early treatment, and control of localized infections
Elective alimentary tract decontamination in selected high-risk patients (?)

**Figure 3-40** Prevention of bacteremia and sepsis. Important considerations for the prevention of bacterial sepsis include risk assessment and vaccine administration to elderly and immunocompromised patients (*eg*, pneumococcal vaccine). Physicians must limit unnecessary use of invasive devices, including catheters, and all efforts must be made to protect the integument and mucosal barriers that limit bacterial invasion. Some patients, such as those with prolonged granulocytopenia, might benefit from attempts to minimize their gastrointestinal bacterial load with oral antibacterial agents.

# REFERENCES

1. Centers for Disease Control and Prevention: Increase in national hospital discharge survey rates for septicemia–United States, 1979–1987. *MMWR* 1990, 39:31–34.

2. Bone RC: The pathogenesis of sepsis. *Ann Intern Med* 1991, 115:457–469.

3. Brandtzaeg P, Kierulf P, Gaustad P, *et al.*: Plasma endotoxin as a predictor of multi-organ failure and death in systemic meningococcal disease. *J Infect Dis* 1989, 159:195–205.

4. Opal SM, Palardy JE, Marra MN, *et al.*: Relative contributions of endotoxin-binding proteins in body fluids during infection. *Lancet* 1994, 344:429–431.

5. Beutler B, Cerami A: Biology of cachectin/TNF—A primary mediator of the host response. *Annu Rev Immunol* 1989, 7:625–655.

6. Artenstein AW, Cross AS: Serious infections caused by *Pseudomonas aeruginosa*. *J Intensive Care Med* 1994, 9:34–51.

# SELECTED BIBLIOGRAPHY

Artenstein AW, Cross AS: Serious infections caused by *Pseudomonas aeruginosa*. *J Intensive Care Med* 1994, 9:34–51.

Beutler B, Cerami A: Biology of cachectin/TNF—A primary mediator of the host response. *Annu Rev Immunol* 1989, 7:625–655.

Bone RC: The pathogenesis of sepsis. *Ann Intern Med* 1991, 115:457–469.

Brandtzaeg P, Kierulf P, Gaustad P, *et al.*: Plasma endotoxin as a predictor of multi-organ failure and death in systemic meningococcal disease. *J Infect Dis* 1989, 159:195–205.

Opal SM, Palardy JE, Marra MN, *et al.*: Relative contributions of endotoxin-binding proteins in body fluids during infection. *Lancet* 1994, 344:429–431.

# CHAPTER 4

# Streptococcal Infections

Adnan S. Dajani
Patricia Ferrieri

# PATHOGENESIS

| Group A streptococcal suppurative/invasive diseases | |
|---|---|
| Tonsillopharyngitis | Bone/joint infections |
| Soft-tissue infections | Osteomyelitis |
| Impetigo | Pyogenic arthritis |
| Necrotizing fasciitis | Sinusitis |
| Cellulitis | Mastoiditis |
| Lymphangitis | Pulmonary infections |
| Lymphadenitis | Pneumonitis |
| Thrombophlebitis | Empyema |
| Abscess formation | Postpartum infections |
| Septicemia | Puerperal sepsis |
| Toxic shock–like syndrome | Myometritis |
| Meningitis | Breast abscesses |

**FIGURE 4-1**  Group A streptococcal suppurative/invasive diseases.

| Group A streptococcal nonsuppurative diseases |
|---|
| Rheumatic fever |
| Glomerulonephritis |
| Others |
| Toxic shock–like syndrome |
| Scarlet fever |
| Kawasaki syndrome (?) |

**FIGURE 4-2**  Group A streptococcal nonsuppurative diseases.

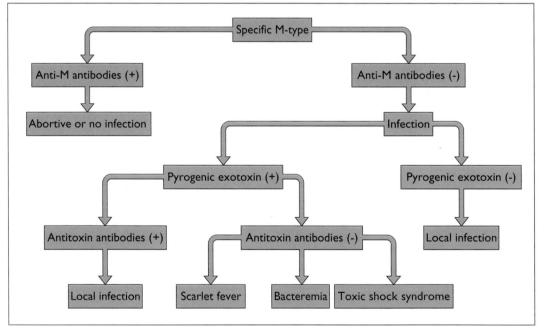

**FIGURE 4-3**  Model for group A streptococcal infections. Group A streptococci contain or produce a number of products that may contribute to disease production. If a human host is exposed to a particular M type of group A streptococci, infection may or may not ensue, depending on the absence or presence of antibodies to the specific M protein. Infection may be localized or may spread; the exact mechanism for invasiveness is not well defined, but invasiveness is associated with certain M types (*eg*, M1, M3). If the infecting strain is capable of producing pyrogenic exotoxins (especially exotoxin A), then scarlet fever, bacteremia, or toxic shock syndrome may occur, particularly if the host lacks antistreptococcal pyrogenic exotoxin antibodies.

**Group A streptococcal constituents or extracellular products that may contribute to pathophysiology of sepsis and shock**

| Constituent/product | Pathogenic property |
|---|---|
| M protein | Antiphagocytic (anti-M antibody promotes bacterial opsonization, uptake, and PMN killing) |
| Pyrogenic exotoxins A, B, C | Pyrogenicity |
| | Suppresses Ig production |
| | Induces monokines (*eg*, interleukin-1β, TNF-α) |
| | T-cell mitogen |
| | Alters reticuloendothelial cell function |
| | Inhibits neutrophil chemotaxis through TNF-α |
| | Enhances delayed hypersensitivity, leading possibly to skin findings |
| Hyaluronidase | Cleaves hyaluronic acid in tissue matrix |
| Protease | Proteolytic, damaging to proteins |
| Streptolysin O | May act synergistically with exotoxin to influence monocyte and macrophage monokine production |

PMN—polymorphonuclear cells; TNF—tumor necrosis factor.

**FIGURE 4-4** Group A streptococcal constituents or extracellular products that contribute to pathophysiology of sepsis and shock. Group A streptococci produce large numbers of extracellular products. Some of these have been shown to play a role in the pathophysiology of disease production.

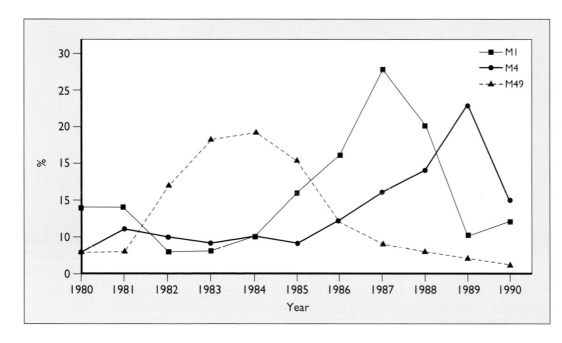

**FIGURE 4-5** Changes in group A streptococcal serotypes in Britain between 1980 and 1990. Extensive epidemiologic investigations of group A streptococcal serotypes in Britain between 1980 and 1990 indicated that some serotypes (such as M3 and M12) showed no great variations from year to year; some other strains caused nationwide epidemics. The figure represents the frequency of three distinct serotypes (M1, M4, and M49) during the observation period. Types M1 and M3 were associated with invasive disease and fatal infections. Type M4 accounted for 50% of erythromycin-resistant strains [1].

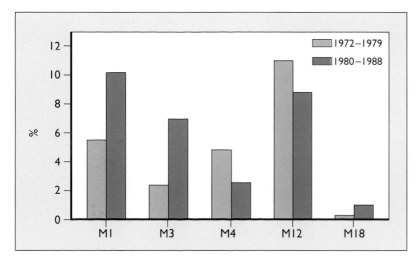

**FIGURE 4-6** Changes in proportion of M types in the United States between 1972 and 1988. The proportions of M types in various parts of the United States vary at different times. The figure compares the frequency of five distinct M types over two periods: 1972 to 1979 and 1980 to 1988. Between 1980 and 1988, a relative increase was noted in types M1, M3, and M18, whereas a relative decrease was observed for types M4 and M12. Types M1 and M3 are known to be associated with invasive (bacteremic) infections. Indeed, an increase in invasive group A streptococcal infections has been observed since the early 1980s in the United States. Type M1, M3, and M18 are all implicated as "rheumatogenic" streptococci [2].

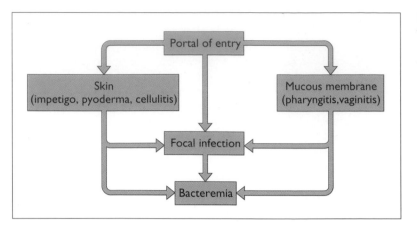

**FIGURE 4-7** Pathogenesis of invasive group A streptococcal infections. Organisms enter via the skin or mucous membranes and may lead to local infection. This may progress to focal infection, or it may spread to systematic bacteremia.

# CLINICAL CONDITIONS

## Impetigo

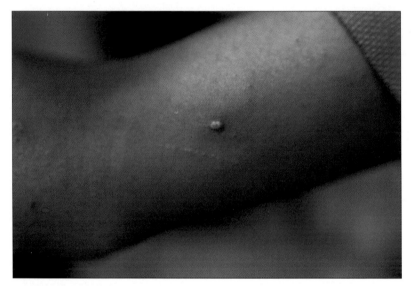

**FIGURE 4-8** Pustular lesion on the skin characteristic of early stages of streptococcal impetigo. During this stage, culture of the lesion usually yields pure growth of group A streptococci. Usually, minimal or no erythema surrounds the lesion. The vesicular stage usually lasts 1 to 2 days.

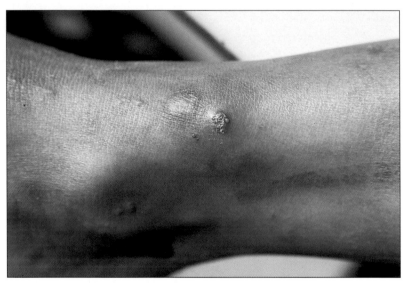

**FIGURE 4-9** Three-day-old lesion of streptococcal impetigo with amber, crumbly crust. Cultures during this stage yield either group A streptococci alone or mixed streptococci and staphylococci.

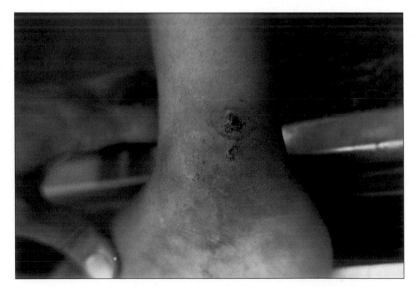

**FIGURE 4-10** One-week-old lesion of streptococcal impetigo with thick, reddish-brown crust. Cultures at this stage usually yield mixtures of group A streptococci and staphylococci.

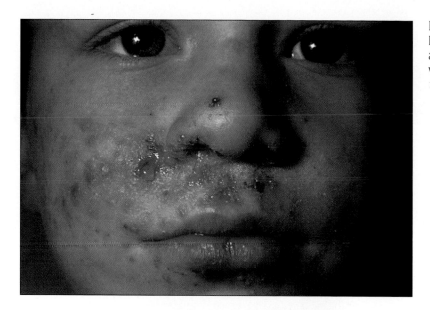

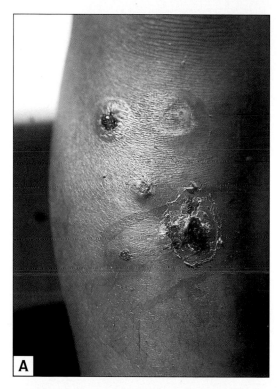

FIGURE 4-11 Facial impetigo 3 days after onset. Serous, oozing, honey-yellow crusts with a "stuck-on" appearance below the nares and pustules below the lips are apparent in this child aged 5 years with classic impetigo. Culture yielded group A streptococci. (*Courtesy of* A.M. Margileth, MD).

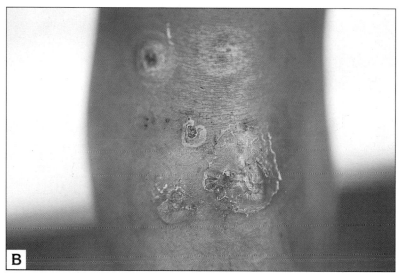

FIGURE 4-12 Stages in the healing process of streptococcal impetigo. **A** and **B**, The same area is shown 5 to 6 days apart. Depigmentation may occur, and peeling of the superficial epidermis surrounding the lesions is common. Depigmentation persists for several weeks, but eventually, the skin returns to its normal color with no permanent scarring.

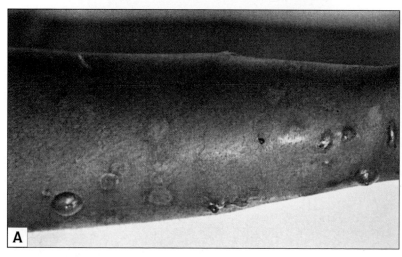

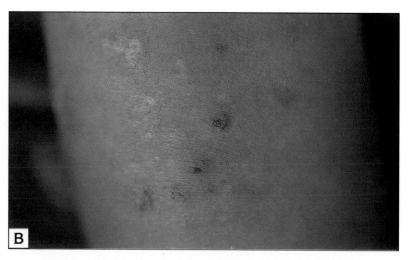

FIGURE 4-13 Staphylococcal impetigo. *Staphylococcus aureus* also may cause impetigo, and recent studies suggest that staphylococcal impetigo may be more common than the streptococcal variety. Clinically, staphylococcal impetigo presents in two forms:

**A**, Bullous impetigo appears as thin-walled, fluid-filled lesions that vary in size from a few millimeters to several centimeters. Bacteria can be recovered from the fluid. **B**, In the second form, lesions have thin, varnishlike, light-brown crusts.

# Ecthyma

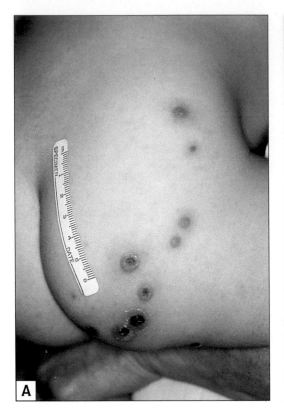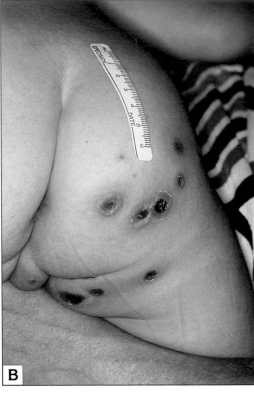

**FIGURE 4-14** Streptococcal ecthyma. **A** and **B**, Ecthyma is a deeper lesion than impetigo. The lesion starts as a pustular eruption, usually seated on a hardened base, and surrounded by an inflammatory area. Pigmented scarring often occurs after healing.

# Cellulitis

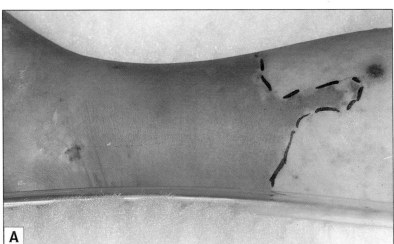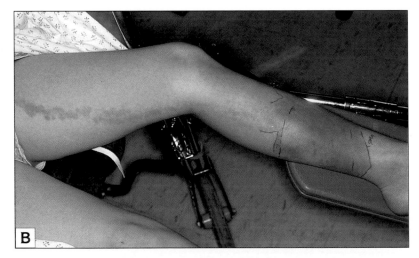

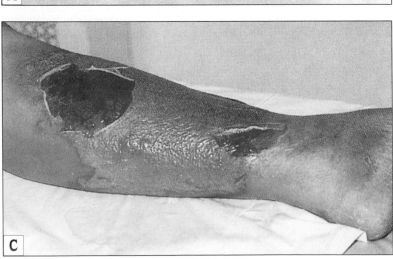

**FIGURE 4-15** Streptococcal cellulitis. Group A streptococci are a common cause of cellulitis. Infection is often secondary to blunt or penetrating injury, usually on exposed skin. **A**, Infection may spread to involve a large area. **B**, Phlebitis or lymphangitis also may be noted. **C**, Infection may be very extensive and results in tissue necrosis and gangrene.

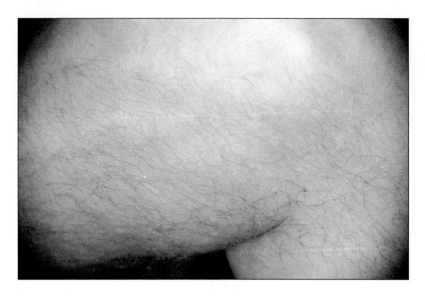

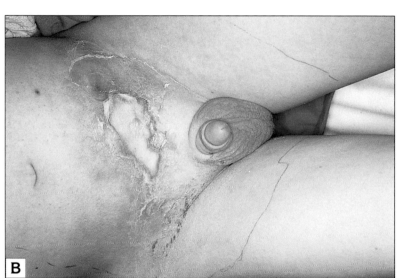

**FIGURE 4-16** Lymphangitis. Reddened streaks extending proximally from an infected wound or cellulitis are invariably caused by group A streptococci. Prompt antibiotic treatment is mandatory because bacteremia and systemic toxicity develop rapidly. (*Courtesy of* D.L. Stevens, MD, PhD.)

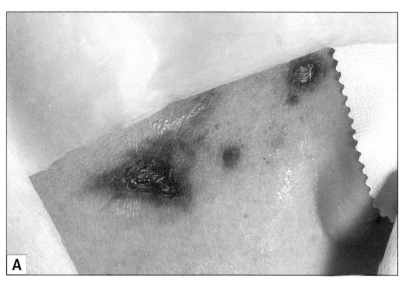

**FIGURE 4-17** Varicella secondarily infected by streptococci. **A** and **B**, Varicella (chickenpox) lesions may sometimes become secondarily infected, and group A streptococci are a very common cause of secondary infection. Such infection may be severe and associated with bacteremia.

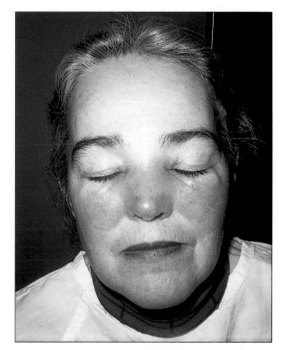

**FIGURE 4-18** Erysipelas. Erysipelas is a form of streptococcal cellulitis that usually occurs on the face. There is commonly a leading edge of the infection as it spreads from the involved area. Constitutional symptoms (fever, malaise, chills) are not uncommon.

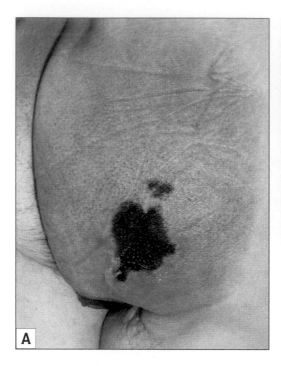

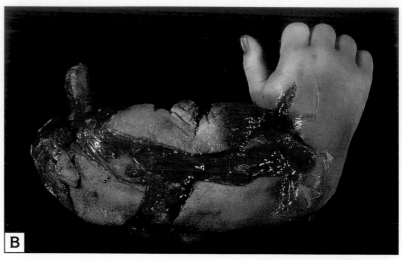

**FIGURE 4-19** Necrotizing fasciitis. **A**, An erythematous, edematous plaque involves the entire buttock, with a rapidly progressing central area of necrosis. **B**, Amputation of an infant's arm following gangrene secondary to group A streptococci infection. (Panel 19A *from* Fitzpatrick *et al.* [3]; with permission.)

# Pharyngitis

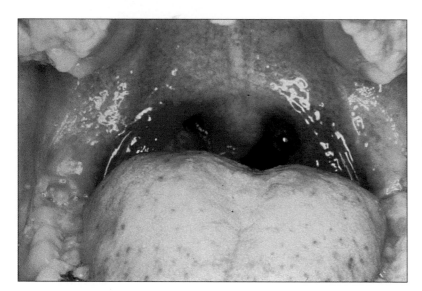

**FIGURE 4-20** Streptococcal pharyngitis. Group A streptococci are the most common cause of bacterial pharyngitis. There is usually tonsillopharyngeal erythema, swelling, and exudate. Soft palate petechiae also may be noted. Anterior cervical adenitis and scarlatiniform rash are other findings. Sore throat usually is sudden and associated with fever, pain on swallowing, and other constitutional symptoms. These findings, however, are not diagnostic. Definitive diagnosis is made by means of a positive rapid streptococcal antigen test or a throat culture.

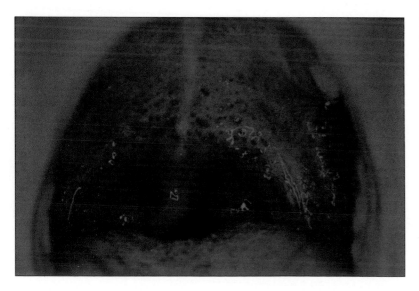

**FIGURE 4-21** Marked petechial stippling of the soft palate in streptococcal pharyngitis. The typical appearance of the pharynx—severe erythema with exudate and palatal petechiae also is seen in scarlet fever. (*From* Stillerman and Bernstein [4]; with permission.)

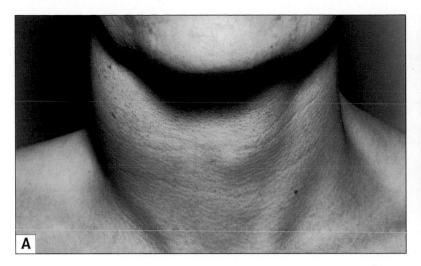
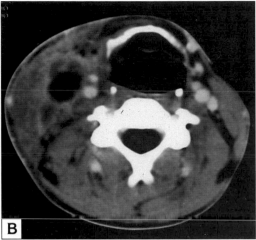

**FIGURE 4-22** Peritonsillar abscess with extension to deep tissues of the neck, complicating streptococcal pharyngitis. **A**, Swelling of the neck with loss of definition of the sternocleidomastoid muscle is shown. **B**, A computed tomography scan of the neck shows a deep collection of inflammatory material. (*Courtesy of* D.L. Stevens, MD, PhD.)

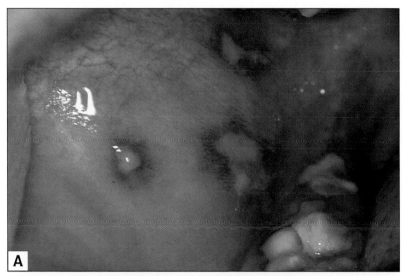
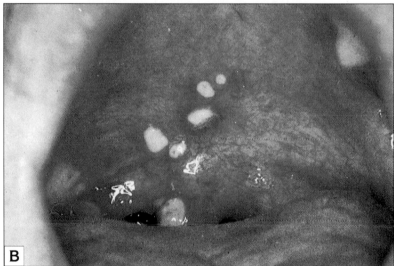
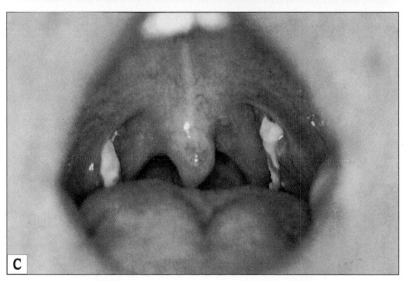

**FIGURE 4-23** Viral causes in the differential diagnosis of streptococcal pharyngitis. Other common causes of pharyngitis include a number of viruses. **A**, Herpes simplex usually causes ulcerative lesions that may involve the tonsils and pharynx, but more commonly these lesions are anterior in the oral cavity.
**B**, Herpangina (caused by many different enteroviruses) appears as ulcerative lesions on the anterior tonsillar pillars, soft palate, tonsils, pharynx, and posterior buccal mucosa. **C**, Infectious mononucleosis is caused by Epstein-Barr virus. In addition to the pharynx, multiple other organs also are involved.

# NONSUPPURATIVE COMPLICATIONS

## Scarlet Fever

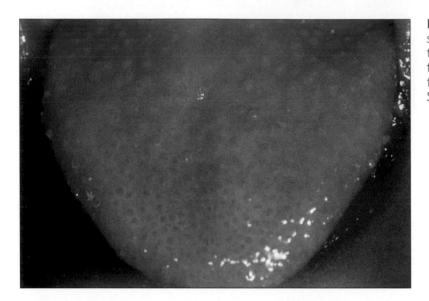

**FIGURE 4-24** Strawberry tongue. Strawberry tongue is sometimes seen in cases of scarlet fever. During the first few days of illness, the tongue is covered with a thick white material through which the enlarged red papillae protrude. The white material peels in a few days, resulting in the red strawberry stage shown here. Strawberry tongue also is seen in patients with Kawasaki disease.

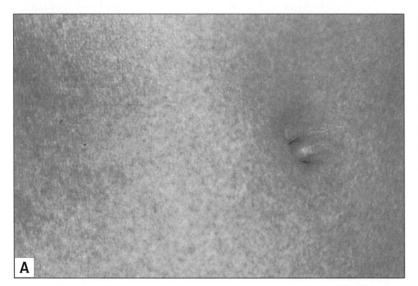

A

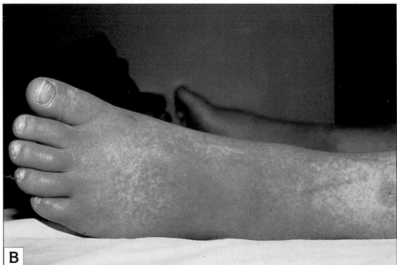

B

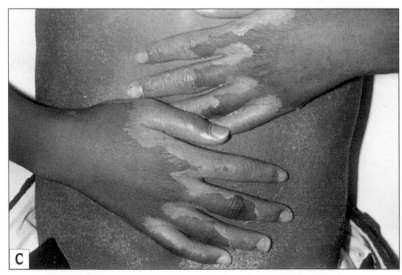

C

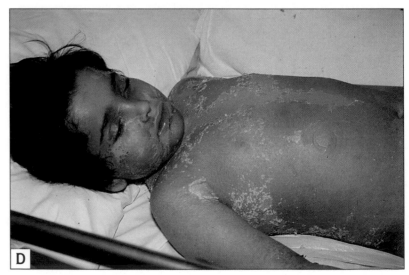

D

**FIGURE 4-25** Rash of scarlet fever. **A** and **B**, The rash of scarlet fever is typically discrete, pinhead-sized, and erythematous, and it may have the feel of sandpaper. The rash blanches on applying pressure to the skin. **C** and **D**, Later in the course of scarlet fever, desquamation occurs.

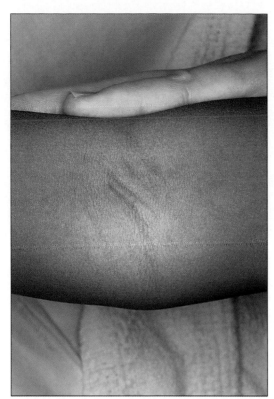

**FIGURE 4-26** Pastia's lines in scarlet fever. The rash of scarlet fever is accentuated in the skin folds, especially the antecubital fossa (as seen here), but also in the neck, axillae, and groin. These lines persist for a day or two after desquamation of the rash.

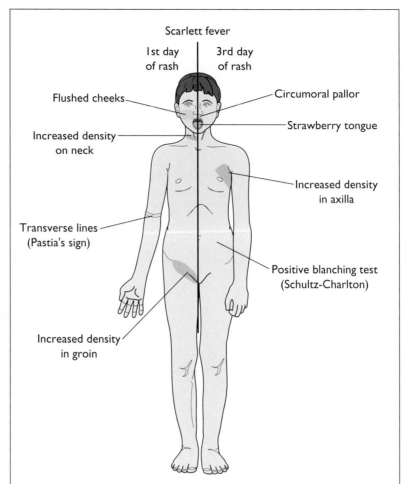

**FIGURE 4-27** Development and distribution of scarlet fever rash. The exanthem of scarlet fever becomes generalized very quickly, usually within 24 hours. The punctate rash commonly does not involve the face, although the forehead and cheeks are red, smooth, and flush. There is an area of paleness around the mouth (circumoral pallor). The tongue changes as the disease progresses, resulting in the distinctive strawberry tongue by the fourth or fifth day. (*Adapted from* Krugman and Ward [5].)

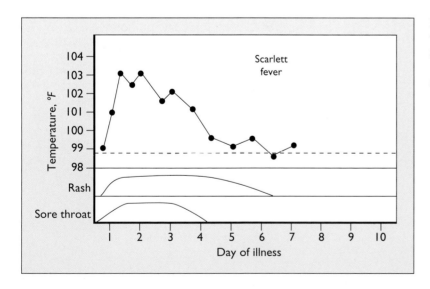

**FIGURE 4-28** Typical course of untreated, uncomplicated scarlet fever. The rash usually appears within 24 hours of onset of fever and sore throat. In the typical case, the fever rises rapidly to 103° F and reaches its peak on the second day. It resolves gradually over 4 to 5 days. (*Adapted from* Krugman and Ward [5].)

# Rheumatic Fever

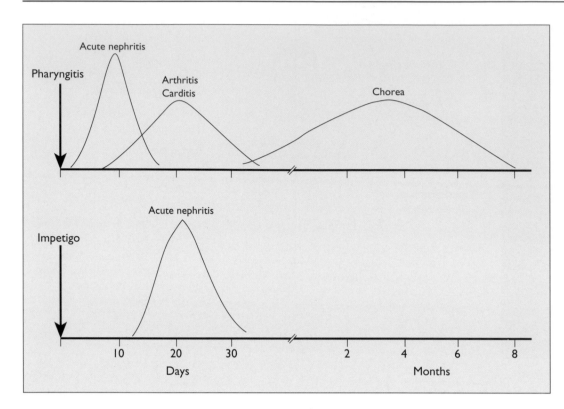

**FIGURE 4-29** Occurrence of complications following group A streptococcal (GAS) infections. The major nonsuppurative complications of GAS infections are rheumatic fever and glomerulonephritis. Acute poststreptococcal nephritis may follow streptococcal pharyngitis or streptococcal impetigo. The latent period for nephritis following pharyngitis is shorter. Rheumatic fever does not occur after impetigo. It may occur in up to 3% of individuals with untreated GAS pharyngitis. Onset of acute rheumatic fever is usually at least 7 to 10 days after the onset of pharyngitis. The latent periods for arthritis and carditis are much shorter than the latent period for chorea.

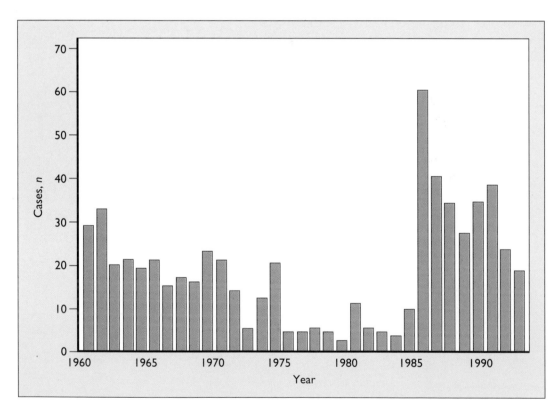

**FIGURE 4-30** Frequency of acute rheumatic fever in Salt Lake City between 1960 and 1992. The incidence of rheumatic fever and prevalence of rheumatic heart disease vary in different countries. At the turn of the century, the incidence of rheumatic fever in the United States was over 100 per 100,000 population, but it declined to 40 to 65 per 100,000 between 1935 and 1960 and is currently estimated at < 2 per 100,000. Data shown in the figure reflect the fluctuations in cases of acute rheumatic fever observed in Salt Lake City between 1960 and 1992. The numbers of cases were declining through the early 1980s, but beginning in 1985, a sharp increase in cases was observed. At about the same time, a similar increase was noted in some other geographic areas in the United States. The increase has been related to the reappearance of specific group A streptococcal serotypes (notably M1, 3, 5, 6, 14, 18, 19, 27, and 29). Rheumatic fever continues to be the major cause of acquired heart disease in many parts of the world, particularly in developing countries [6].

**Guidelines for the diagnosis of initial attack of rheumatic fever (Jones Criteria, updated 1992)**

**Major manifestations**
  Carditis
  Polyarthritis
  Chorea
  Erythema marginatum
  Subcutaneous nodules
**Minor manifestations**
  Clinical findings
    Arthralgia
    Fever
  Laboratory findings
    Elevated acute phase reactants
      Erythrocyte sedimentation rate
      C-reactive protein
    Prolonged PR interval
**Supporting evidence of antecedent group A streptococcal infection**
    Positive throat culture or rapid streptococcal antigen test
    Elevated or rising streptococcal antibody titer

**FIGURE 4-31** Modified Jones criteria for rheumatic fever. Because there is no single pathognomonic feature for the diagnosis of rheumatic fever, a set of diagnostic guidelines were developed by Jones in 1944, and these have been updated regularly by the American Heart Association, most recently in 1992. The diagnosis of an initial attack of acute rheumatic fever is strongly suggested in patients with two major or one major and two minor criteria and documentation of recent streptococcal infection (positive throat culture or elevated serum streptococcal antibodies) [7].

# Streptococcal Toxic Shock Syndrome

**Features of streptococcal toxic shock syndrome**

Hypotension/shock
Fever
Rash—diffuse erythroderma (may be absent)
Desquamation, 1–2 wks after onset of illness
Involvement of ≥ 3 organ systems:
  Gastrointestinal (vomiting and/or diarrhea)
  Mucous membrane (erythema)
  Renal
  Hepatic
  Hematopoietic (coagulopathy)
  Musculocutaneous (soft-tissue necrosis)
  Central nervous system
  Pulmonary (acute respiratory distress syndrome)
Isolation of group A streptococci from a normally sterile site
  (definite) or nonsterile site (probable)

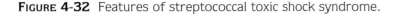

**FIGURE 4-32** Features of streptococcal toxic shock syndrome.

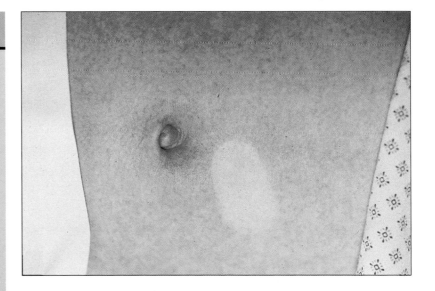

**FIGURE 4-33** Blanching of petechial rash in streptococcal toxic shock syndrome. Sudden onset of high fever (to 40° C, 104° F), erythroderma, petechial rash, conjunctival hemorrhages, pharyngitis, and abdominal pain is typical of toxic shock syndrome, as seen in this girl aged 13 years 6 hours after onset. Shock may develop along with hypotension, very poor capillary filling, marked malaise, lethargy, and jaundice. In this patient, a throat culture was positive for group A streptococci and her antistreptolysin titer was elevated to 1:1360 (although most cases of toxic shock syndrome are due to *Staphylococcus aureus*). Desquamation of her fingers and toes developed after 3 to 7 days on antibiotic therapy, with recover following. (*Courtesy of* A.M. Margileth, MD.)

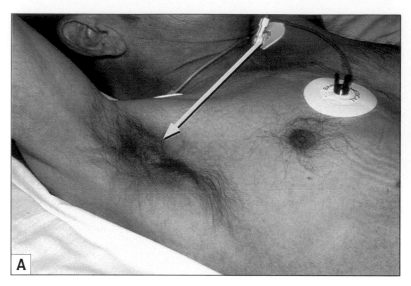

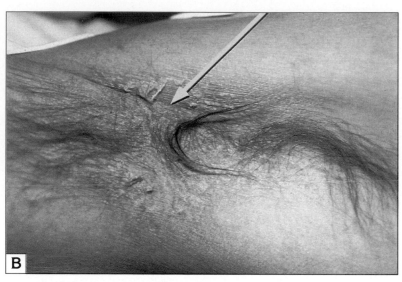

**FIGURE 4-34** Erythematous rash in streptococcal toxic shock syndrome. The rash (*arrows*) may occur anywhere and is transient. **A**, Erythema of the axillae in a patient. **B**, Desquamation of the erythematous skin 10 to 14 days after the rash appeared. (*Courtesy of* D.L. Stevens, MD, PhD.)

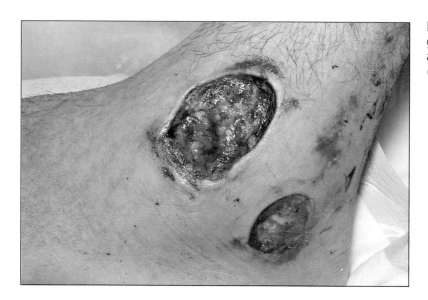

**FIGURE 4-35** Localized cutaneous gangrene in a patient with group A streptococcal bacteremia. The well-circumscribed necrotic areas are likely due to vascular occlusion and tissue infarction. (*Courtesy of* D.L. Stevens, MD, PhD.)

# DIAGNOSIS AND TREATMENT

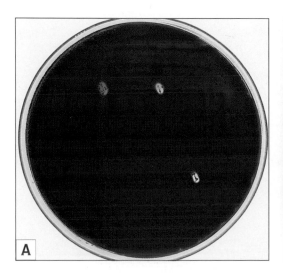

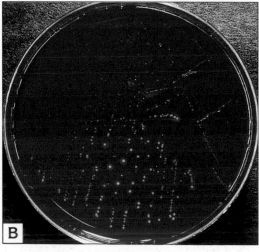

**FIGURE 4-36** Throat cultures for group A streptococci (GAS). The "gold standard" for diagnosing GAS pharyngitis is to obtain an appropriate throat culture. A swab of both tonsils and the posterior pharynx should be plated on a blood agar plate (5% sheep blood in trypticase soy agar), the plate streaked and "stabbed," and incubated at 35° to 37° C for 18 to 24 hours. **A**, GAS colonies are usually small and slightly whitish and are surrounded by a clear zone of hemolysis (β-hemolysis). Sometimes, the hemolysis is accentuated or occurs only in subsurface growth (where the agar had been stabbed). **B**, Single β-hemolytic colonies are then picked and streaked onto a fresh blood agar plate to obtain a pure culture.

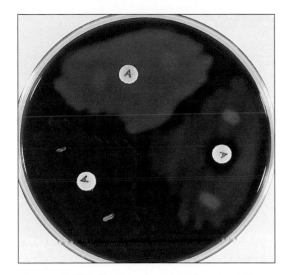

**FIGURE 4-37** Bacitracin inhibition test for group A streptococci (GAS). GAS can be differentiated from other β-hemolytic colonies by determining if they are inhibited by an "A" disc (disc containing 0.02 units of bacitracin) after an additional overnight incubation. Strains inhibited by the bacitracin disc are presumptively identified as group A; strains not inhibited by bacitracin are presumed to be nongroup A. Alternatively, serologic tests may be performed to identify GAS.

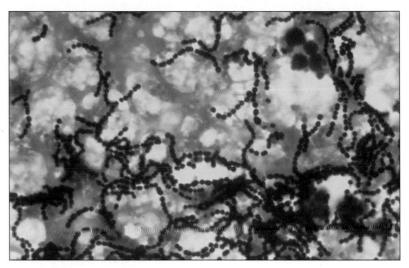

**FIGURE 4-38** Gram stain of group A streptococci (GAS). GAS can be suspected when a Gram stain of material obtained from normally sterile body site or of pus shows gram-positive cocci in chains. The identity of the organisms should be confirmed by appropriate cultures. Gram stains of material obtained from the respiratory (throat, pharynx), gastrointestinal, or genitourinary tracts or from the skin are less helpful because other organisms (α-hemolytic streptococci, enterococci, pneumococci) may resemble GAS on Gram smears.

---

**Choice of antibiotics in the treatment of group A streptococcal infections**

**First choice**
Penicillin
**Other acceptable choices**
Other penicillins (ampicillin, amoxicillin, oxacillin, etc.)
Cephalosporins
Macrolides (erythromycin, azithromycin, clarithromycin)
Clindamycin
**Unacceptable**
Tetracyclines
Chloramphenicol
Sulfonamides, including trimethoprim-sulfamethoxazole

**FIGURE 4-39** Choice of antibiotics in the treatment of group A streptococcal infections. Macrolides and clindamycin are recommended for individuals allergic to penicillin. Cephalosporins should not be used in individuals with immediate (anaphylactic-type) hypersensitivity to penicillin.

---

**Usual doses for penicillin for the treatment of group A streptococcal infections**

**Streptococcal pharyngitis**
Penicillin V, 250–500 mg 2–3 times daily orally × 10 days, *or*
Benzathine penicillin, 600,000 U im once for children < 60 lbs *or* 1.2 MU for patients > 60 lbs
**Other infections**
Penicillin G, 50,000–100,000 U/kg/day (im or iv)
Duration of treatment depends on illness and clinical response

im—intramuscularly; iv—intravenously.

**FIGURE 4-40** Usual dosages for penicillin for group A streptococcal infections. Duration of treatment depends on an individual's severity of illness and clinical response.

# REFERENCES

1. Colman G, Tanna A, Efstratiou A, Gaworzewska E: The serotypes of *Streptococcus pyogenes* present in Britain during 1980–1990 and their association with disease. *J Med Microbiol* 1993, 39:165–178.

2. Schwartz B, Facklam RR, Breiman RF: Changing epidemiology of group A streptococcal infection in the USA. *Lancet* 1990, 336:1167–1171.

3. Fitzpatrick TB, Johnson RA, Polano MK, *et al.*: *Color Atlas and Synopsis of Clinical Dermatology: Common and Serious Diseases*, 2nd ed. New York: McGraw-Hill; 1992.

4. Stillerman M, Bernstein SH: Streptococcal pharyngitis: Evaluation of clinical syndromes in diagnosis. *Am J Dis Child* 1961, 101:476–489.

5. Krugman S, Ward R: *Infectious Diseases of Children and Adults*, 5th ed. St. Louis: Mosby; 1973.

6. Veasey LG, Tani LY, Hill HR: Persistence of acute rheumatic fever in the intermountain area of the United States. *J Pediatr* 1994, 124:9–16.

7. Dajani AS, Ayoub E, Bierman FZ, *et al.*: Guidelines for the diagnosis of rheumatic fever: Jones criteria, 1992 update. *JAMA* 1992, 268:2069–2073.

# SELECTED BIBLIOGRAPHY

Cleary PP, Kaplan EL, Handley JP, *et al.*: Clonal basis for resurgence of serious *Streptococcus pyogenes* disease in the 1980s. *Lancet* 1992, 339:518–521.

Dajani AS, Ayoub E, Bierman FZ, *et al.*: Guidelines for the diagnosis of rheumatic fever: Jones criteria, 1992 update. *JAMA* 1992, 268:2069–2073.

Dajani AS, Taubert K, Ferrieri P, *et al.*: Treatment of acute streptococcal pharyngitis and prevention of rheumatic fever: A statement for health professionals. *Pediatrics* 1995, 96:758–764.

Schwartz B, Facklam RR, Breiman RF: Changing epidemiology of group A streptococcal infection in the USA. *Lancet* 1990, 336:1167–1171.

Stevens DL: Invasive group A streptococcus infections. *Clin Infect Dis* 1992, 14:2–13.

# CHAPTER 5

## *Staphylococcus aureus* Infections

Neil Barg
Barney Graham
Clark Gregg
David Gregory

# PATHOGENESIS AND ETIOLOGY

### Conditions predisposing to staphylococcal infection

Trauma
Surgical wounds
Diabetes mellitus
Intravenous drug abuse
Chronic lymphedema
Close living quarters (*eg*, barracks, college dormitories)

**FIGURE 5-1** Conditions predisposing to staphylococcal infection.

### A. Staphylococcal virulence factors: Cell-wall associated

| | |
|---|---|
| Surface receptors | Attach to host tissues |
| Laminin | |
| Collagen type II, IV | |
| Fibronectin | |
| Vitronectin | |
| Protein A | Protects against host defenses |
| Coagulase | |
| Peptidoglycan | Precipitates shock |

### B. Staphylococcal virulence factors: Exoproteins

| | |
|---|---|
| Hemolysins | Damage host cell membranes |
| $\alpha, \beta, \delta, \gamma$ | |
| Enterotoxins | Food poisoning, septic shock |
| A, B, $C_{1,2,3}$, D, E | |
| Toxic shock syndrome toxin–I | Toxic shock syndrome |
| Exfoliatins | Staphylococcal scalded skin syndrome |

**FIGURE 5-2** Staphylococcal virulence factors. **A**, Cell-wall associated factors. **B**, Exoproteins.

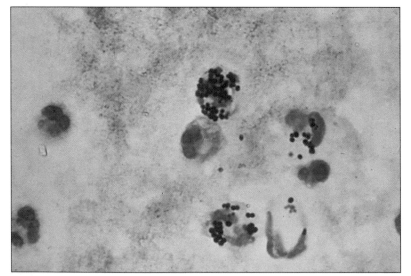

**FIGURE 5-3** Gram stain of *Staphylococcus aureus* colonies. Within purulent material obtained from an abscess caused by *S. aureus*, it is common to find numerous gram-positive cocci in clusters, often within neutrophils. Staphylococci eventually lyse the neutrophil.

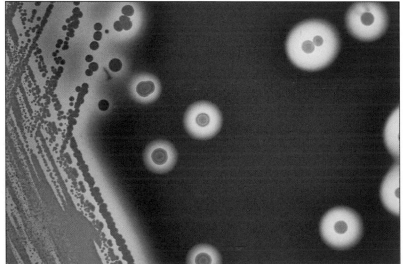

**FIGURE 5-4** Culture plate showing *Staphylococcus aureus* colonies. *S. aureus* colonies typically appear buff- or golden-colored and produce a zone of clear hemolysis on blood agar plates. The zone of hemolysis differentiates *S. aureus* from coagulase-negative species. Of course, *S. aureus* are coagulase-positive. Rarely, highly mucoid colonies of *S. aureus* may be recovered and initially test as coagulase-negative.

# HEAD AND NECK INFECTIONS

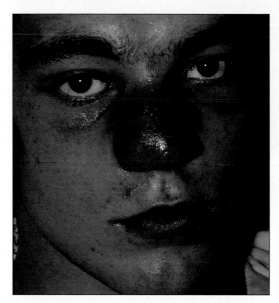

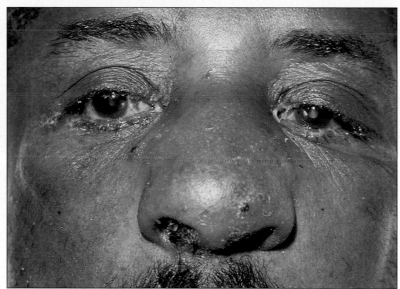

**FIGURE 5-5** Nasal abscess in an adolescent boy. The patient initially noted a small acneiform lesion at the end of his nose, which he manipulated with his fingers. Erythema and swelling increased over the next 4 days, after which he sought the assistance of a physician. Gram stain of purulent drainage near the original pimple showed gram-positive cocci in clusters, and the material cultured grew *Staphylococcus aureus*. Simple drainage of this abscess was sufficient for cure. However, it did heal with a scar. Lack of manipulation and either topical or oral antibiotic treatment will sometimes accelerate healing and produce a more cosmetic result.

**FIGURE 5-6** Nasal abscess in a patient aged 48 years undergoing renal dialysis. The patient developed irritation in his left nostril, and subsequently his nose became tender, erythematous, and indurated. He was febrile. Blood cultures grew *Staphylococcus aureus*. Dialysis patients have a higher risk of infection with *S. aureus*. A high proportion of these patients are nasal carriers of this organism, and because these patients frequently are traumatized by needles, *S. aureus* have easy access to the vascular system. Bacteremic complications, such as metastatic infection and endocarditis, may occur. Three to 4 weeks of effective therapy is often necessary to treat an uncomplicated bacteremia in these patients in order to prevent such complications.

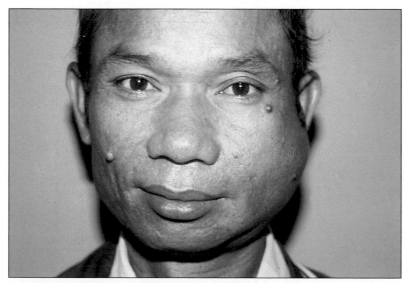

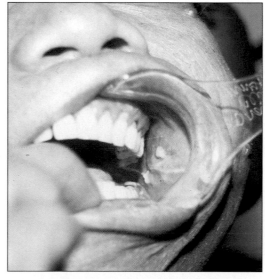

**FIGURE 5-7** Acute staphylococcal parotitis. This disorder usually is hospital-acquired in debilitated patients but occasionally occurs in an ambulatory patient whose parotid gland duct system is unobstructed. Drying of oral secretions by anticholinergic drugs or other conditions that decrease the salivary output of the glands, such as head and neck irradiation or Sjögren's syndrome, may predispose to these abrupt infections. For patients having these problems, frequent drinking of liquids or sucking on hard candies maintains salivary flow and prevents the illness.

**FIGURE 5-8** Acute staphylococcal parotitis showing purulent drainage from the opening of Stensen's duct. Gram stain of this exudate often will provide an immediate diagnosis. Prompt antimicrobial treatment usually is effective without surgical drainage. Antistaphylococcal antibiotics, such as nafcillin, oxacillin, or first- or second-generation of cephalosporins are sufficient to treat this infection.

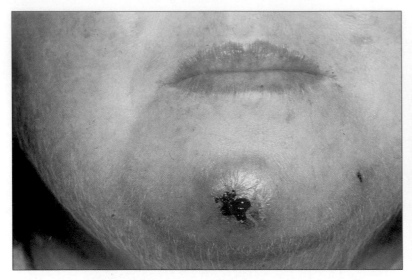

**FIGURE 5-9** Chin furuncle. A woman aged 40 years presented with an unresolved furuncle on her chin and with fever. A complete blood count and bone marrow revealed a new diagnosis of acute myelomonocytic leukemia. Blood cultures grew *Staphylococcus aureus*. Acute leukemia sometimes presents as an unresolved, unusually severe staphylococcal infection. Cutaneous *S. aureus* infection would normally be sequestered by the host defenses and form an abscess, but in this patient with leukemia, early bacteremia was the result.

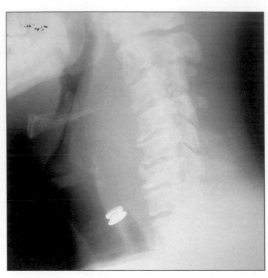

**FIGURE 5-10** Retropharyngeal abscess in a man with diabetes. The patient, aged 39 years, was a type II diabetic (insulin-dependent) injecting drug user with a 1-week history of sore throat and 1 day of muffled speech and neck swelling. A lateral radiograph of the neck soft tissue shows a retropharyngeal space infection. Incision and drainage yielded free pus, which grew a pure culture of *Staphylococcus aureus*. Subsequently the patient developed osteomyelitis of the anterior body of the fifth cervical vertebra, with an abscess in the prevertebral space. Both diabetics who use insulin and drug abusers who inject drugs are subjected to *S. aureus* infections by the use of needles. Particularly in drug abusers, bacteremia often leads to right-sided endocarditis. Sustained bacteremia associated with right-sided endocarditis is probably the cause of metastatic infections. Diabetics are more likely to succumb to serious *S. aureus* infections. Sustained elevations of serum glucose qualitatively diminish neutrophil function, the primary defense against *S. aureus* infections.

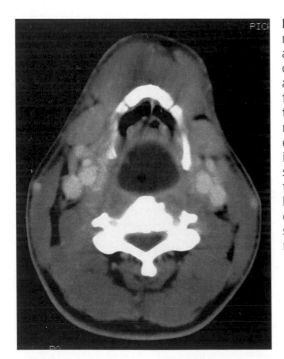

**FIGURE 5-11** Transverse computed tomography (CT) scan showing a retropharyngeal abscess. A CT scan of the neck at the level of hyoid bone shows a large soft-tissue abscess, which appears as a low-density fluid collection, in the midline anterior to the vertebral body. Both CT and magnetic resonance imaging are excellent tests for evaluating infections in the neck. Surgical intervention will be aided by either of these studies. In addition, extension of the infection into the mediastinum may be detected by these studies. If discovered, this grave complication would require a more extensive surgical procedure than would a simple retropharyngeal abscess.

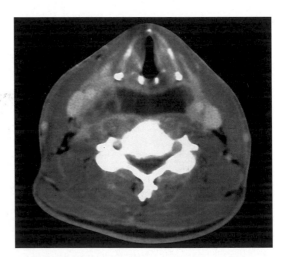

**FIGURE 5-12** Transverse computed tomography scan of neck at the level of the cricoid cartilage showing the retropharyngeal abscess between the vertebral body and larynx. Complications associated with these infections, in addition to mediastinal extension, include internal jugular thrombosis and septic pulmonary embolization, vertebral osteomyelitis, paravertebral abscess, and epidural abscess.

# INFECTIONS OF THE TORSO

## Sternal Wound Infections and Osteomyelitis

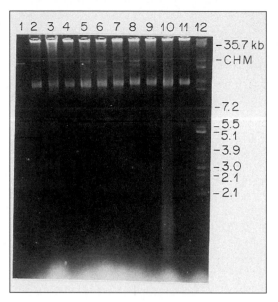

**FIGURE 5-13** Plasmid profiles of 11 *Staphylococcus aureus* strains isolated from patients with postoperative sternal wound infections. Over a 3-month period, almost a dozen patients developed postoperative wound infections—an unusually high rate. All infections occurred in patients undergoing thoracic surgery, and several were life threatening. On plasmid profiles, identical bands seen prominently below the CHM mark (chromosome) indicate the presence of the same plasmid in each strain. This pattern implies that the strains are the same and spread from one patient to the other or that they originated from a common source. *S. aureus* is the most common cause of postoperative wound infection. The use of perioperative prophylactic antibiotics has greatly reduced the incidence of these infections. Despite the wide use of antibiotics in this fashion, postoperative wound infections still occur, even with strains of *S. aureus* that are susceptible to the administered antibiotics. The complications of surgical wound infections can be life threatening. Trivial infections may result in bacteremia and secondary infections in these patients.

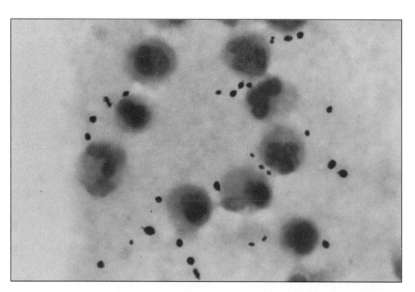

**FIGURE 5-14** Gram stain of pericardial fluid aspirated during debridement of an infected sternal wound. Cultures grew *Staphylococcus aureus*, indicating that the infection included the pericardial sack and most likely the mediastinum. Deep sternal wound infections are life threatening and require aggressive surgical intervention. Adjunctive antibiotic therapy also is required, sometimes for durations of 3 to 6 weeks.

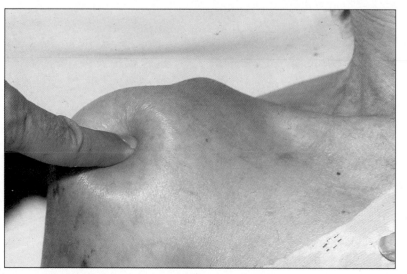

**FIGURE 5-15** Septic arthritis affecting the right shoulder. This patient's coronary artery bypass surgery was complicated by a staphylococcal sternal wound infection. A few weeks later, she was readmitted with fever, right shoulder pain, and lumbar back pain. A radiograph of her lumbar spine showed erosion and sclerosis of two adjacent lumbar vertebrae with disc-space narrowing. Needle aspiration of the right shoulder and of the intervertebral disc revealed staphylococci. The patient was treated with repeated aspiration of the joint and 6 weeks of intravenous oxacillin, 2 g every 4 hours. Radiographs repeated 4 weeks later showed no further destruction of the bony structures.

**FIGURE 5-16**
Lumbar radiograph showing vertebral osteomyelitis and discitis. Patients may complain of pain overlying the abnormal area. Punch tenderness is easily elicited. Radiologic changes indicative of infection typically cross the disc space and involve both vertebral bodies. Tumors rarely cross the vertebral endplate. It is not uncommon for this type of infection to be accompanied by a paravertebral abscess or an epidural abscess. If an epidural abscess is suspected, computed tomography scan or magnetic resonance imaging should be done urgently, because this condition represents a potential neurosurgical emergency.

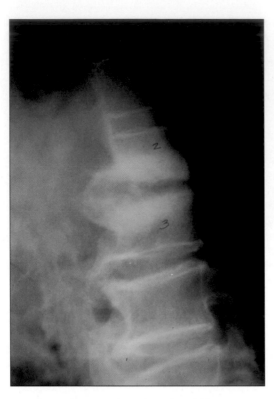

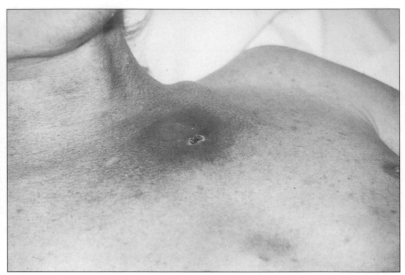

**FIGURE 5-17**  Sternoclavicular osteomyelitis and arthritis. This patient developed a chest wall infection in the setting of intravenous drug abuse and staphylococcal bacteremia. The chest wall likely became infected by contiguous spread of infection from a septic sternoclavicular arthritis and osteomyelitis. If symptoms persist after 10 to 15 days of antibiotics, surgical resection of the sternoclavicular joint may be required.

# Other Infections

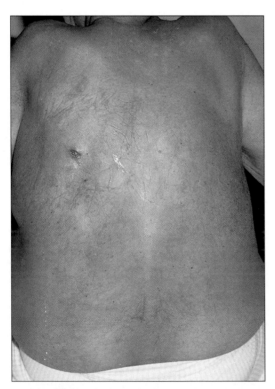

**FIGURE 5-18**  Back abscess. An elderly man with metastatic carcinoma of the penis presented with a large fluctuant periscapular mass. It was a classic cold abscess without redness or warmth. The pus obtained from the site of spontaneous drainage showed gram-positive cocci in clusters and grew *Staphylococcus aureus*. Large abscesses such as this one should be drained surgically and packed. Abscesses of this type probably result from trivial trauma that inoculates *S. aureus* in the subcutaneous area. Antibiotics can be used if there is surrounding erythema. However, superficial abscesses often respond to simple surgical drainage.

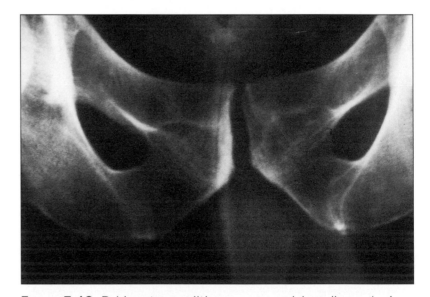

**FIGURE 5-19**  Pubic osteomyelitis seen on a pelvic radiograph. A young male athlete who had increasing difficulty in walking and pain in the perineal region presented with fever of 102° F. There was erosion of the cortical margins and enlargement of the pubic symphysis. Blood cultures were positive for *Staphylococcus aureus*. This type of osteomyelitis frequently occurs in healthy, active young people. The diagnosis is often missed even though the patients are quite ill. Patients are often bacteremic but respond rapidly to any antistaphylococcal antibiotics. Treatment should continue for a total of 6 weeks. The most sensitive test for making the diagnosis is bone scan of this area. The sedimentation rate is usually elevated and will decrease with serial determinations when therapy is effective.

# SKIN RASHES AND INFECTIONS

**FIGURE 5-20** Toxic epidermal necrolysis presenting with a large bullous skin lesion on the thigh. Impetigo and cellulitis are two common cutaneous infections caused by *Staphylococcus aureus*. However, there are three illnesses that appear quite different clinically that are caused by specific staphylococcal strains that produce an exfoliative toxin. The most feared manifestation is Ritter's disease, or toxic epidermal necrolysis. Although usually a disease of childhood, adults may be affected. Bullous impetigo, in which localized bullae are noted in contrast to Ritter's disease, and staphylococcal scarlet fever are the other two diseases caused by the exfoliatin-producing *S. aureus*. Bullous impetigo and staphylococcal scarlet fever are less severe diseases than Ritter's disease.

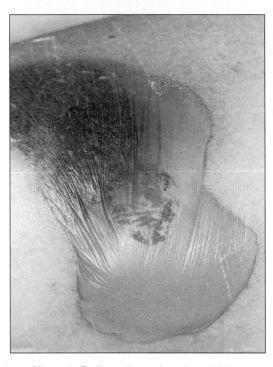

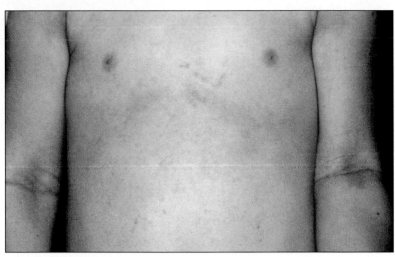

**FIGURE 5-21** Staphylococcal scarlet fever. Staphylococcal scarlet fever is typified by a diffuse erythroderma during the acute illness, followed by superficial desquamation 2 to 4 days later. In this patient, the redness is accentuated in the skinfolds of the antecubital area. Staphylococcal scarlet fever, along with bullous impetigo and Ritter's disease, are grouped under the staphylococcal scalded skin syndrome. (*Courtesy of* J. Hirschmann, MD.)

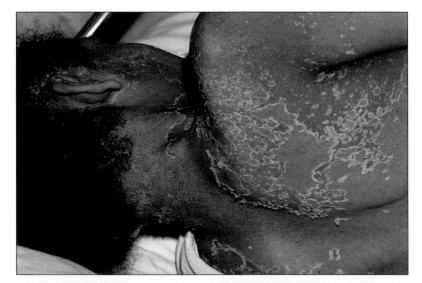

**FIGURE 5-22** Exfoliative rash postinfection. This patient, after a high fever related to staphylococcal bacteremia, developed exfoliation of the superficial layers of the epidermis. No hypotension or other organ dysfunction was observed. This is an example of staphylococcal scarlet fever. Treatment of the underlying staphylococcal infection is sufficient to permit recovery. Staphylococcal strains isolated from these patients may elaborate exfoliative toxins.

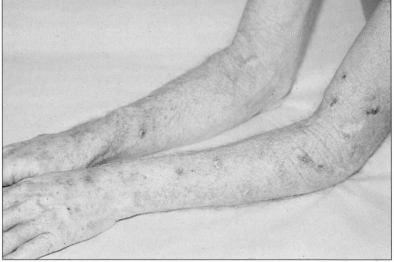

**FIGURE 5-23** Long-standing impetigo in an elderly man. The patient had a crusting, oozing rash for 6 months. The neighborhood children made fun of him, and his grandchildren were no longer allowed to visit. After several visits to physicians, a Gram stain and culture were done, which confirmed the diagnosis of staphylococcal impetigo. Formerly, impetigo was caused mostly by group A streptococci, but now the majority of cases are due to *Staphylococcus aureus*. Topical antimicrobials, particularly mupirocin, are effective against this infection. Spread of the organism from the wound to fingers to uninvolved skin disseminates the illness to other areas of the patient's skin and to other patients. Eradicating the organism from the infected site treats the primary disease and interrupts transmission of the bacteria.

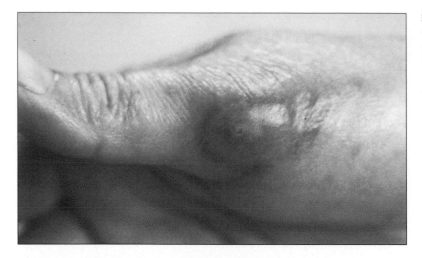

**FIGURE 5-24** Hemorrhagic bulla on the hand. A middle-aged woman developed a red crusty rash on her hands. When it persisted, she applied a topical steroid cream and then put on tight-fitting rubber gloves. The next morning she had a fever of 102° F and this hemorrhagic bullous lesion on her hand. The aspirate from this lesion and her blood grew *Staphylococcus aureus*. Because of her systemic symptoms, this patient required treatment with intravenous antistaphylococcal antibiotics.

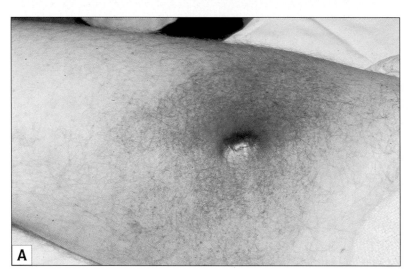

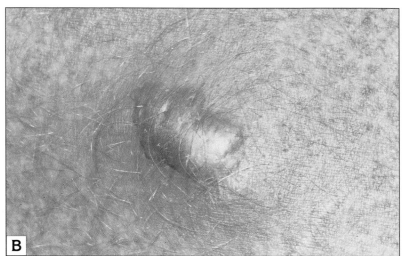

**FIGURE 5-25** Ecthyma-like skin lesion on the thigh. **A**, A woman aged 35 years with acute myelomonocytic leukemia and neutropenia following chemotherapy developed a large ecthyma-like lesion on her thigh. Blood and exudate cultures grew *Staphylococcus aureus*. The presentation of this infection was identical to that seen with early ecthyma gangrenosum from *Pseudomonas* bacteremia in neutropenic hosts. Because of this woman's immunocompromised state secondary to her leukemia and neutropenia, a high-grade staphylococcal bacteremia probably resulted. Because of this high-grade bacteremia, there was seeding of the vasculature of the skin and likely other organs. Without the host immune response to confine the infection, *Staphylococcus* lodge in the endothelium of the small vessels, where they multiply and damage the vessels, causing thrombosis, necrosis, and eventually ecthyma. **B**, Close-up view of the same lesion. The necrotic lesion is probably due to a combination of staphylococcal toxins and vascular insufficiency to this area. Pseudomonal exotoxins have a similar effect on the tissue, which might explain the similar appearances of lesions caused by either organism in this type of patient.

# Toxic Shock Syndrome

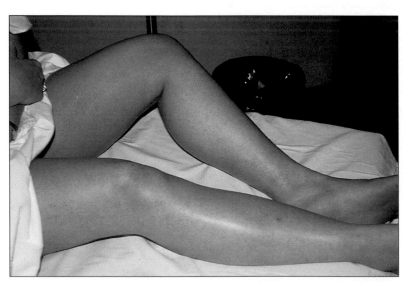

**FIGURE 5-26** Sunburnlike rash on the legs due to toxic shock syndrome (TSS). An acutely ill young woman with TSS presented with diarrhea, fever, hypotension, diffuse erythema, and a sunburnlike rash. TSS is most often caused by *Staphylococcus aureus* toxic shock syndrome toxin. This toxin alone can reproduce the disease in animals. The protein is not directly toxic to cells but rather stimulates the immune cells to secrete massive amounts of cytokines. The cytokine production results in the clinical syndrome manifested by fever, hypotension, erythematous rash, and multiorgan failure. Both tampon-associated and wound-associated cases occur. Supportive care, including fluid resuscitation, ventilatory support, and dialysis, may be required in addition to treatment with antistaphylococcal antibiotics. Intravenous immunoglobulins administered early in the course of the illness may alleviate the severe organ damage and hypotension that accompany the most severe cases.

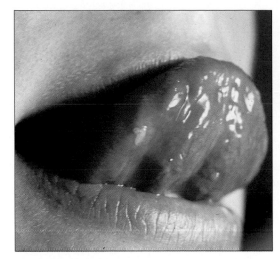

**FIGURE 5-27** Ulceration on the underside of the tongue in toxic shock syndrome (TSS). A young woman who developed TSS in association with tampon use has acute ulceration of her tongue. Elimination of super-absorbent tampons has reduced the incidence of tampon-associated TSS. This type of tampon probably provided a suitable environment in which TSS toxin–producing strains of *Staphylococcus aureus* could multiply.

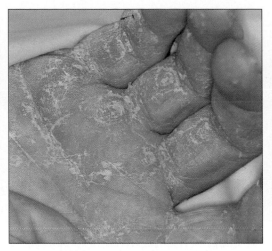

**FIGURE 5-28** Skin desquamation on the palms related to toxic shock syndrome. A man with scabies developed superficial desquamation of the palmar surface 2 weeks after admission to the intensive care unit with hypotension and acute renal failure. Excoriations of infested areas became secondarily infected with *Staphylococcus aureus*, perhaps a toxic shock syndrome toxin-1–producing strain.

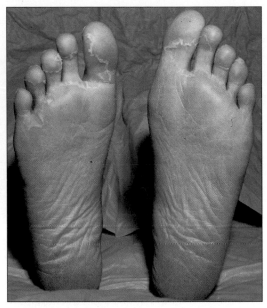

**FIGURE 5-29** Desquamative rash of the soles in toxic shock syndrome. Such a rash affecting the soles (and palms) is characteristic of toxic shock syndrome. The rash is notable for peeling in the creases of the palms and soles and occurs 10 to 14 days after the acute illness. This is in contrast to the rash of staphylococcal scarlet fever, in which rash occurs 2 to 4 days after the acute illness.

# INFECTIONS OF THE EXTREMITIES

## Catheter-Related Infections

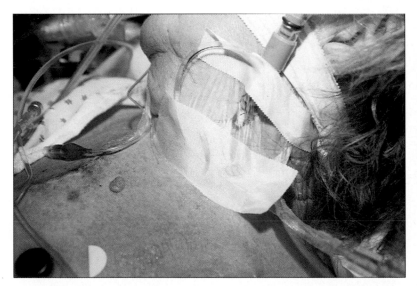

**FIGURE 5-30** Introducer inserted in the left internal jugular for the placement of a Swan-Ganz catheter. Care of the line site was suboptimal. The transparent occlusive dressing was not properly applied and the line was inadequately anchored. After 72 hours the site became erythematous and tender. The patient was febrile. Four blood cultures grew *Staphylococcus aureus*. Gram-positive cocci are the most common cause of catheter-related infections. *S. epidermidis* and the other coagulase-negative staphylococci are the most frequent causes of these infections. *S. aureus* infections are the next most common; however, in contrast to the mild illness caused by coagulase-negative species, *S. aureus* catheter infections may cause severe illness. As with staphylococcal bacteremias, *S. aureus* line-related infections can precipitate secondary infections in many sites.

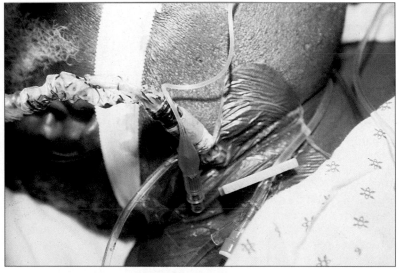

**FIGURE 5-31** Poorly maintained central venous catheter. The instability of the line and lack of occlusion of the dressing lead to colonization and subsequent infection of this site. The internal jugular vein in this case thrombosed and was easily palpated beside the sternocleidomastoid muscle. Removal of the line is necessary with this complication. Note that povidone iodine, a fluid that is not necessarily sterile, has been injected into the flexible introducer sheath surrounding the catheter.

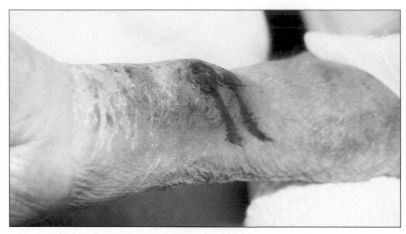

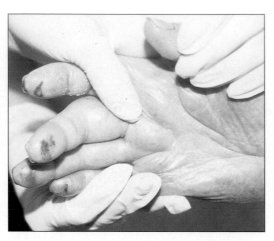

**FIGURE 5-32** Mycotic aneurysm in the forearm. This arterial aneurysm, due to methicillin-resistant *Staphylococcus aureus*, complicated use of an arterial monitoring catheter in an intensive care unit. Infection of arterial lines is uncommon and probably results from aggressive manipulations of these lines or inadequate preparations during placement. Unlike intravenous lines, intra-arterial lines cause an arteritis and may result in either embolization or thrombosis and occlusion of the vessel. Thus, the degree of tissue damage is often greater than with a venous line-related infection. Treatment of these infections often requires excision of the infected area and/or embolectomy; bypass of the site with a venous graft or prosthetic graft may be required in a few cases.

**FIGURE 5-33** Arterial emboli and ischemia of digits distal to a mycotic aneurysm. These lesions, which occurred in the patient shown in Figure 5-32, appear similar to septic emboli seen in left-sided endocarditis.

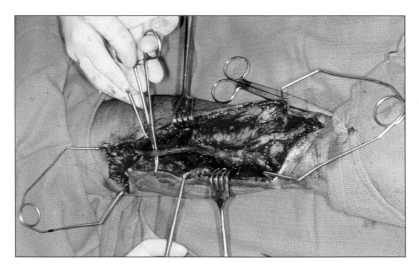

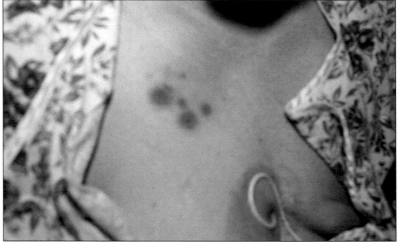

**FIGURE 5-34** Surgical exploration of septic thrombophlebitis of the antecubital vein secondary to prolonged use of an indwelling catheter. Occasionally, venous catheter-related infections cause thrombosis of the vessel. With *Staphylococcus aureus* and other organisms such as *Candida* and gram-negative rods, the infections may progress to the point where surgical excision of the infected vein is necessary for cure. Patients who require surgical excision often have persistent fever and bacteremia despite the administration of effective antimicrobials. If thrombosis is suspected, it is vitally important that the catheter be removed and antibiotics started through another site. Some clinicians may add heparin to decrease venous inflammation, but its use in septic thrombosis (other than in the pelvic veins) is not well established.

**FIGURE 5-35** Hickman-Broviac catheter in a patient with leukemia with erythematous nodules above the catheter exit site. Surface cultures of these lesions and blood cultures grew *Staphylococcus aureus*. Despite treatment with vancomycin, bacteremia persisted until the catheter was removed. The skin lesions near the catheter tunnel suggested tunnel infection. Central indwelling lines are occasionally treated with antibiotics alone. This modality of treatment is more often successful when the organisms are coagulase-negative staphylococci. *S. aureus*, yeast, and gram-negative organisms causing catheter-related infections may require removal of the catheter to effect cure. In addition to evidence of venous thrombosis, signs of a tunnel infection or failure to observe a rapid clinical response to intravenous antimicrobials also suggest that the line should be removed.

# Other Infections of the Extremities

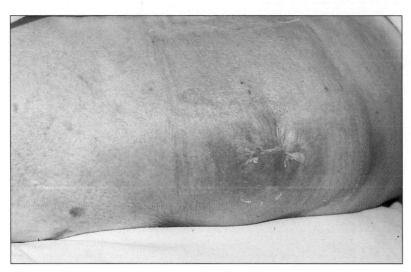

**FIGURE 5-36** Prepatellar bursitis. A few weeks after falling and bruising her knee, an elderly woman developed a painful, red joint. There was no joint effusion, but there was a fluctuant area immediately over the patella. A needle aspirate yielded purulent material, from which grew a pure culture of *Staphylococcus aureus*. This is an extreme example of housemaid's knee. Bursae infections often require surgical drainage and in severe cases excision of the bursa. This patient was treated with antistaphylococcal antibiotics for 3 weeks and healed without surgical drainage.

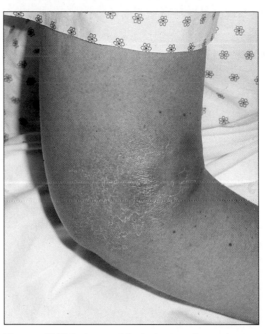

**FIGURE 5-37** Antecubital abscess in an intravenous drug abuser. A young woman came in with a high fever and blood cultures positive for *Staphylococcus aureus*. She had a painful, red abscess in the right antecubital fossa that contained *S. aureus*. Drug abusers suffer from a variety of staphylococcal infections. The most severe of these is endocarditis. However, based on the sites of injection, drug abusers may have cutaneous infections ranging from cellulitis, abscess, or even necrotizing faciitis. Long-term intravenous drug abusers may inject into proximal veins, such as the neck or femoral triangle, and often hit larger arteries in the process. Pseudoaneurysms and arteritis may result from injection in these areas. It is important to realize that vascular anomalies may exist in these areas, and exploration or aspiration should occur with the assistance of a surgeon. Once drained, repaired, and treated with antistaphylococcal antibiotics, these lesions usually heal without complication.

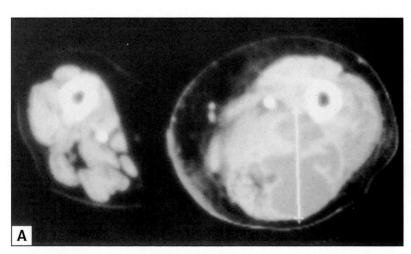

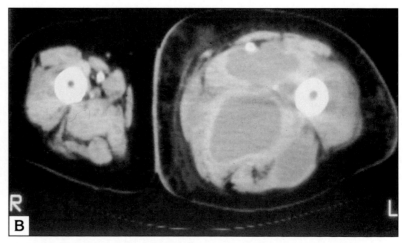

**FIGURE 5-38** Computed tomography (CT) scans showing pyomyositis of the thigh. An elderly woman had staphylococcal bacteremia complicated by multifocal pyomyositis of left thigh musculature. **A,** Transverse CT scans at the level of the upper thigh show large, low-density fluid collections within the bodies of the major thigh muscles. Pyomyositis is an interesting staphylococcal infection in that large amounts of purulent material collect within the muscle groups, but little or no tissue damage result from this infection. In tropical climates, this infection may result from the migration of filarial organisms through the muscle, carrying skin flora (*Staphylococcus aureus*) with them as they migrate. In temperate zones, the disease appears to be spontaneous, with no distinct precipitating cause. The initial onset of the illness may be subtle, but eventually patients can become quite toxic. Extensive surgical drainage is often required in combination of antistaphylococcal antibiotics. **B,** CT of distal thigh in this patient shows extension of fluid collections. Aspiration of the most dorsal fluid collection yielded purulent material and grew *S. aureus*. Treatment of this infection required a series of oblique incisions in the skin of the lateral thigh. More than 5 L of purulent material was drained. The patient received 4 weeks of oxacillin, 2 g every 4 hours.

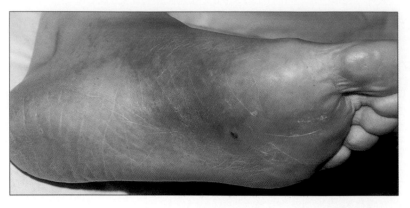

**FIGURE 5-39** Nail puncture of the foot. A man aged 56 years with diabetes stepped on a nail while working on his house. The nail pierced his wet work boot and sock, and he could feel the resistance of the nail sticking in his tissue as he withdrew it from his foot. Seven days later, he developed pain, redness, and swelling in the area. Surprisingly, the culture of pus at the time of debridement yielded a pure growth of *Staphylococcus aureus*. This type of infection presenting this long after the injury is usually caused by *Pseudomonas aeruginosa*. *S. aureus* more commonly complicates nail puncture wounds within 48 to 72 hours. Because there was likely traumatic injury to the bone with a contaminated object, the patient was administered 6 weeks of antistaphylococcal antibiotics.

# ENDOCARDITIS

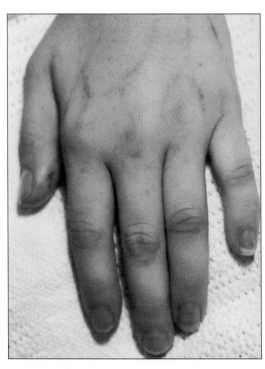

**FIGURE 5-40** Osler's nodes and splinter hemorrhages on the hand of a woman with bacterial endocarditis. This woman, who had been a long-term user of intravenous drugs, has an Osler's node on the thumb and several splinter hemorrhages, which are evidence of bacterial endocarditis. Early in her hospital course, she complained of increasing shortness of breath and orthopnea. She rapidly decompensated and could not be stabilized for surgery. Staphylococcal endocarditis of the aortic or mitral valve can rapidly progress, as shown by this case. Early surgery and effective antimicrobials are indicated when there is cardiac decompensation.

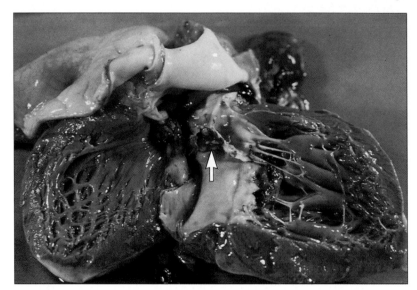

**FIGURE 5-41** Gross autopsy view of a heart with bacterial endocarditis. On autopsy, the heart of the woman pictured in Figure 5-40 showed vegetations at the base of the mitral valve (*arrow*). During her hospitalization, she developed a lengthening PR interval on electrocardiography and a loud continuous murmur. Rapidly changing murmurs may occur with *Staphylococcus aureus* endocarditis. These are probably caused by accelerated valvular damage and often lead to cardiac decompensation necessitating surgery. Because these changing murmurs may be noticed within hours of a normal examination, repeated bedside auscultation may be necessary to detect the change in murmur before the hemodynamic changes become severe. Serial electrocardiograms also are indicated. As was the case in this patient, the lengthening PR interval was a clue of a valve ring abnormality.

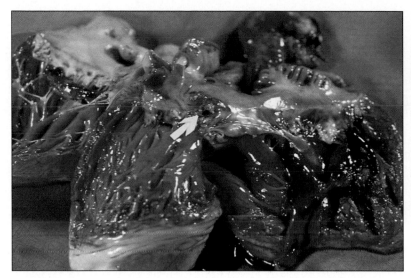

**FIGURE 5-42** Autopsy view of a valve ring abscess in bacterial endocarditis. The conduction abnormality in the woman shown in Figures 5-40 and 5-41 suggested that she had a valve ring abscess, and the continuous murmur was caused by a rupture of the abscess between the left atrium and right ventricle (*arrow*). A valve ring abscess is a known complication of *Staphylococcus aureus* endocarditis, although valve rupture and valve perforation occur more commonly. Valve ring abscess also may be suspected if a patient's fever and leukocytosis fail to return to normal. Along with these laboratory abnormalities, the sedimentation rate may remain persistently elevated. Valve ring abscesses do not respond to antibiotics alone and probably should be drained surgically.

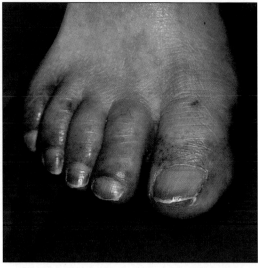

**FIGURE 5-43** Digital infarctions of the foot due to thromboembolic complications of bacterial endocarditis. The petechial character of the lesions on this man's foot are secondary to the immune complex or thromboembolic complications of aortic valve endocarditis. The distal part of each toe shows discoloration, perhaps caused by digital artery occlusion by embolization and subsequent tissue infarction. Repeated embolization is an ominous sign of *Staphylococcus aureus* endocarditis. It suggests that the vegetation on the valve is large and that the patient is at risk for a cerebral or myocardial embolism. Serial transthoracic echocardiograms or transesophageal echocardiography may show an increasing size of the vegetation if there is ongoing embolization. Despite the recommendation in most infectious disease textbooks to operate in patients with recurrent major embolization, many surgeons are reluctant to operate for this condition. Other indications for valve surgery include fungal endocarditis, persistent bacteremia, and decompensated congestive heart failure.

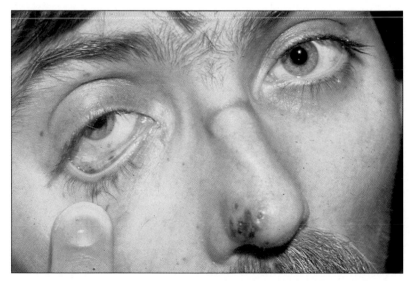

**FIGURE 5-44** Conjunctival hemorrhage in a patient with staphylococcal endocarditis. Hemorrhages of this nature often indicate high-grade and sustained staphylococcal bacteremia. A fundoscopic examination in such patients would be prudent, because endophthalmitis can occur with sustained bacteremia.

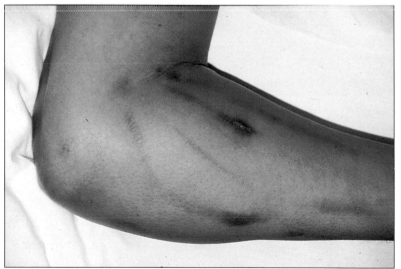

**FIGURE 5-45** Septic arthritis of the elbow due to infective endocarditis. This patient, whose sclerosal veins indicate his intravenous drug use, developed septic arthritis of the elbow and infective endocarditis. It is not unusual for patients with staphylococcal endocarditis to develop septic arthritis in one or more joints. Septic arthritis may occur despite adequate antibiotic therapy. The proper treatment of joints infected with *Staphylococcus aureus* includes repeated aspiration or surgical drainage. Without surgical drainage, the joint may be destroyed, even with the administration of appropriate antibiotics.

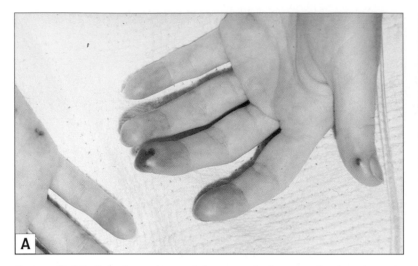

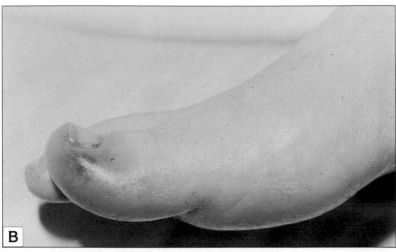

**FIGURE 5-46** Osler's nodes and Janeway lesions on the hands and feet in a patient with infective endocarditis. **A**, A young woman, experiencing her fifth episode of staphylococcal endocarditis secondary to intravenous drug abuse, developed painful Osler's nodes on her digits. Also note the Janeway lesion on her right palm. Osler's nodes and Janeway lesions are not commonly seen in the antibiotic era, but patients with a significant delay in the onset of effective antimicrobial therapy are likely to exhibit these manifestations of endocarditis. **B**, An Osler's node on the great toe. Osler's nodes could be easily confused with digital infarcts caused by septic embolization. Often, septic embolization will develop into a pustule or subcutaneous abscess.

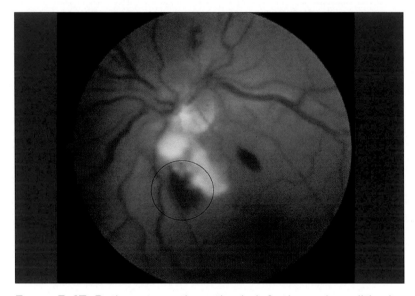

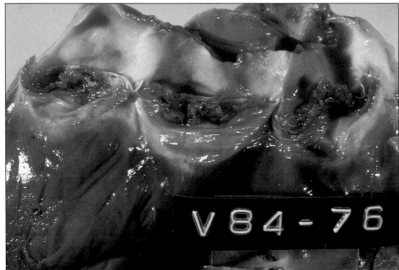

**FIGURE 5-47** Roth spots on the retina in infective endocarditis. A Roth spot, or retinal hemorrhage, is seen in a patient with a 2-week history of fever, rigor, and night sweats. The patient was acutely ill and in congestive heart failure. A grade 4/6 systolic ejection murmur and an early diastolic blow were auscultated at the second right interspace. An echocardiogram showed aortic insufficiency and vegetations on the aortic valve, confirming the diagnosis of acute aortic valve endocarditis. Six of 6 admission blood cultures grew *Staphylococcus aureus*. It is unusual to see these lesions in patients who are treated earlier in the course of their illness. Patients with left-sided endocarditis should be treated with 6 weeks of a first-line antistaphylococcal antibiotic, *ie*, nafcillin or oxacillin. Penicillin-allergic patients should receive vancomycin. Failures have been reported with use of clindamycin or cefazolin and other cephalosporins. Quinolone antibiotics also should not be used to treat left-sided endocarditis.

**FIGURE 5-48** Pathologic specimen showing vegetations on the cusp of an aortic valve in staphylococcal endocarditis. The luxuriant vegetations seen in this specimen show the extent of involvement with staphylococcal endocarditis. Embolization from such lesions would not be unusual. Aortic vegetations may embolize into coronary arteries and cause acute myocardial infarction. Myocardial damage plus valvular insufficiency may cause cardiac decompensation and congestive heart failure.

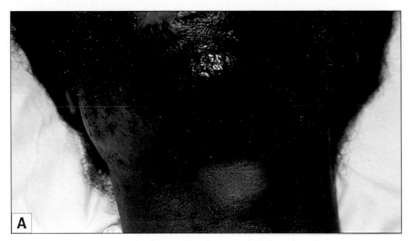

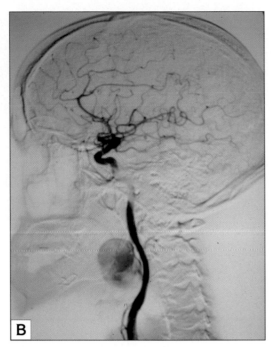

**FIGURE 5-49** Mycotic aneurysm of the carotid artery in infective endocarditis. **A,** A patient with staphylococcal endocarditis secondary to intravenous drug abuse developed a painful swelling of the right side of his neck while receiving intravenous nafcillin. Mycotic aneurysms of the large arteries are often seen in intravenous drug abusers who inject into the veins adjacent to these arteries. Such aneurysms are subject to sudden rupture and can result in rapid death of the patient. Carotid artery aneurysms may be particularly difficult to treat if the location does not permit operative intervention. **B,** Contrast arteriography of the carotid artery showing the mycotic aneurysm. Arteriograms also may show cerebral mycotic aneurysms. Because of the risk of operation, cerebral mycotic aneurysms are rarely repaired unless there is an acute cerebral bleed. Often after therapy, repeat angiograms show resolution or marked improvement in the size of the aneurysms.

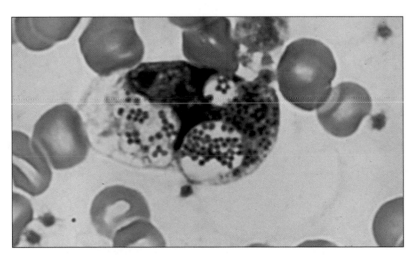

**FIGURE 5-50** Gram stain of peripheral blood smear in staphylococcal bacteremia. If a Gram stain of a peripheral blood smear is done in the setting of high-grade staphylococcal bacteremia, it is possible that organisms could be recognized, either free or in phagocytic cells as in this case. Gram stain or Wright's stain of the peripheral blood in patients with high-grade bacteremia may provide a rapid diagnosis that could lead to the early institution of appropriate therapy. Especially in patients with endocarditis or in patients after splenectomy with severe sepsis, this smear may be positive.

# THERAPY

| Treatment of *Staphylococcus aureus* infections |
| --- |
| **Serious illness** |
| Oxacillin, nafcillin (2 g every 4 hrs) |
| Vancomycin (1 g every 12 hrs) |
| **Mild illness** |
| Dicloxacillin (500 mg 4 times daily) |
| First- or second-generation cephalosporin |
| Trimethoprim-sulfamethoxazole |
| Clindamycin |
| Macrolide |

**FIGURE 5-51** Treatment of *Staphylococcus aureus* infections. Serious illness is defined as that involving severe toxemia, shock, or extensive involvement of tissue. Gentamicin and/or rifampin may be added to either of the listed regimens for the treatment of critically ill patients. In milder illness, in addition to the listed agents, a macrolide antibiotic (*eg,* erythromycin, clarithromycin, or azithromycin) may be used if the isolate is susceptible. Note that vancomycin is uniformly active against methicillin-resistant *S. aureus.* When susceptibilities permit, trimethoprim-sulfamethoxazole can be used. Quinolone resistance is now widespread, limiting the use of these agents for *S. aureus* infections.

## Mechanisms of antibiotic resistance

| Resistance factor | Drugs affected |
|---|---|
| β-Lactamase | Penicillin |
| Altered penicillin-binding proteins | Methicillin, oxacillin, nafcillin |
| Novel dihydrofolate reductase | Trimethoprim |
| Aminoglycoside-modifying enzyme | Gentamicin |
| Altered efflux pump | Tetracycline, quinolone |
| Ribosomal alteration | Erythromycin, clindamycin |
| RNA polymerase alteration | Rifampin |

**FIGURE 5-52** Mechanisms of antibiotic resistance.

# SELECTED BIBLIOGRAPHY

Bailey CJ, Lockhart BP, Redpath MB, Smith TP: The epidemolytic (exfoliative) toxins of *Staphylococcus aureus*. *Med Microbiol Immunol (Berl)* 1995, 184:53–61.

Bergdoll MS, Reiser RF, Crass BA, *et al.*: Toxic shock syndrome—the role of the toxin. *Postgrad Med J* 1985, 61(suppl 1):35–38.

Cohen ML: *Staphylococcus aureus*: Biology, mechanisms of virulence, epidemiology. *J Pediatr* 1986, 108:796–799.

Gemmell CG: Staphylococcal scalded skin syndrome. *J Med Microbiol* 1995, 43:318–327.

Muder RR, Brennen C, Wagener MM, Goetz AM: Bacteremia in a long-term-care facility: A 5-year prospective study of 163 consecutive episodes. *Clin Infect Dis* 1992, 14:647–654.

Sheagren JN: *Staphylococcus aureus*: The persistent pathogen (pts I and II). *N Engl J Med* 1984, 310:1368–1373, 1437–1442.

# CHAPTER 6

## Lyme Disease

Janine Evans
Stephen Malawista

# EPIDEMIOLOGY

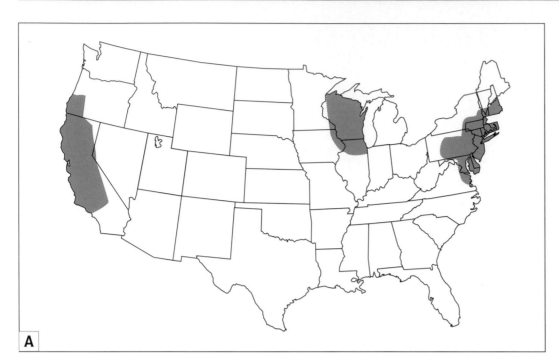

**A**

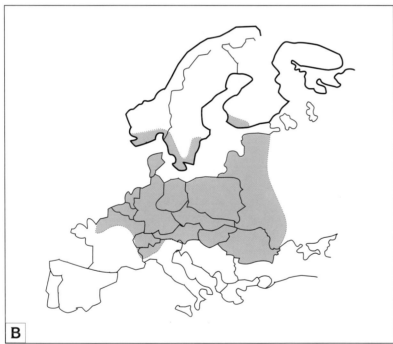

**B**

**FIGURE 6-1** Map showing geographic distribution of Lyme disease. The distribution of Lyme disease is worldwide, primarily in temperate climates. The figures show endemic foci of Lyme disease in the United States and Europe. The predominant vectors are tiny, hard ticks belonging to the *Ixodes ricinus* complex. **A**, Endemic foci of Lyme disease in the United States. **B**, Endemic foci of Lyme disease in Europe.

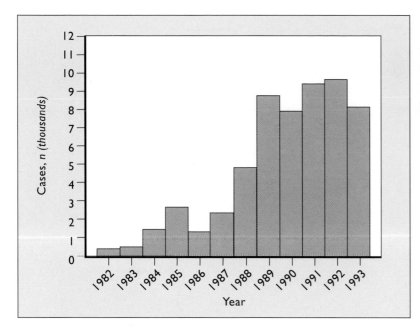

**FIGURE 6-2** Annual reported cases of Lyme disease in the United States between 1982 and 1993. In 1982, 11 states reported cases of Lyme disease. By 1993, 8185 cases fulfilling the Centers for Disease Control and Prevention's criteria of Lyme disease were reported by 44 state health departments. Despite the large number of states reporting this disease, Lyme disease risks remain geographically limited. Most cases are reported from the northeast, mid-Atlantic, north central, and Pacific coastal regions, areas previously identified as endemic for Lyme disease (*Adapted from* Centers for Disease Control and Prevention [1].)

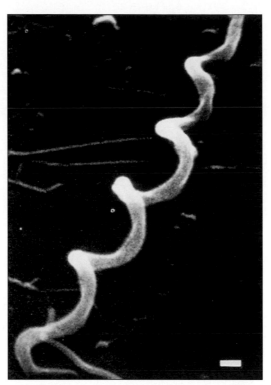

**FIGURE 6-3** Scanning electron micrograph of the spirochete, *Borrelia burgdorferi*, the causative agent of Lyme disease. Note the left-handed coiling of the spirochete. Several strains of *B. burgdorferi* have been isolated, which may account for some differences in disease expression in the United States and Europe. (Bar=0.5 μm.) (*From* Johnson *et al.* [2]; with permission.)

# ETIOLOGIC AGENT AND TRANSMISSION

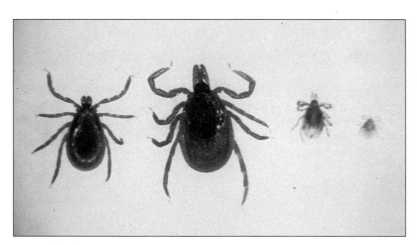

**FIGURE 6-4** Larva, nymph, and adult female and male *Ixodes dammini* ticks (from *right* to *left*). The larva (*far left*) is approximately 1 mm in diameter. *I. dammini* is the principal vector for transmission of Lyme disease in the eastern and midwestern United States. (*From* Rahn [3]; with permission.)

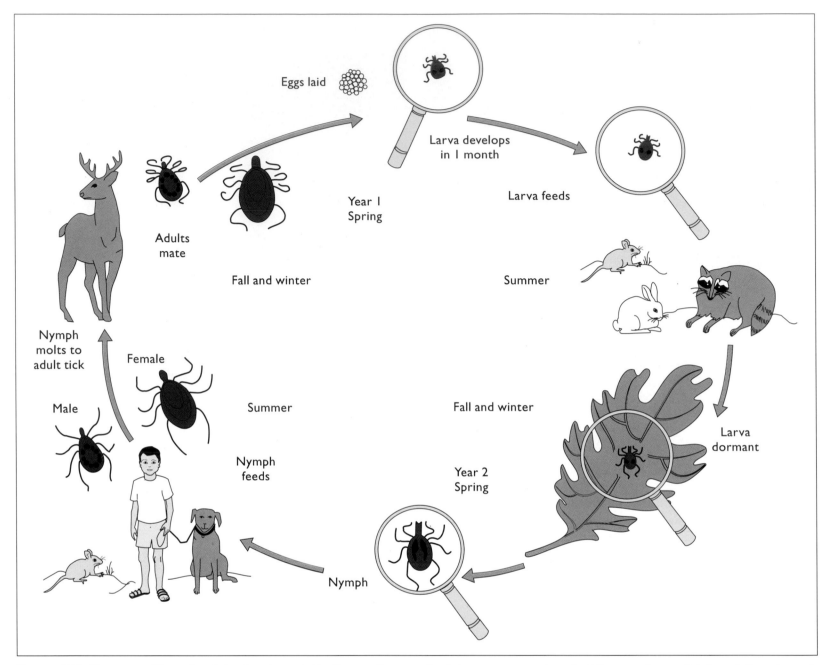

**FIGURE 6-5** Two-year life cycle of *Ixodes dammini* in the north-eastern United States. Larvae are born in the spring uninfected and acquire *Borrelia burgdorferi* after feeding on their preferred host, the white-footed mouse. The following spring, larvae molt into nymphs that feed once again on small mammals (or occasionally humans), transmitting the infection to naive hosts. In the late summer and early fall, nymphs molt into adult male and female ticks. Adults mate in early fall, and eggs are laid. Humans and other animals are incidental hosts for *I. dammini* and not required for maintenance of the tick's life cycle. (*Adapted from* Rahn and Malawista [4].)

# CLINICAL MANIFESTATIONS

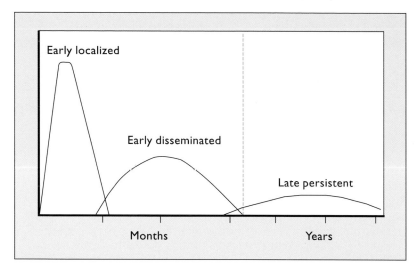

**FIGURE 6-6** Clinical stages of Lyme disease. Clinical features of Lyme disease are typically divided into three general stages, termed *early localized*, *early disseminated*, and *late persistent*. Overlap of these stages may occur, and most patients do not exhibit all stages. Early localized disease occurs 3 to 32 days (mean, 7 days) after a tick bite. Symptoms of early disseminated disease appear several weeks after initial infection and coincide with hematologic and lymphatic dissemination of the spirochete. Late persistent infection typically begins months to several years following a tick bite.

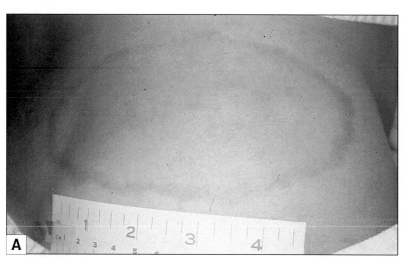

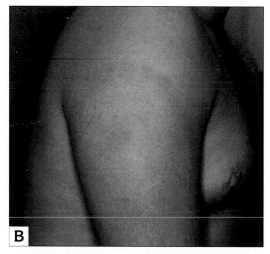

**FIGURE 6-7** Erythema (chronicum) migrans. **A** and **B**, Erythema migrans (EM), the pathognomonic skin lesion of Lyme disease, appears as an expanding erythematous lesion, often with central clearing, around the site of the tick bite. Rare lesions of EM can have erythematous and indurated centers resembling streptococcal cellulitis or vesicular and necrotic centers. EM is reported in 60% to 80% of patients. Common sites are the thigh, groin, trunk, and axilla. (Panel 7A *from* Steere *et al.* [5]; panel 7B *from* Klempner [6]; with permission.)

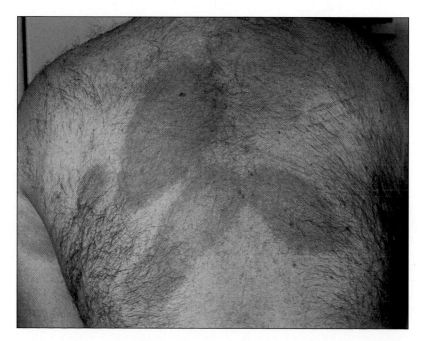

**FIGURE 6-8** Multiple secondary skin lesions in erythema migrans (EM). Multiple secondary skin lesions occur in some patients within days of EM and represent hematogenous dissemination of *Borrelia burgdorferi*. They are similar in appearance to EM but generally are smaller, expand less, and lack central induration. They may accompany musculoskeletal flulike symptoms, another characteristic early finding. (*From* Steere *et al.* [5]; with permission.)

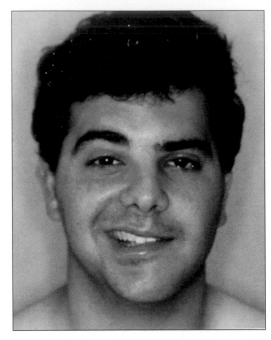

**Neurologic abnormalities in Lyme disease**

| Early disseminated disease | Late persistent disease |
| --- | --- |
| Lymphocytic meningitis | Progressive *Borrelia* encephalomyelitis |
| Meningoencephalitis | Neuropsychologic impairment |
| Cranial nerve palsies | Peripheral neuropathy |
| Peripheral neuritis | Demyelinating syndromes mimicking multiple sclerosis |
| Radiculoneuritis | |

**FIGURE 6-10** Neurologic manifestations of Lyme disease. Acute neurologic manifestations such as meningitis and cranial neuropathies in Lyme disease typically respond promptly to antibiotic therapy and full recovery occurs in the majority of patients. Chronic neurologic features resolve more slowly to antibiotic treatment, often taking months and incomplete recovery due to permanent neurologic damage occurs more frequently.

**FIGURE 6-9** Left facial palsy (Bell's palsy) in early Lyme disease. The left facial droop reflects a seventh nerve palsy (Bell's palsy), an early neurologic manifestation of Lyme disease, and one that may be bilateral. Other neurologic manifestations include lymphocytic meningitis or meningoencephalitis and other cranial or peripheral neuritis. They typically occur 2 to 8 weeks after infection. (*From* Klempner [6]; with permission.)

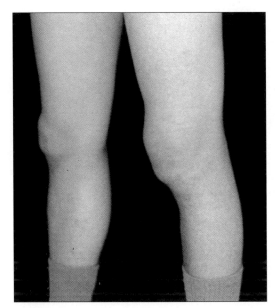

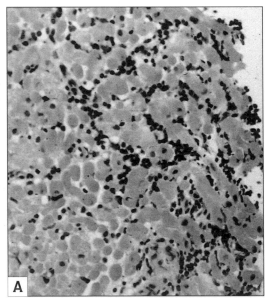

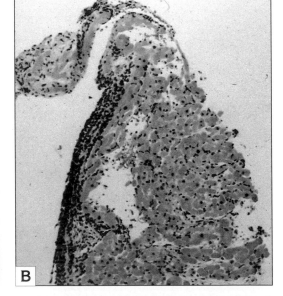

**FIGURE 6-11** Lyme arthritis affecting a unilateral knee. Lyme arthritis occurs in 60% of untreated patients with Lyme disease. The most common presentation is intermittent inflammatory arthritis of one or more large joints, particularly the knee, occurring months to years after erythema migrans. Approximately 10% of these patients develop chronic arthritis. (*From* Steere [7]; with permission.)

**FIGURE 6-12 A** and **B**, Endomyocardial biopsy specimen demonstrating Lyme myocarditis. A characteristic bandlike endocardial infiltration of lymphocytes and plasma cells is seen. Spirochetes compatible with *Borrelia burgdorferi* have been demonstrated near lymphoid cells and in the endocardium. (Hematoxylin-eosin stain.) (*From* Duray [8]; with permission.)

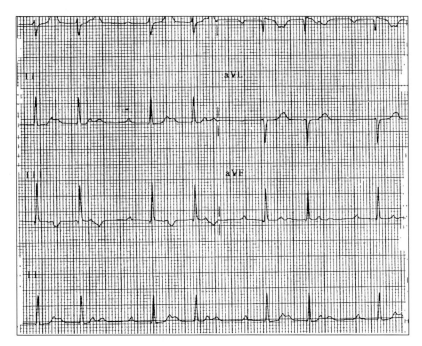

FIGURE 6-13 Electrocardiogram of Mobitz type 1 second-degree heart block in Lyme disease. Cardiac involvement in Lyme disease occurs in 4% to 8% of untreated individuals with erythema migrans. The most common abnormalities of Lyme carditis are conduction disturbances manifested by varying degrees of heart block and myocarditis.

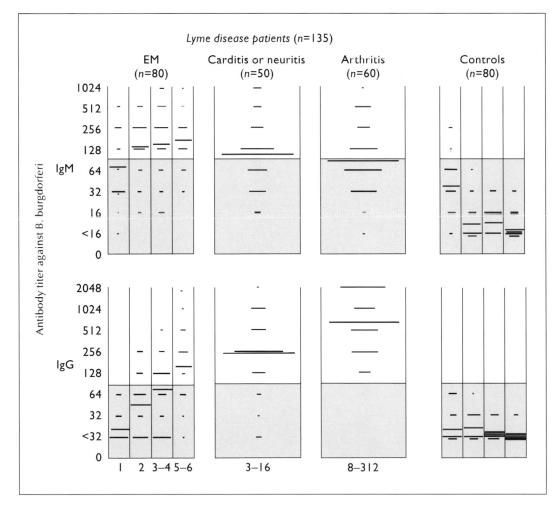

FIGURE 6-14 Serum antibody titers against *Borrelia burgdorferi* patients with Lyme disease. Serum samples were tested from 135 patients with different clinical manifestations of Lyme disease and from 80 control subjects. The *red bars* show the geometric mean titer for each group; the *shaded areas* indicate the range of values measured in the control group. Anti–*B. burgdorferi* antibodies appear in the serum within 4 to 6 weeks in untreated individuals. The first response is a rise in the IgM antibodies that peak during early phases of Lyme disease and then decline. Later, IgG antibody levels rise and are typically present during late stages of Lyme disease. (EM—erythema migrans.) (*Adapted from* Steere *et al.* [9]; with permission.)

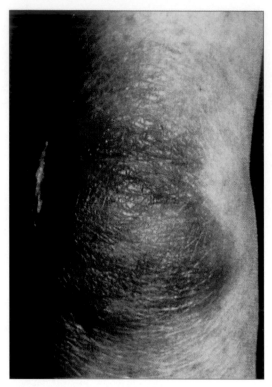

**Figure 6-15** Acrodermatitis chronica atrophicans affecting the elbow. A late manifestation of Lyme disease, acrodermatitis chronica atrophicans appears as an indurated plaque, which may progress to an atropic phase. This condition is more common in European patients and is rarely seen in US populations. (*From* Weber *et al.* [10]; with permission.)

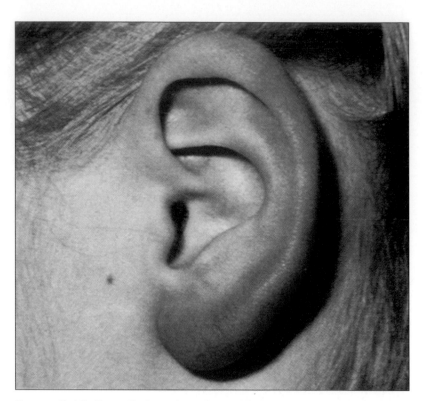

**Figure 6-16** Borrelia lymphocytoma. This rare cutaneous manifestation of Lyme disease appears as a tumorlike nodule at the base of the earlobe or on the nipple. The histologic characteristics of the nodules resemble those of lymph node follicles, consisting of small and large lymphocytes. Macrophages, plasma cells, and eosinophils may also be seen in follicular and nonfollicular structures. Borrelia lymphocytoma is seen more commonly in Europe (*From* Weber *et al.* [10]; with permission.)

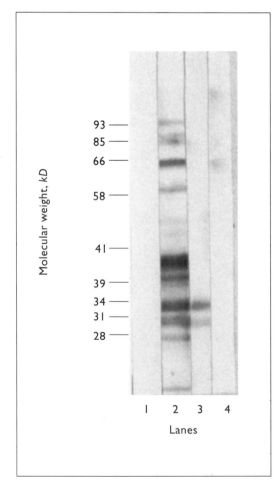

**Figure 6-17** Immunoblot (Western blot) of *Borrelia burgdorferi* extracts. Lanes *1* and *2* identify IgG antibodies, lanes *3* and *4* identify IgM antibodies. Sera used in lanes *1* and *4* are negative control sera; in lanes *2* and *3* is serum obtained from a patient with late persistent Lyme disease. The Centers for Disease Control and Prevention (CDC) has made recommendations for interpretation of immunoblots. An IgM blot is considered positive if two of the following bands are present: 24(Osp C), 39, and 41(flagellin) kDa. Once antibodies are developed to the 37-kDa antigen, this protein could be considered as an additional band for IgM criteria (> 2 of 4 bands). An IgG blot is considered positive if 5 of the following 10 bands are present: 18, 21(Osp C), 28, 30, 39, 41(flagellin), 45, 58, 68, and 93 kDa. In this figure, according to the CDC criteria, the IgG blot would be considered positive and the IgM not positive.

# DIAGNOSIS AND TREATMENT

## A. Treatment recommendations in Lyme disease: Early Lyme disease

| | |
|---|---|
| Amoxicillin | 500 mg three times a day × 21 days |
| Doxycycline | 100 mg twice a day × 21 days |
| Cefuroxime axetil | 500 mg twice a day × 21 days |
| Azithromycin | 500 mg every day × 7 days |

## B. Treatment recommendations in Lyme disease: Neurologic manifestations

Bell's palsy (no other neurologic abnormalities)
  Oral regimens for early disease suffice
Meningitis (± radiculoneuropathy or encephalitis)

| | |
|---|---|
| Ceftriaxone | 2 g/d × 14–28 days |
| Penicillin G | 20 MU/d × 14–28 days |
| Doxycycline | 100 mg twice a day, orally or intra-venously, × 14–28 days |
| Chloramphenicol | 1 g four times a day × 14–28 days |

## C. Treatment recommendations in Lyme disease: Lyme arthritis

| | |
|---|---|
| Amoxicillin + probenecid | 500 mg four times a day × 30 days |
| Doxycycline | 100 mg twice a day × 30 days |
| Ceftriaxone | 2 g/d × 14–28 days |
| Penicillin G | 20 MU/d × 14–28 days |

## D. Treatment recommendations in Lyme disease: Lyme carditis

| | |
|---|---|
| Ceftriaxone | 2 g/d × 14 days |
| Penicillin G | 20 MU/d × 14 days |
| Doxycycline | 100 mg orally twice a day × 21 days |
| Amoxicillin | 500 mg three times a day × 21 days |

## E. Treatment recommendations in Lyme disease: Pregnancy

Localized early disease
  Amoxicillin   500 mg three times a day × 21 days
Disseminated disease, any manifestation
  Penicillin G 20 MU/d × 14–28 days
Asymptomatic seropositivity
  No treatment necessary

FIGURE 6-18 Treatment recommendations in Lyme disease. **A**, Early Lyme disease. Recommendations apply to Lyme disease without neurologic, cardiac, or joint involvement. For early Lyme disease limited to a single erythema migrans lesions, 10 days is sufficient duration of treatment, rather than the usual 21 days. In addition to amoxicillin, some experts advise the addition of probenecid, 500 mg three times a day. Azithromycin is considered less effective than other agents, but experience with this agent is limited; the optimal duration of therapy is unclear. **B**, Neurologic manifestations. Optimal duration of therapy in meningitis has not been established; there are no controlled trials of therapy longer than 4 weeks for any manifestation of Lyme disease. There is no published experience in the United States with doxycyclin for treating meningitis. **C**, Arthritis. In patients with Lyme arthritis, an oral regimen should be selected only if there is no neurologic involvement. Amoxicillin is generally, administered three times a day, but the only trial of this agent in Lyme arthritis used a four-times-daily regimen. **D**, Lyme carditis. Oral regimens have been reserved for mild carditis limited to first-degree heart block with a PR interval < 30 seconds and normal ventricular function. **E**, Pregnancy. (*Adapted from* Rahn and Malawista. [11].)

# REFERENCES

1. Centers for Disease Control and Prevention: Lyme disease: United States, 1993. *JAMA* 1994, 272:1164.

2. Johnson RC, *et al.*: Taxonomy of the Lyme disease spirochetes. *Yale J Biol Med* 1984:13–21.

3. Rahn D: Lyme disease: Clinical manifestations, diagnosis, and treatment. *Semin Arthritis Rheum* 1991, 20:201–218.

4. Rahn D, Malawista SE: Clinical judgment in Lyme disease. *Hosp Pract* 1990, 25(Mar 30):39–56.

5. Steere AC, *et al.*: The early clinical manifestations of Lyme disease. *Ann Intern Med* 1983, 99:76-82.

6. Klempner MS: Lyme disease [images in clinical medicine]. *N Engl J Med* 1992, 327:1793.

7. Steere AC: Lyme disease: *In* Kelley WN, Harris ED, Ruddy S, Sledge CB (eds.): *Textbook of Rheumatology*, 4th ed. Philadelphia: W.B. Saunders; 1993:1484–1493.

8. Duray PH: Histopathology of clinical phases of human Lyme disease. *Rheum Dis Clin North Am* 1989, 15:691–710.

9. Steere AC, *et al*: The spirochetal etiology of Lyme disease. *N Engl J Med* 1983, 308:733–742.

10. Weber K, *et al.*: European erythema migrans disease and related disorders. *Yale J Biol Med* 1984:13–21.

11. Rahn DW, Malawista SE: Treatment of Lyme disease. *In* Rogers DE, Bone R, Clin MJ, *et al.* (eds.): *1994 Year Book of Medicine*. St. Louis: Mosby-Year Book; 1995:xxi–xxxvi.

# SELECTED BIBLIOGRAPHY

Barbour AB, Fish D: The biological and social phenomenon of Lyme disease. *Science* 1993, 260:1610–1615.

Bockenstedt LK, Malawista SE: Lyme disease. *In* Rich RR (ed.): *Clinical Immunology*. St. Louis: Mosby-Year Book; 1996:1234–1249.

Finkel MJ, Halperin JJ: Nervous system Lyme borreliosis—Revisited. *Arch Neurol* 1992, 49:102–107.

Rahn D, Malawista SE: Lyme disease: Recommendations for diagnosis and treatment. *Ann Intern Med* 1991, 114:472–481.

Steere AC, Bartenhagen NH, Craft JE, *et al.*: The early clinical manifestations of Lyme disease. *Ann Intern Med* 1983, 99:76-82.

Steere AC, Schoen RT, Taylor E: The clinical evolution of Lyme arthritis. *Ann Intern Med* 1987, 107:725–731.

# CHAPTER 7

## Ehrlichiosis and Babesiosis

J. Stephen Dumler
David H. Persing

# Monocytic and Granulocytic Ehrlichiosis

### Classification of ehrlichiae by 16S ribosomal genotype and/or serologic groups

| Genetic group | Major host(s) | Predominant host cell | *In vitro* cultivation | Vector | Geographic distribution | Diagnostic tests |
|---|---|---|---|---|---|---|
| ***Ehrlichia canis* group** | | | | | | |
| *E. canis* | Dogs | Mononuclear cells | Yes | Tick | Worldwide | Serology, peripheral blood smear |
| *E. chaffeensis* | Humans | Mononuclear cells | Yes | Tick | North America, Europe (?), Africa (?) | Serology, PCR, immunohistology |
| *E. ewingii* | Dogs | Granulocytes | No | Tick (?) | North America | Serology, peripheral blood smear |
| *E. muris* | Mice | Mononuclear cells | Yes | ? | Japan | |
| *Cowdria ruminantium* | Cattle, goats | Endothelial cells | Yes | Tick | Africa, Caribbean | Serology, brain biopsy |
| ***E. phagocytophila* group** | | | | | | |
| *E. phagocytophila* | Sheep, goats, cattle | Granulocytes | No | Tick | Europe, Asia (?), Africa (?) | Peripheral blood smear, serology |
| *E. equi* | Horses, dogs | Granulocytes | Yes | Tick (?) | North America, Europe (?) | Peripheral blood smear, serology, ELISA |
| Human granulocytic *Ehrlichia* | Humans | Granulocytes | Yes | Tick (?) | North America, Europe | Peripheral blood smear, serology, PCR, immunohistology |
| *E. platys* | Dogs | Platelets | No | ? | North America | Serology, ELISA, DFA |
| *Anaplasma marginale* | Cattle | Erythrocytes | Yes | Tick | Africa, North America, Europe | Peripheral blood smear |
| ***E. sennetsu* group** | | | | | | |
| *E. sennetsu* | Humans | Mononuclear cells | Yes | ? | Japan, Malaysia | Serology, culture |
| *E. risticii* | Horses | Mononuclear cells | Yes | ? | North America, Europe (?) | Serology, ELISA, PCR |
| *Neorickettsia helminthoeca* | Dogs, bears | Mononuclear cells | Yes | Fluke (?) | North America | |

DFA—direct fluorescent antibody; ELISA—enzyme-linked immunosorbent assay; PCR—polymerase chain reaction.

**Figure 7-1** Classification of ehrlichiae by 16S ribosomal genotype and/or serologic groups. Until 1987, infections by members of the genus *Ehrlichia* were recognized mainly in animals, especially dogs (canine ehrlichiosis), and in humans only in foci in the Orient (sennetsu ehrlichiosis, in western Japan and Malaysia). Human ehrlichiosis was first recognized in the United States in 1986, in a man aged 51 years who became ill 12 to 14 hours after tick bites in rural Arkansas.

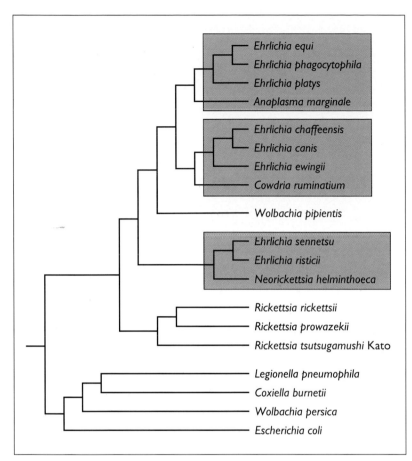

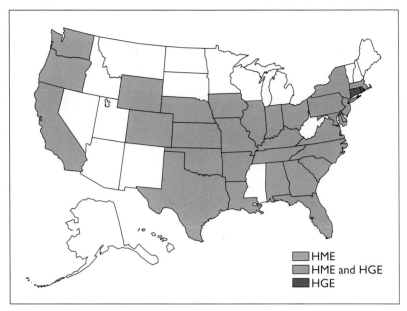

**FIGURE 7-2** Phylogenetic tree depicting relationships among the genus *Ehrlichia* and closely related genera. The evolutionary relationships as determined by 16S ribosomal RNA comparisons indicate that *Ehrlichia* and *Rickettsia* evolved from a related common ancestor. Within the genus *Ehrlichia*, analysis shows three distinctive and closely related groups (genogroups), as indicated by the *yellow boxes*. Species within each genogroup are also more antigenically similar than out-of-group species. Some members of the genus *Rickettsia*, the obligate intracellular bacteria *Coxiella burnetii*, *Wolbachia persica*, the facultative intracellular bacteria *Legionella pneumophila*, and *Escherichia coli* are included for out-of-group comparison.

**FIGURE 7-3** Geographic distribution of recognized cases of human monocytic ehrlichiosis (*Ehrlichia chaffeensis* infection) and human granulocytic ehrlichiosis (*E. equi*–like agent) in the United States through 1994. Most cases of human monocytic ehrlichiosis (HME) occur in areas where Rocky Mountain spotted fever is frequently recognized, whereas human granulocytic ehrlichiosis (HGE) occurs mostly where Lyme borreliosis and deer ticks (*Ixodes* spp) are also frequent. The distribution of HME cases overlaps the geographic distribution of the Lone Star tick, *Amblyomma americanum*, the probable major vector of human monocytic ehrlichiosis in the United States. (HME data *courtesy of* J.E. Dawson.)

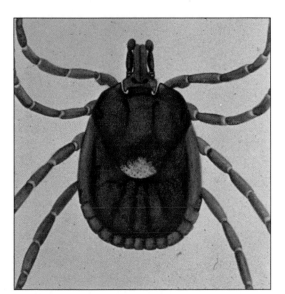

**FIGURE 7-4** The Lone Star tick, *Amblyomma americanum*. *A. americanum* is known to harbor *Ehrlichia chaffeensis* and is probably the major vector of monocytic ehrlichiosis in the United States. This tick is often recognized by the prominent, light-colored "Lone Star" spot located centrally on the dorsal surface of the tick. The presence of *E. chaffeensis* infections in regions outside the range of this tick implicates additional tick vectors, including the American dog tick *Dermacentor variabilis*. Both adult *A. americanum* and *D. variabilis* will bite large and medium-sized animals, and suspected mammalian reservoirs include deer, foxes, and perhaps other canids including dogs [1]. (*Courtesy of* D. Sonenshine, PhD.)

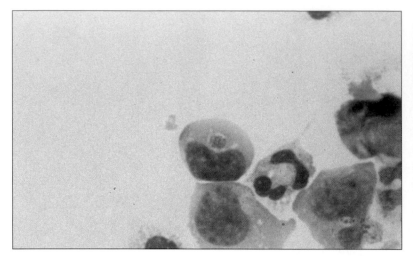

**FIGURE 7-5** *Ehrlichia chaffeensis* morula within a mononuclear cell present in the cerebrospinal fluid of a patient with monocytic ehrlichiosis. The morula measures approximately 3 to 7 µm in diameter and is composed of a phagosome containing multiple ehrlichial bacteria, which stain basophilic with Wright-Giemsa stains. Although patients infected with *E. chaffeensis* may have morulae present in peripheral blood leukocytes, especially monocytes, these are infrequently detected in stained blood smears. *E. chaffeensis* rarely infects granulocytes. The diagnosis is best achieved by the demonstration of a seroconversion in convalescence or by polymerase chain reaction amplification of specific *E. chaffeensis* nucleic acids present in acute phase blood or leukocytes [2]. (Wright stain; original magnification, × 1200.)(*Courtesy of* B.E. Dunn, MD.)

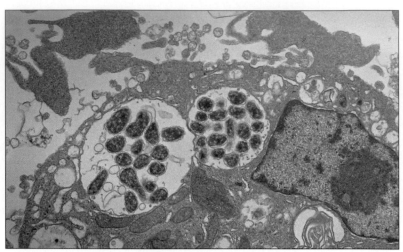

**FIGURE 7-6** *Ehrlichia chaffeensis* within a DH82 canine macrophage-like tissue culture cell. Ultrastructural studies of *E. chaffeensis* and all other species in the genus indicate that these obligate intracellular bacteria have gram-negative–type cell walls and live within a vacuole in the cytoplasm of host mammalian leukocytes or platelets. The ehrlichiae may be coccoid or coccobacillary and very pleomorphic, most measuring < 2 µm in maximum dimension. The ehrlichiae within the phagosome divide by binary fission to form an aggregate recognized by light microscopy as a morula. (Original magnification, × 15,000.)

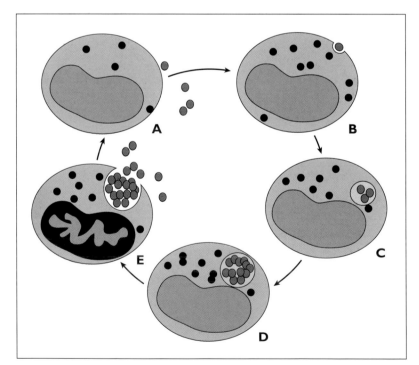

**FIGURE 7-7** Schematic diagram depicting the course of infection of phagocytic cells by ehrlichiae. The depicted cell represents a monocyte or macrophage but could easily be represented by a neutrophil. Ehrlichiae attach to the cell surface via bacterial and host cell protein ligands (*A*). The attached ehrlichia is engulfed (*B*) and inhibits phagolysosome fusion by active bacterial protein synthesis (*C* and *D*). After proliferation, the ehrlichiae are released from the dying cell to infect other susceptible cells (*E*). Active replication of ehrlichiae may be abrogated by interferon-γ, which is probably a necessary component of intact host immunity to recovery and reinfection [3].

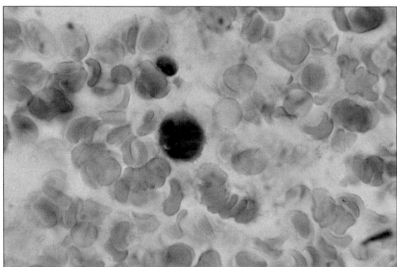

**FIGURE 7-8** Bone marrow biopsy with immunohistologic demonstration of *Ehrlichia chaffeensis* in mononuclear cells. Many patients with ehrlichiosis become leukopenic, lymphopenic, thrombocytopenic, or pancytopenic. Bone marrow examination usually reveals a normocellular or hypercellular marrow [4]. (Immunoalkaline phosphatase with hematoxylin counterstain; original magnification, × 1200.)

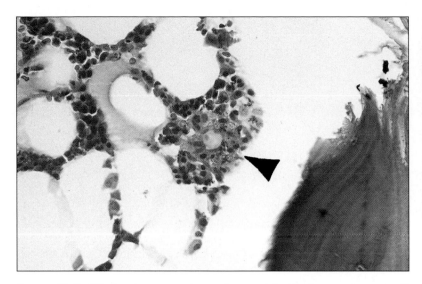

**FIGURE 7-9** Fibrin-ring granuloma (*arrow*) in the bone marrow of a patient with monocytic ehrlichiosis. The bone marrow examination often reveals evidence of proliferation of mononuclear phagocytes, and in nonfatal monocytic ehrlichiosis, this includes ring granulomas and small noncaseating granulomas. Ring granulomas may be seen in many other infections, including Q fever, Epstein-Barr virus infections, cytomegalovirus infections, leishmaniasis, boutonneuse fever, and toxoplasmosis [4]. (Hematoxylin-eosin stain; original magnification, × 480.)

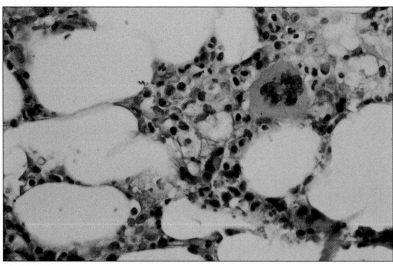

**FIGURE 7-10** Foamy histiocytes (macrophages) in the bone marrow of a patient with fatal monocytic ehrlichiosis. Similar infiltrates of foamy macrophages or hemophagocytic macrophages are present in other tissues of the mononuclear phagocyte system, including liver, spleen, and lymph node. (Hematoxylin-eosin stain; original magnification, × 480.)

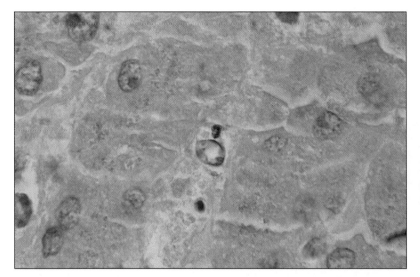

**FIGURE 7-11** Immunohistologic localization of *Ehrlichia chaffeensis* within sinusoidal Kupffer cells of the liver in a patient with fatal monocytic ehrlichiosis. Note the morula within the cytoplasm of the cell. Despite the frequency with which elevated serum hepatic transaminase levels are observed in ehrlichiosis, relatively little hepatitis is present. Focal necrotic hepatocytes, Kupffer cell hyperplasia, infiltrates of foamy macrophages, and granulomas may also be seen. (Immunoalkaline phosphatase with hematoxylin counterstain; original magnification, × 480.)

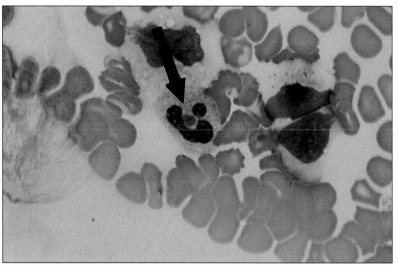

**FIGURE 7-12** Peripheral blood band neutrophil with a morula (*arrow*) from a patient with fatal granulocytic ehrlichiosis. The specific identity of this agent is not known, but it is very closely related to the granulocytic ehrlichiae *Ehrlichia phagocytophila* (in Europe) and *E. equi* (in the United States) only known to cause veterinary diseases. Unlike monocytic ehrlichiosis, ehrlichiae that infect granulocytes may appear in large numbers in peripheral blood. Infection is predominantly restricted to neutrophils and bands. Diagnosis is strongly suggested when morulae are observed only in peripheral blood neutrophils or bands. The diagnosis may be confirmed by polymerase chain reaction amplification of specific granulocytic ehrlichia nucleic acids from acute phase blood; by immunocytologic demonstration of granulocytic ehrlichiae with *E. equi* antibodies in peripheral blood, buffy coat smears, or tissues; or by the demonstration of a serologic reaction with *E. equi* in convalescence [5,6]. (Wright stain; original magnification, × 1200.)

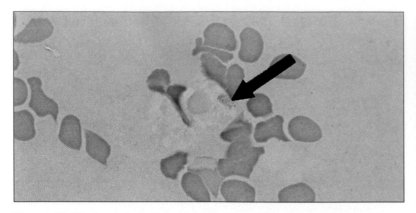

**FIGURE 7-13** Immunocytologic detection of human granulocytic ehrlichiae in a morula (*arrow*) within the cytoplasm of an infected peripheral blood band neutrophil. This method distinguishes the rare granulocyte infected by *Ehrlichia chaffeensis* from granulocytic ehrlichiosis. (Immunoalkaline phosphatase with hematoxylin counterstain; original magnification, × 1200.)

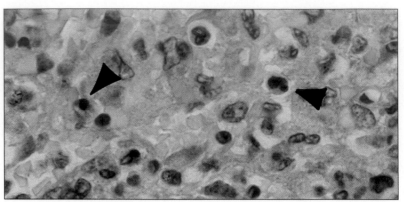

**FIGURE 7-14** Immunohistologic demonstration of human granulocytic ehrlichia in postmortem spleen from a patient with granulocytic ehrlichiosis. Note the small morulae (*arrowheads*) present in granulocytes circulating throughout the splenic cords and sinuses. Other pathologic findings in granulocytic ehrlichiosis frequently include opportunistic pathogens [6]. (Immunoalkaline phosphatase with hematoxylin counterstain; original magnification, × 1200.)

**FIGURE 7-15** Comparison of epidemiologic features of human monocytic versus granulocytic ehrlichiosis [7,8].

## Comparison of epidemiologic features of human monocytic versus granulocytic ehrlichioses

| | Monocytic ehrlichiosis | Granulocytic ehrlichiosis |
|---|---|---|
| Etiologic agent | *Ehrlichia chaffeensis* | Species closely related or identical to *E. phagocytophila* and *E. equi* |
| Tick exposure | 83% | 90% |
| Tick bites | 68% | 73% |
| Suspected tick vectors | *Amblyomma americanum* (Lone Star tick) | *Ixodes scapularis* (deer or black-legged tick) |
| Median age of infected patients | 44 yrs | 60 yrs |
| Competent mammalian hosts | Horses, deer, dogs | Horses, dogs, ruminants (?), wild rodents, deer (?) |
| Potential reservoir hosts | Deer | Wild rodents, deer |

**FIGURE 7-16** Symptoms and signs seen in ehrlichioses. The percentage of patients with ehrlichioses who had the specific symptom or sign at any time during the course of illness is presented. The clinical picture is generally of a mild to severe multisystemic illness, with approximately 40% of patients requiring hospitalization. Presentations range from subclinical to fatal [7–9].

## Symptoms and signs seen in ehrlichioses

| | Monocytic ehrlichiosis, % (*n*=156–211) | Granulocytic ehrlichiosis, % (*n*=29–41) |
|---|---|---|
| Fever | 97 | 97–100 |
| Malaise | 84 | 38–98 |
| Myalgia | 68 | 38–98 |
| Headache | 81 | 76–85 |
| Rigor | 61 | 98 |
| Diaphoresis | 53 | 98 |
| Nausea | 48 | 39 |
| Vomiting | 37 | 34 |
| Cough | 26 | 29 |
| Arthralgias | 41 | 27 |
| Rash | 36 | 2 |
| Confusion | 20 | 17 |

## Abnormal laboratory findings in ehrlichiosis

| | Monocytic ehrlichiosis, % | Granulocytic ehrlichiosis, % |
|---|---|---|
| Leukopenia | 60–74 | 53 |
| Thrombocytopenia | 72 | 88 |
| Anemia (hemoglobin or hematocrit) | 50 | 38 |
| Elevated serum AST | 86–88 | 92 |

AST—asparate aminotransferase.

**FIGURE 7-17** Abnormal laboratory findings in ehrlichiosis. The percentage of patients with ehrlichiosis who developed specific laboratory abnormalities at any time during the course of illness is presented. Important laboratory features are mild to moderate leukopenia, thrombocytopenia, and elevated serum hepatic transaminases [7,8,10].

## Differential diagnosis of human monocytic and granulocytic ehrlichiosis

| | |
|---|---|
| Viral syndromes | Lyme borreliosis |
| Rocky Mountain spotted fever | Brucellosis |
| Meningococcemia | Collagen-vascular diseases |
| Viral meningitis | Acute respiratory distress syndrome |
| Murine typhus | |
| Bacterial sepsis | Hematopoietic neoplasms, leukemia |
| Bacterial endocarditis | |
| Toxic shock syndrome | Kawasaki disease |
| Influenza | Infectious mononucleosis |
| Viral hepatitis | Tularemia |
| Q fever | Babesiosis |
| Typhoid fever | Relapsing fever |
| Leptospirosis | Colorado tick fever |

**FIGURE 7-18** Differential diagnosis of human monocytic and granulocytic ehrlichiosis. Early in the course of disease, when the patient presents with fever, headache, myalgia, and malaise, the differential diagnosis includes a wide variety of syndromes. Patients presenting with these symptoms plus a history of recent tick bite in endemic areas from May to September should be considered as possibly having ehrlichiosis [11,12].

## Suggested therapeutic regimens for monocytic and granulocytic ehrlichiosis

| | |
|---|---|
| **Adults** | |
| Tetracycline | 25 mg/kg/d in four divided doses |
| Doxycycline | 200 mg/d in two divided doses |
| **Children** | |
| Tetracycline | 25 mg/kg/d in four divided doses |
| Doxycycline | 4–5 mg/kg/d (maximum 200 mg/day) in two divided doses |

**FIGURE 7-19** Suggested therapeutic regimens for monocytic and granulocytic ehrlichiosis. Tetracycline and doxycycline have been used successfully to treat both forms of ehrlichiosis. For human monocytic ehrlichiosis, therapy should be continued for 3 to 5 days after defervescence. For human granulocytic ehrlichiosis, the duration of therapy should be extended for a total of 14 days if Lyme borreliosis is also suspected.

# HUMAN BABESIOSIS AND PIROPLASMOSIS

## Comparison of epidemiologic features of human babesiosis, piroplasmosis, and Lyme disease

|  | Babesiosis | Piroplasmosis | Lyme disease |
|---|---|---|---|
| Causative agent | *Babesia microti* (United States), *Babesia divergens* (Europe) | WA1 and related *Theileria*-like protozoal organisms | *Borrelia burgdorferi* |
| Geographic distribution | Europe, Northeast, Great Lakes, Pacific Northwest United States | Pacific Northwest United States | Europe, Northeast, Great Lakes, Pacific Northwest United States |
| Tick vector | *Ixodes dammini* (scapularis) | Unknown | *Ixodes dammini* (scapularis) White-footed mouse (*P. leucopus*) |
| Reservoir host | White-footed mouse (*Peromyscus leucopus*) | Unknown | |
| Diagnosis | Blood smear; serology; PCR | Blood smear examination | Serology; culture; PCR |

PCR—polymerase chain reaction.

FIGURE 7-20 Comparison of epidemiologic features of human babesiosis, piroplasmosis, and Lyme disease.

## Comparison of clinical features in Lyme disease and babesiosis

| | Lyme disease (n=224) | Babesiosis (n=10) | Both (n=26) |
|---|---|---|---|
| Fatigue | 49 | 60 | 81 |
| Headache | 42 | 60 | 77 |
| Erythema migrans | 85 | 0 | 62 |
| Fever | 42 | 80 | 58 |
| Sweats | 11 | 20 | 46 |
| Chills | 23 | 50 | 42 |
| Myalgia | 31 | 20 | 38 |
| Anorexia | 14 | 10 | 31 |
| Arthralgia | 36 | 50 | 27 |
| Emotional lability | 7 | 0 | 23 |
| Nausea | 5 | 10 | 23 |
| Neck stiffness | 21 | 30 | 23 |
| Multiple erythema migrans | 14 | 0 | 19 |
| Cough | 10 | 20 | 15 |
| Sore throat | 9 | 20 | 15 |
| Conjunctivitis | 3 | 0 | 12 |
| Splenomegaly | 0 | 10 | 8 |
| Vomiting | 4 | 0 | 8 |
| Joint swelling | 3 | 0 | 4 |

FIGURE 7-21 Comparison of clinical features in Lyme disease and babesiosis. Babesiosis may vary widely in clinical presentation, from a potentially life-threatening hemolytic disease in persons predisposed to severe infection by old-age, asplenia, or immune suppression, to an occult disease process with few known sequelae that occurs in younger, normosplenic, immunocompetent persons. Little is known about the course of subclinical infection during which the numbers of circulating parasites is likely to be much lower than in clinically apparent cases. A history of tick bite is not consistently obtained from infected patients, but in most cases, a history of travel to an endemic area is present. In addition, because patients with serologically confirmed Lyme disease are, by definition, at increased risk for concurrent babesiosis, patients failing to respond to antimicrobial agents directed at *Borrelia burgdorferi* may be suffering from underlying babesial infection. (*Adapted from* Krause *et al.* [13].)

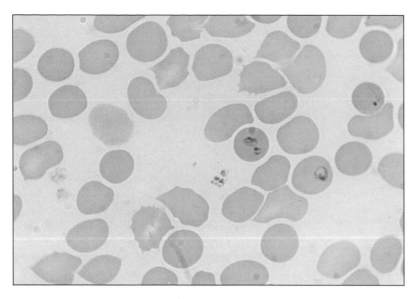

**FIGURE 7-22** Peripheral smear of human red blood cells infected with *Babesia microti*. The patient was a man aged 62 years from Minnesota with a several-week history of severe fatigue, malaise, weight loss, and night sweats [14].

| Therapy for human babesiosis | | |
| --- | --- | --- |
| **Proven effective** | **Possibly effective** | **Probably ineffective** |
| Clindamycin plus quinine | Azithromycin | Chloroquine |
| | Atovaquone | Tetracycline |
| | Trimethoprim/sulfamethoxazole | Primaquine |
| | Pentamidine | Sulfadiazine |
| | Clindamycin (alone) | Pyrimethamine |
| | | Spirogermanium |
| | | Ciprofloxacin |

**FIGURE 7-23** Therapy for human babesiosis. Most patients with human babesiosis have subclinical or mild illness and recover without treatment.

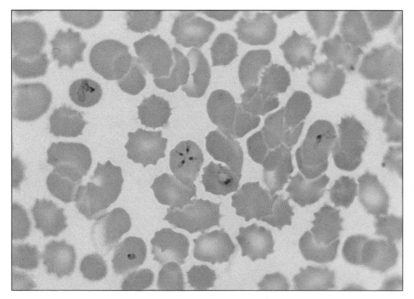

**FIGURE 7-24** Peripheral smear of human red blood cells containing a newly identified piroplasm acquired in the Western United States. The patient, an asplenic man aged 41 years, had a several-day history of fever, chills, sweats, headache, body aches, nausea, fatigue, and dark urine. This organism is morphologically similar to *Babesia microti* (*see* Fig. 7-22) but is genetically and antigenically distinct [15]. This infection is caused by an unnamed organism genetically related to the WA1 piroplasms [16,17] and *Babesia gibsoni*, a cause of severe hemolytic anemia in dogs that is often confused with autoimmune hemolytic anemia. This group of related organisms is also phylogenetically related to members of the genus *Theileria*, even to the exclusion of some members of the genus *Babesia* itself [13].

# REFERENCES

1. Anderson BE, Sims KG, Olson JG, *et al.*: *Amblyomma americanum*: A potential vector of human ehrlichiosis. *Am J Trop Med Hyg* 1993, 49:239–244.

2. Dawson JE, Anderson BE, Fishbein DB, *et al.*: Isolation and characterization of an *Ehrlichia* sp. from a patient diagnosed with human ehrlichiosis. *J Clin Microbiol* 1991, 29:2741–2745.

3. Rikihisa Y: The tribe *Ehrlichiae* and ehrlichial diseases. *Clin Microbiol Rev* 1991, 4:286–308.

4. Dumler JS, Dawson JE, Walker DH: Human ehrlichiosis: Hematopathology and immunohistologic detection of *Ehrlichia chaffeensis*. *Hum Pathol* 1993, 24:391–396.

5. Chen SM, Dumler JS, Bakken JS, Walker DH: Identification of a granulocytotropic *Ehrlichia* species as the etiologic agent of human disease. *J Clin Microbiol* 1994, 32:589–595.

6. Bakken JS, Dumler JS, Chen SM, *et al.*: Human granulocytic ehrlichiosis in the upper Midwest United States: A new species emerging? *JAMA* 1994, 272:212–218.

7. Fishbein DB, Dawson JE, Robinson LE: Human ehrlichiosis in the United States, 1985 to 1990. *Ann Intern Med* 1994, 120:736–743.

8. Bakken JS, Dumler JS: Human granulocytic ehrlichiosis (HGE): Clinical and laboratory characteristics of 41 patients from Minnesota and Wisconsin. *JAMA* 1996, 275:199–205.

9. Wormser G, McKenna D, Aguero-Rosenfeld M, *et al.*: Human granulocytic ehrlichiosis—New York, 1995. *MMWR* 1995, 44:593–595.

10. Eng TR, Harkness JR, Fishbein DB, *et al.*: Epidemiologic, clinical, and laboratory findings of human ehrlichiosis in the United States, 1988. *JAMA* 1990, 264:2251–2258.

11. Everett ED, Evans KA, Henry RB, McDonald G: Human ehrlichiosis in adults after tick exposure: Diagnosis using polymerase chain reaction. *Ann Intern Med* 1994, 120:730–735.

12. Dumler JS, Bakken JS: Ehrlichial diseases of humans: Emerging tick-borne infections. *Clin Infect Dis* 1995, 20:1102–1110.

13. Krause PJ, Telford SR III, Persing DH, *et al.*: Increased severity of Lyme disease due to concurrent babesiosis (in press).

14. Pruthi RK, Marshall WF, Wiltsie JC, Persing DH: Human babesiosis. *Mayo Clin Proc* 1995, 70:853–862.

15. Persing DH, Herwaldt BL, Glaser C, *et al.*: Infection with *Babesia*-like organisms in northern California. *N Engl J Med* 1995, 332:298–303.

16. Quick RE, Herwaldt BL, Thomford JW, *et al.*: Babesiosis in Washington State: A new species of *Babesia*? *Ann Intern Med* 1993, 119:284–290.

17. Thomford JW, Conrad PA, Telford SR, *et al.*: Cultivation and phylogenetic characterization of a newly recognized human pathogenic protozoan. *J Infect Dis* 1994, 169:1050–1056.

# SELECTED BIBLIOGRAPHY

Dumler JS, Bakken JS: Ehrlichial diseases of humans: Emerging tick-borne infections. *Clin Infect Dis* 1995, 20:1102–1110.

Fishbein DB, Dawson JE, Robinson LE: Human ehrlichiosis in the United States, 1985 to 1990. *Ann Int Med* 1994, 120:736–743.

Persing DH, Herwaldt BL, Glaser C, *et al.*: Infection with *Babesia*-like organisms in northern California. *N Engl J Med* 1995, 332:298–303.

Pruthi RK, Marshall WF, Wiltsie JC, Persing DH: Human babesiosis. *Mayo Clin Proc* 1995, 70:853–862.

# CHAPTER 8

## *Bartonella* Infections

David A. Relman
Philip E. LeBoit

# CLASSIFICATION

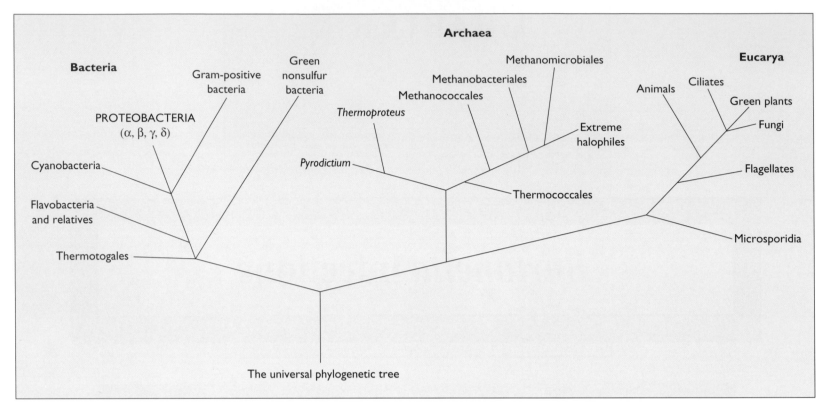

**FIGURE 8-1** Universal phylogenetic tree with the three domains, Bacteria, Archaea, and Eucarya. The evolutionary relationships represented in this tree are inferred from the analysis of small subunit ribosomal RNA sequences. The agents of bacillary angiomatosis and cat scratch disease belong to the Proteobacteria division of Bacteria [1,2].

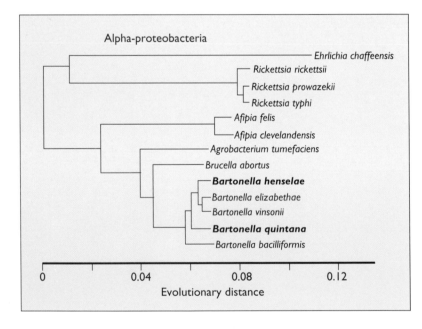

**FIGURE 8-2** Phylogenetic tree of the Proteobacteria, alpha subdivision. This subdivision encompasses many of the rickettsia and rickettsia-like organisms that are pathogenic for humans, including the agents associated with nearly all cases of bacillary angiomatosis and cat scratch disease (*Bartonella henselae* and *B. quintana*). Many of these organisms establish a close endosymbiotic relationship with their host. Members of the former *Rochalimaea* genus, including *R. henselae* and *R. quintana*, are now reclassified as members of *Bartonella* [3,4]. At present, *Afipia felis* does not appear to be a significant pathogen in humans.

**FIGURE 8-3** *Bartonella*-associated diseases.

### Bartonella-associated diseases

| Clinical syndrome | B. henselae | B. quintana | B. elizabethae |
|---|---|---|---|
| Recurrent/persistent fever and bacteremia | x | x | |
| Trench fever | | x | |
| Endocarditis | x | x | x |
| Bacillary angiomatosis | x | x | |
| Bacillary peliosis | x | x | |
| Cat scratch disease | x | | |

### Microbiologic and clinical features associated with pathogenic *Bartonella* species

| | B. henselae | B. quintana | B. bacilliformis |
|---|---|---|---|
| Clinical syndrome | BA, BP, BE, bacteremia/fever, cat scratch disease | Trench fever, bacteremia/fever, BA, BE, BP | Bartonellosis (Oroya fever, verruga peruana) |
| Vector | ? | Louse | Sandfly |
| Reservoir | Cats | ? | ? |
| Detection | Cell-free growth, serum IFA, PCR, immunohistochemistry | Cell-free growth, serum IFA, PCR, immunohistochemistry | Cell-free growth, PCR |
| Treatment | Macrolides, doxycycline | Macrolides, doxycycline, others | Tetracycline, penicillin |

BA—bacillary angiomatosis; BE—bacterial endocarditis; BP—bacillary peliosis; IFA—immunofluorescent assay; PCR—polymerase chain reaction.

**FIGURE 8-4** Microbiologic and clinical features associated with pathogenic *Bartonella* species. Both *B. henselae* and *B. quintana* have been associated with bacillary angiomatosis; *B. henselae* is also associated with most cases of cat scratch disease [5]. Bacillary angiomatosis (only *B. henselae*–associated cases) and cat scratch disease are associated with cat scratches and bites, because cats are a reservoir for *B. henselae* [6]. It is unclear whether transmission of bacillary angiomatosis is also dependent on an arthropod vector (possibly cat fleas). *B. quintana* has been responsible for some outbreaks of "urban trench fever" in the past few years associated with chronic alcoholism [7].

# BACILLARY ANGIOMATOSIS

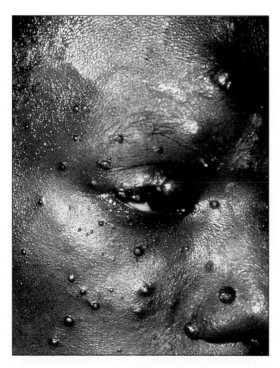

**FIGURE 8-5**
Disseminated cutaneous papules in cutaneous bacillary angiomatosis. The range of appearances of cutaneous bacillary angiomatosis is broad. This patient with HIV disease and disseminated cutaneous papules has many lesions clustered on the skin of the eyelids. This distribution is also seen in the disseminated papular form of bartonellosis, called *forma milliar.*

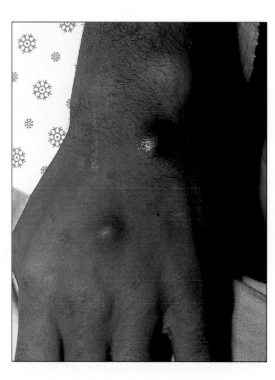

**FIGURE 8-6**
Deep red nodules of bacillary angiomatosis on the wrist of an HIV-infected patient. Biopsy of these lesions revealed the concomitant presence of *Mycobacterium avium* complex. Whereas all lesions of bacillary angiomatosis contain *Bartonella*, other pathogens can be found in lesional tissue, including cryptococci, Epstein-Barr virus, and cytomegalovirus.

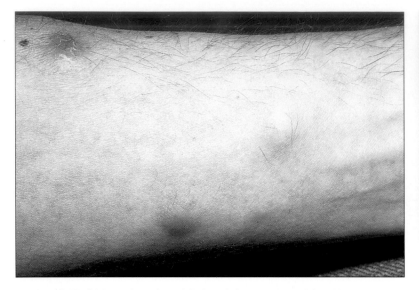

**FIGURE 8-7**  Skin-colored and light pink papules of bacillary angiomatosis on the volar wrist and forearm.

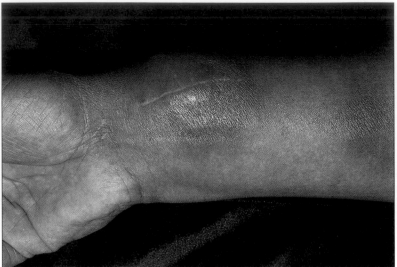

**FIGURE 8-8**  Deep nodular lesion of bacillary angiomatosis with eroded underlying bone. The linear scar is from an attempted incision and drainage procedure. The lesion responded to treatment with oral antibiotics.

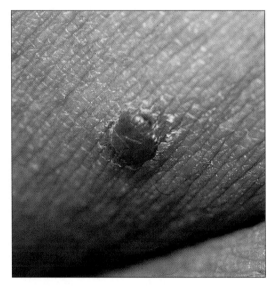

**FIGURE 8-9**  Cutaneous bacillary angiomatosis lesion on an HIV-seropositive hispanic man. This lesion is older and has a "collarette" of scale around the periphery.

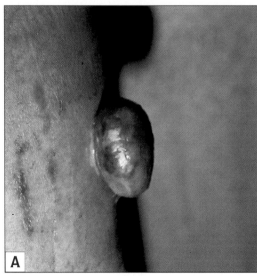

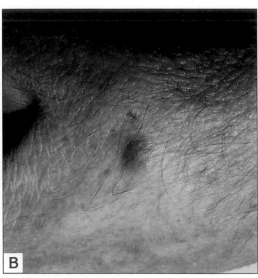

**FIGURE 8-10  A** and **B**, A pedunculated cutaneous lesion of bacillary angiomatosis on an HIV-seropositive patient. Pedunculation is a less frequent feature of cutaneous lesions.

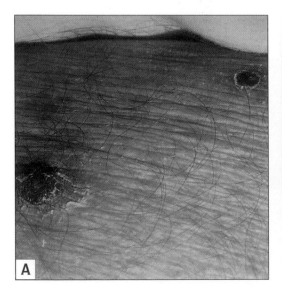

**FIGURE 8-11**  Comparison of bacillary angiomatosis and Kaposi's sarcoma. Vascular lesions in an immunosuppressed patient should not be assumed to be Kaposi's sarcoma without a biopsy. Even though Kaposi's sarcoma is far more common than bacillary angiomatosis, the two conditions can closely resemble each other in their clinical appearances. **A**, Papules of bacillary angiomatosis. At one time, the collarettes of scale were believed to favor a diagnosis of bacillary angiomatosis, but these can be seen in Kaposi's sarcoma also. **B**, Lesions of Kaposi's sarcoma. Kaposi's sarcoma is closely associated with a newly discovered herpesvirus, HHV-8 [8]. (*From* Berger *et al.* [9]; with permission.)

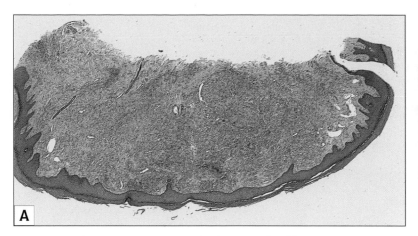

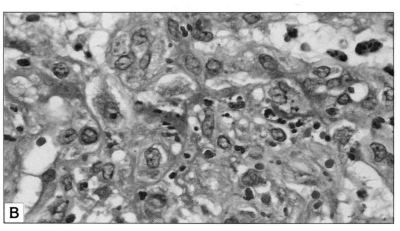

**FIGURE 8-12** Histopathology of cutaneous bacillary angiomatosis. **A**, A low-magnification photomicrograph displays the pedunculated configuration of a lesion (hematoxylin-eosin stain). **B**, At higher magnification, endothelial cells can be seen with large clear nuclei that have irregular nuclear membranes. The presence of small purplish clusters of bacilli surrounded by neutrophils and

neutrophilic nuclear dust is a valuable clue to the pathologist who otherwise could mistake these changes for those of a vascular neoplasm. Histopathologic criteria can distinguish bacillary angiomatosis from Kaposi's sarcoma, pyogenic granuloma, angiosarcoma, and angiolymphoid hyperplasia with eosinophilia [10]. (Hematoxylin-eosin stain.)

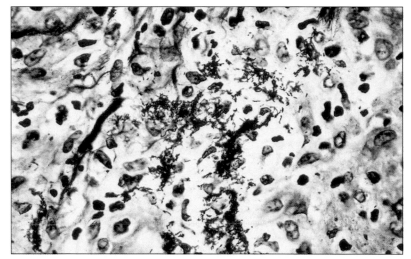

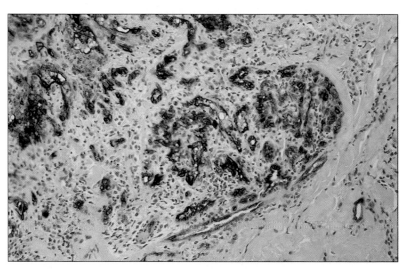

**FIGURE 8-13** Warthin-Starry silver stain of cutaneous bacillary angiomatosis demonstrating tangled masses of bacilli. Note that the nuclei of cells in the background are delicately outlined by silver; this "internal control" is useful in determining the technical adequacy of the stain. Warthin-Starry and related silver stains are technically difficult to perform, and without optimal background staining of cells, the absence of bacteria should not be interpreted as ruling out the disease.

**FIGURE 8-14** Immunoperoxidase staining for factor VIII–related antigen in bacillary angiomatosis. The vascular nature of the proliferation in cutaneous bacillary angiomatosis is confirmed by immunoperoxidase staining for factor VIII–related antigen (von Willebrand's factor), which is expressed by blood vascular endothelial cells in this routinely processed tissue. In contrast, the cells of Kaposi's sarcoma show only weak factor VIII–related antigen expression, supporting lymphatic rather than blood vascular differentiation.

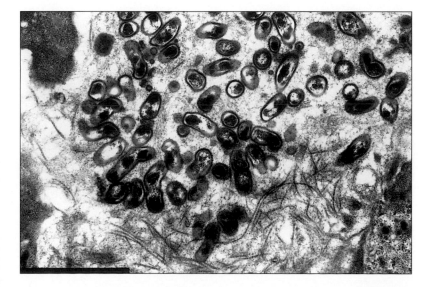

**FIGURE 8-15** Electron microscopic appearance of one of the organisms of bacillary angiomatosis, *Bartonella henselae*. There is a mass of bacteria with trilaminar cell walls, whose structure is consistent with that of gram-negative organisms.

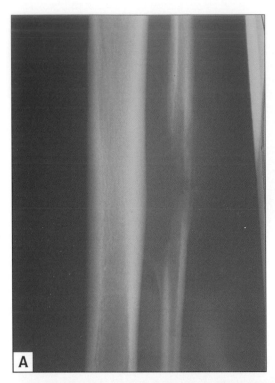

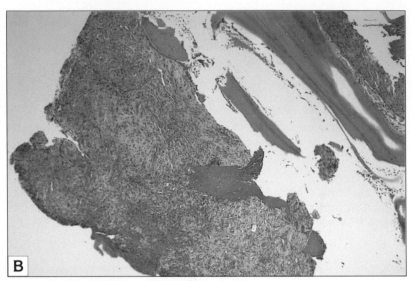

**FIGURE 8-16** Deep lesion of bacillary angiomatosis. **A,** Soft-tissue masses of bacillary angiomatosis can erode underlying bone. A large mass in the lower leg of this patient resulted in a lytic defect in the fibula. This patient was scheduled for amputation prior to review of the slides by one of the authors. **B,** Bony trabecula are separated by a granulation tissuelike proliferation of capillaries. (Hematoxylin-eosin stain.) **C,** The pink granular material between vessels is a massive growth of bacilli. Unlike the case in cutaneous bacillary angiomatosis, deep bacillary angiomatosis lesions often have very few neutrophils. (Hematoxylin-eosin stain.) **D,** Warthin-Starry silver stain demonstrates large black masses of bacilli. The mass involuted following therapy with erythromycin.

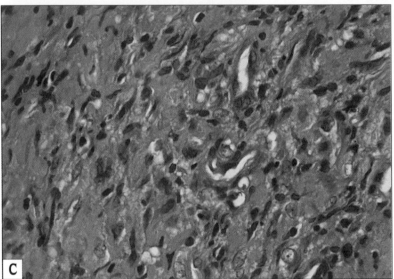

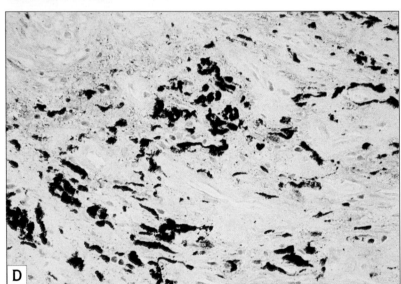

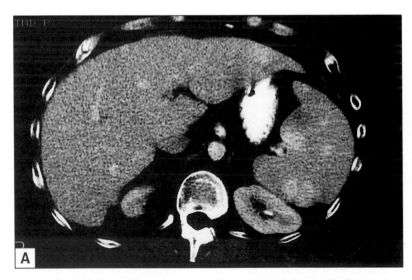

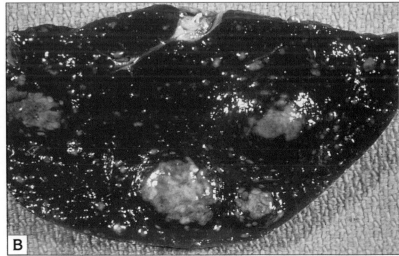

**FIGURE 8-17** Visceral lesions of bacillary angiomatosis. **A,** Computed tomography scan of the abdomen demonstrating lesions of bacillary angiomatosis. The patient was a woman aged 38 years receiving chronic immunosuppressive medications. Numerous lesions of the spleen and liver enhance with contrast [11]. **B,** Cross-section of spleen shows lobular, flesh-colored lesions varying from 0.1 to 3.0 cm in diameter. Visceral bacillary angiomatosis may involve nearly any site but most often involves the liver, spleen, lymphatic system, and bone marrow. (*continued*)

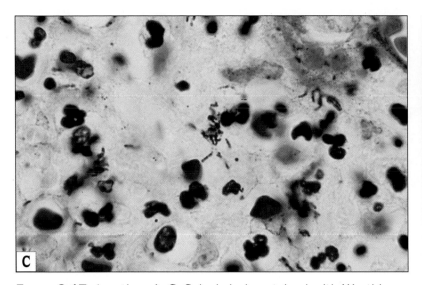

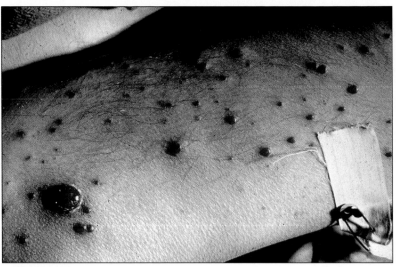

**FIGURE 8-17** (*continued*) **C,** Splenic lesion stained with Warthin-Starry silver stain. *Bartonella henselae,* one of the etiologic agents of bacillary angiomatosis, are visible at the center of the picture as single bacillary rods and in clumps. This organism was originally identified directly from this tissue using a novel approach that does not rely on microbial cultivation [12]. (Original magnification, × 1000.) (*Courtesy of* D. Regula, MD.)

**FIGURE 8-18** Bacillary angiomatosis–like lesions in the absence of HIV infection. Is bacillary angiomatosis a new disease? Several reports dating prior to the HIV epidemic described patients suffering from advanced malignancies who had disseminated, pyogenic, granuloma-like vascular lesions, such as those pictured here. Unfortunately, tissue from many of these cases is no longer available [13]. Bacillary angiomatosis due to *Bartonella* has been confirmed in a number of patients seronegative for HIV, including some with no detectable evidence of immunosuppression [14]. (*Courtesy of* E. Omura, MD.)

# BACILLARY PELIOSIS

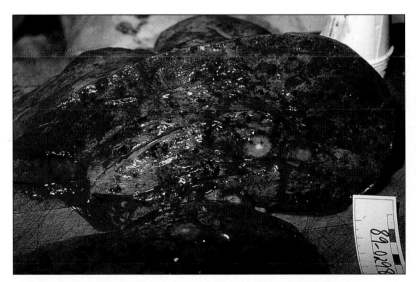

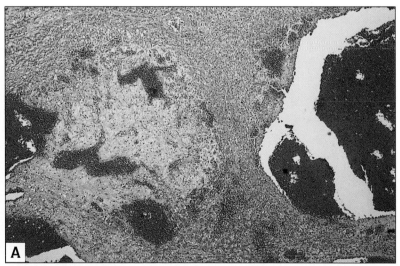

**FIGURE 8-19** Bacillary peliosis hepatis seen at autopsy as large and small, blood-filled and mucoid-appearing cysts in the liver. Bacillary peliosis is a form of disseminated *Bartonella henselae* and *B. quintana* infection that is manifest by variant angioproliferative pathology. *Peliosis* means "dark purple" in ancient Greek, referring to the color of the blood-filled cysts. In general, peliosis hepatis and splenis have been associated with a variety of etiologic factors, including anabolic steroids, inanition, tuberculosis, and widespread malignancy, but in immunosuppressed patients it is often associated with infection by *Bartonella.* (*From* Perkocha *et al.* [15]; with permission.)

**FIGURE 8-20** Tissue cross-section of bacillary peliosis hepatis. **A,** A photomicrograph shows blood-filled spaces, areas of myxoid stroma, and residual hepatic parenchyma. (Hematoxylin-eosin stain.) (*continued*)

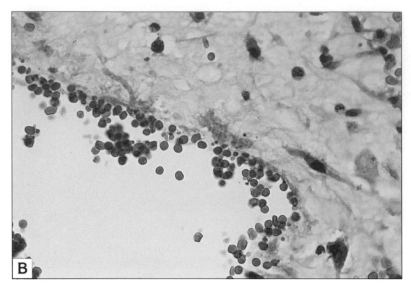

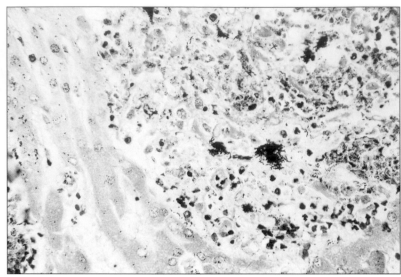

**Figure 8-20** (*continued*)  **B,** Within myxoid stroma at the edge of a peliotic space is a clump of purplish granules, representing a colony of bacilli. (Hematoxylin-eosin stain.)

**Figure 8-21** Warthin-Starry silver stain of myxoid stroma in bacillary peliosis hepatis. Several tangled masses of bacilli are seen within an area of myxoid stroma near a peliotic space.

# OTHER *BARTONELLA* INFECTIONS

## Disease Due to *Bartonella bacilliformis*

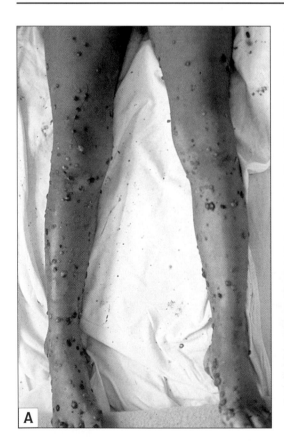

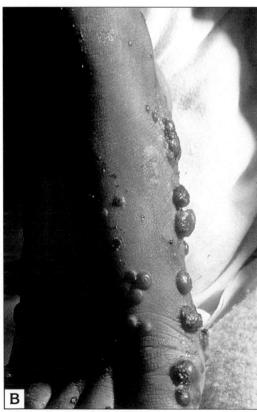

**Figure 8-22** Verruga peruana. **A** and **B,** The cutaneous vascular papules and nodules due to infection with *Bartonella bacilliformis* are astonishingly similar to those of bacillary angiomatosis in their clinical appearance, reflecting the close phylogenetic relationship of the organisms (*see* Fig. 8-2). *B. bacilliformis* and its associated disease have only been detected in the Andean regions of South America.

# Cat Scratch Disease

## Epidemiologic features of cat scratch disease

Most common *Bartonella*-associated disease in United States
(~ 22,000 cases/yr)
Peak incidence occurs age < 14 yrs, September–January
Risk: intimate cat (kitten) exposure
*B. henselae* antibody–positive in 84%–95% of cases
DNA-positive in 60%–95% of cases
Cats: 28% seropositive in United States, up to 70%; 41%
bacteremic in one study (*B. henselae*, not *B. quintana*)

**FIGURE 8-23** Epidemiologic features of cat scratch disease. Antibody-positive indicates a positive test result for circulating antibodies; DNA-positive refers to a positive polymerase chain reaction test result for *Bartonella henselae* DNA.

## Clinical features of cat scratch disease

Most common presentation is solitary cervical or axillary
lymphadenopathy, with stellate necrotizing granulomatous
response; duration, 2 wks–8 mos
Preceding inoculation papule
Oculoglandular syndrome of Parinaud seen in 2%–10%
Complications: central nervous system seizures, encephalitis;
hepatitis; bone marrow involvement; optic neuritis, retinitis

**FIGURE 8-24** Clinical features of cat scratch disease.

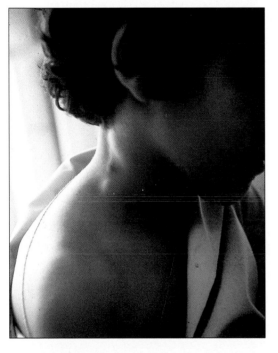

**FIGURE 8-25** Child with posterior cervical lymphadenopathy typical of cat scratch disease. The cervical region is the second most common site for the development of regional lymphadenopathy in cat scratch disease; the axilla is the most common site.

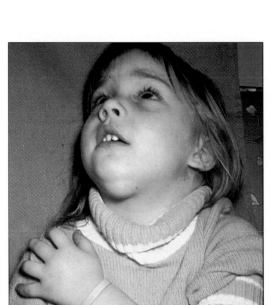

**FIGURE 8-26** Submental lymphadenopathy in a girl aged 3 years with cat scratch disease. There had been a preceding inoculation papule in the center of her chin. Her lymphadenopathy resolved spontaneously after approximately 6 weeks. In roughly 2% to 10% of cases, there is suppuration of affected lymph nodes, sometimes requiring needle aspiration. (*Courtesy of* A.M. Margileth, MD.)

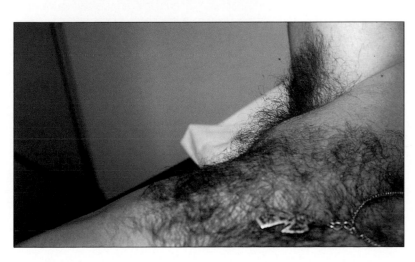

**FIGURE 8-27** Axillary lymphadenopathy in a patient with cat scratch disease. (*Courtesy of* E.J.C. Goldstein, MD.)

**FIGURE 8-28** Cat scratch disease in a young woman. A papule is often evident at the site of the bite or scratch, seen here on the skin of the eyelid. Lymphadenopathy generally follows approximately 2 weeks later. Inoculation site papules are not always present, and patients some-

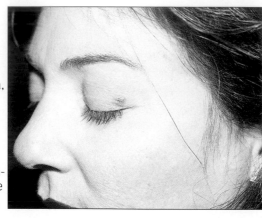

times present with adenopathy in the absence of cutaneous lesions. Systemic complications, such as pleuritis, encephalitis, transverse myelitis, osteomyelitis, and splenomegaly, occur in < 2% of patients [16]. Serologic, molecular, and culture-based evidence suggest that *Bartonella henselae* is the cause of most cases of cat scratch disease.

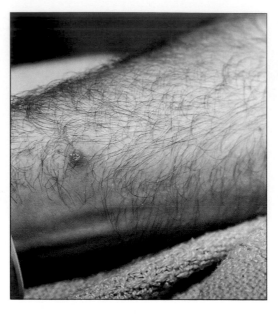

**FIGURE 8-29** Primary inoculation papule of cat scratch disease. (*Courtesy of* E.J.C. Goldstein, MD.)

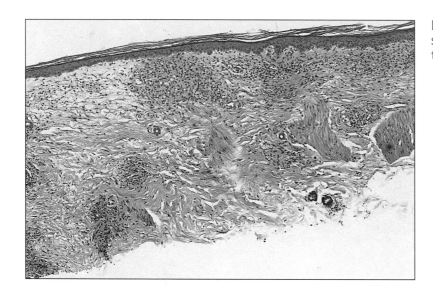

**FIGURE 8-30** Histopathology of an inoculation site papule of cat scratch disease. The dermis contains palisaded granulomatous infiltrates that surround the suppurative foci containing the bacteria.

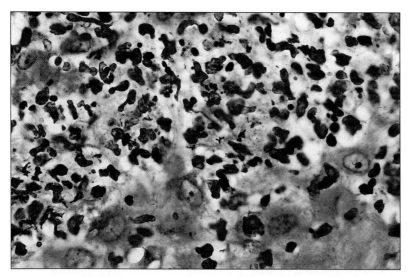

**FIGURE 8-31** Warthin-Starry silver stain of a histologic section of an inoculation site papule. Individual bacilli are visible among the neutrophils seen at top. The cells with large nuclei at the bottom are macrophages. The cause of cat scratch disease was in dispute for decades, with both viral and bacterial organisms suggested as candidates. The identification of bacteria in most cases of cat scratch disease by silver staining in 1983 settled this preliminary issue [17]. Conventional special stains used to demonstrate bacteria, such as the Brown-Brenn modification of the Gram stain, do not reveal the bacilli of cat scratch disease, and acid-fast stains are similarly ineffective. Silver stains, such as the Warthin-Starry, Levaditi, and Dieterle methods, will all stain the bacilli of cat scratch disease (and those of bacillary angiomatosis as well); however, these stains are not specific, *ie,* they will stain almost all bacteria. A positive stain only indicates cat scratch disease when coupled with negative conventional special stains.

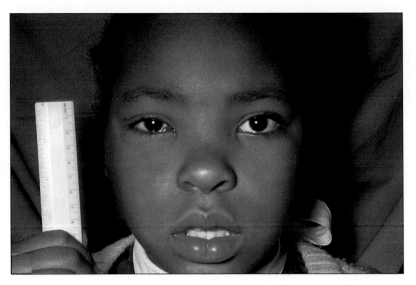

**Figure 8-32** Oculoglandular syndrome of Parinaud, secondary to cat scratch disease. A girl aged 8 years developed a conjunctival lesion and preauricular lymphadenopathy secondary to cat scratch disease inoculation into the eye. The resulting clinical picture, the oculoglandular syndrome of Parinaud, occurs in 2% to 10% of cat scratch disease cases; however, Parinaud's syndrome can occur in the setting of other infections, such as tularemia. (*Courtesy of* A.M. Margileth, MD.)

# DIAGNOSTIC EVALUATION

**Diagnosis of *Bartonella*-associated disease**

Clinical findings and histology ± Warthin-Starry silver stain

Serology: immunofluorescent assay or enzyme-linked immunoassay (4 × ↑ or ↓)

Polymerase chain reaction, immunohistochemistry, culture (research/reference)

**Figure 8-33** Diagnosis of *Bartonella*-associated disease. The diagnosis in many cases can be made with clinical and histologic findings alone. Serologic techniques (immunofluorescent antibody or enzyme-linked immunoassay) can be used to corroborate these findings, especially when a concurrent fourfold or greater rise or fall in antibody titer is documented. Polymerase chain reaction assays, immunohistochemistry tests, or culture methods are available in reference or research laboratories only at present [18].

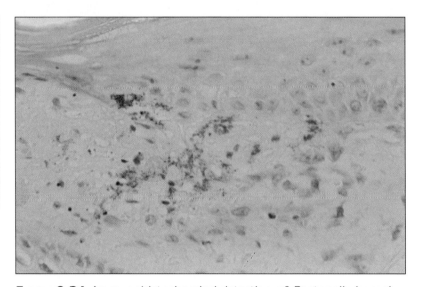

**Figure 8-34** Immunohistochemical detection of *Bartonella henselae* in a formalin-fixed, paraffin-embedded section from a cutaneous bacillary angiomatosis lesion. This procedure is based on primary binding with a specific polyclonal antisera directed against *B. henselae*, followed by detection with a biotinylated secondary antibody and an avidin-alkaline phosphatase conjugate. Organisms appear red. Preadsorbed primary antisera can distinguish between *B. henselae* and *B. quintana*. *In situ* detection of the agents of bacillary angiomatosis and cat scratch disease with either immunochemical or nucleic acid hybridization techniques may lead to a more rapid diagnosis of these disorders [19]. (*Courtesy of* K.-W. Min, MD, J. Reed, MD, and L. Slater, MD.)

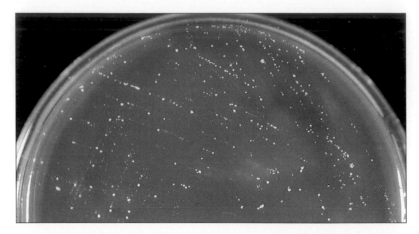

**FIGURE 8-35** Cultivation of *Bartonella henselae* on Columbia-rabbit blood agar. As with many of the initial laboratory isolates, this organism was grown from a blood sample that was processed by lysis-centrifugation. Pelleted material was then incubated on blood-containing plates in an elevated $CO_2$ atmosphere for as many as 21 days. The relative frequencies of isolation of *B. henselae* and *B. quintana* seem to vary according to geographic region or laboratory [20,21]. (*Courtesy of* L. Slater, MD.)

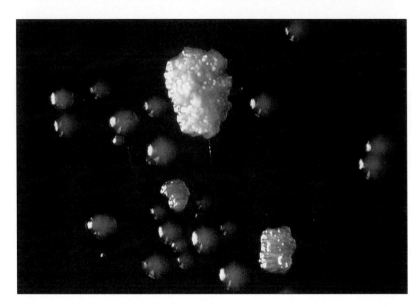

**FIGURE 8-36** Variable colony morphology of *Bartonella henselae*. Two colony morphotypes are commonly observed: whitish, dry, crumbly-appearing colonies of heterogeneous size that pit the agar surface (at center) and round, dull, smooth, mucoid colonies (at periphery). Pitting probably reflects the expression of type IV pili. Fresh clinical isolates most often display the first morphotype; after serial laboratory passage, the second morphotype becomes progressively more dominant. *B. quintana* usually displays a brownish version of the second morphotype on initial laboratory growth [22]. (*Courtesy of* L. Slater, MD.)

# THERAPY

**Treatment of *Bartonella*-associated disease**

| | |
|---|---|
| **Cat scratch disease** | |
| Localized (immunocompetent) | None |
| Disseminated or immunocompromised | Gentamicin, 5 mg/kg/d, *or* ciprofloxacin, 500 mg twice a day (*or* rifampin, TMP-SMX?) × 10–14 days |
| **Other *Bartonella* infection** | |
| Bacteremia, bacterial endocarditis, bacillary angiomatosis, bacillary peliosis | Erythromycin, 500–1000 mg four times a day; *or* tetracycline, 500 mg four times a day; *or* doxycycline, 100 mg twice a day (*or* azithromycin, clarithromycin, rifampin?) |
| For cutaneous bacillary angiomatosis | Given orally, × 2–3 mos |
| For visceral or relapsing disease | Given intravenously or orally, 4+ mos |

TMP-SMX—trimethoprim-sulfamethoxazole.

**FIGURE 8-37** Treatment of *Bartonella*-associated disease. Uncomplicated cat scratch disease is a self-limited infection and does not require treatment, whereas systemic disease usually requires treatment. Gentamicin and ciprofloxacin are effective therapies, with rifampin and trimethoprim-sulfamethoxazole as possible alternatives [23]. Systemic *Bartonella* disease in an immunocompromised host always requires antibiotic therapy, sometimes for prolonged periods.

# REFERENCES

1. Woese CR: Bacterial evolution. *Microbiol Rev* 1987, 51:221–271.

2. Woese CR, Kandler O, Wheelis ML: Towards a natural system of organisms: Proposal for the domains Archaea, Bacteria, and Eucarya. *Proc Natl Acad Sci U S A* 1990, 87:4576–4579.

3. Relman DA, Lepp PW, Sadler KN, Schmidt TM: Phylogenetic relationships among the agent of bacillary angiomatosis, *Bartonella bacilliformis*, and other alpha-proteobacteria. *Mol Microbiol* 1992, 6:1801–1807.

4. Brenner DJ, O'Connor SP, Winkler HH, Steigerwalt AG: Proposals to unify the genera *Bartonella* and *Rochalimaea*, with descriptions of *Bartonella quintana* comb. nov., *Bartonella vinsonii* comb. nov., *Bartonella henselae* comb. nov., and *Bartonella elizabethae* comb. nov., and to remove the family *Bartonellaceae* from the order *Rickettsiales. Int J Syst Bacteriol* 1993, 43:777–786.

5. Regnery RL, Perkins BA, Olson JG, Bibb W: Serological response to "Rochalimaea henselae" antigen in suspected cat scratch disease. *Lancet* 1992, 339:1443–1445.

6. Koehler JE, Glaser CA, Tappero JW: *Rochalimaea henselae* infection: A new zoonosis with the domestic cat as reservoir. *JAMA* 1994, 271:531–535.

7. Spach DH, Kanter AS, Dougherty MJ, *et al.: Bartonella (Rochalimaea) quintana* bacteremia in inner-city patients with chronic alcoholism. *N Engl J Med* 1995, 332:424–428.

8. Chang Y, *et al.*: Identification of herpesvirus-like DNA sequences in AIDS associated Kaposi's sarcoma. *Science* 1994, 266:1865–1869.

9. Berger TG, Tappera JW, Kaymen A, LeBoit PE: Bacillary (epithelioid) angiomatosis and concurrent Kaposi's sarcoma in AIDS. *Arch Dermatol* 1989, 125:1543–1547.

10. LeBoit PE, Berger TM, Egbert BM, *et al.*: Bacillary angiomatosis: The histopathology and differential diagnosis of a pseudoneoplastic infection in patients with human immunodeficiency virus disease. *Am J Surg Pathol* 1989, 13:909–920.

11. Kemper CA, Lombard CM, Deresinski SC, Tompkins LS: Visceral bacillary epithelioid angiomatosis: Possible manifestations of disseminated cat scratch disease in the immunocompromised host: A report of two cases. *Am J Med* 1990, 89:216–222.

12. Relman DA, Loutit JS, Schmidt TM, *et al.*: The agent of bacillary angiomatosis: An approach to the identification of uncultured pathogens. *N Engl J Med* 1990, 323:1573–1580.

13. Omura EF, Omura GA: Human immunodeficiency virus-associated skin lesions [letter]. *JAMA* 1989, 261:991.

14. Tappero JW, Koehler JE, Berger TG, *et al.*: Bacillary angiomatosis and bacillary splenitis in immunocompetent adults. *Ann Intern Med* 1993, 118:363–365.

15. Perkocha LA, Geaghan SM, Yen TS, *et al.*: Clinical and pathological features of bacillary peliosis hepatis in association with human immunodeficiency virus infection. *N Engl J Med* 1990, 323:1581–1586.

16. Margileth AM, Wear DJ, English CK: Systemic cat scratch disease: Report of 23 patients with prolonged or recurrent severe bacterial infection. *J Infect Dis* 1987, 155:390–402.

17. Wear DJ, Margileth AM, Hadfield TL, *et al.*: Cat scratch disease: A bacterial infection. *Science* 1983, 221:1403–1405.

18. Dalton MJ, Robinson LE, Cooper J, *et al.*: Use of *Bartonella* antigens for serologic diagnosis of cat-scratch disease at a national referral center. *Arch Intern Med* 1995, 155:1670–1676.

19. Reed JA, Brigati DJ, Flynn SD, *et al.*: Immunocytochemical identification of *Rochalimaea henselae* in bacillary (epithelioid) angiomatosis, parenchymal bacillary peliosis, and persistent fever with bacteremia. *Am J Surg Pathol* 1992, 16:650–657.

20. Slater LN, Welch DF, Hensel D, Coody DW: A newly recognized fastidious gram-negative pathogen as a cause of fever and bacteremia. *N Engl J Med* 1990, 323:1587–1593.

21. Koehler JE, Quinn FD, Berger TG, *et al.*: Isolation of *Rochalimaea* species from cutaneous and osseous lesions of bacillary angiomatosis. *N Engl J Med* 1992, 327:1625–1631.

22. Welch DW, *et al.*: *Rochalimaea henselae* sp. nov., a cause of septicemia, bacillary angiomatosis, and parenchymal bacillary peliosis. *J Clin Microbiol* 1992, 30:275–280.

23. Margileth AM: Antibiotic therapy for cat-scratch disease: Clinical study of the therapeutic outcome in 268 patients and a review of the literature. *Pediatr Infect Dis J* 1992, 11:474–478.

# SELECTED BIBLIOGRAPHY

Carithers HA: Cat-scratch disease: An overview based on a study of 1,200 patients. *Am J Dis Child* 1985, 139:1124–1133.

Carithers HA, Carithers CM, Edwards RO Jr: Cat scratch disease: Its natural history. *JAMA* 1969, 207:312–316.

Cockerell CJ, LeBoit PE: Bacillary angiomatosis: A newly characterized, pseudoneoplastic, infectious, cutaneous vascular disorder. *J Am Acad Dermatol* 1990, 22:501–512.

Relman DA: Bacillary angiomatosis and *Rochalimaea* species. *In* Remington JS, Swartz MN (eds.): *Current Clinical Topics in Infectious Diseases*, vol 14. Boston: Blackwell Scientific Publications; 1994:205–219.

Relman DA: The identification of uncultured microbial pathogens. *J Infect Dis* 1993, 168:1–8.

Koehler JE, Tappero JW: Bacillary angiomatosis and bacillary peliosis in patients infected with human immunodeficiency virus. *Clin Infect Dis* 1993, 17:612–624.

# CHAPTER 9

## Leprosy

Bruce H. Clements
David M. Scollard

# ETIOLOGY

## Major sites of involvement in leprosy

1. Skin
2. Peripheral nerves
3. Eyes
4. Mucous membranes

**FIGURE 9-1** Definition and major sites of involvement in leprosy. Leprosy (Hansen's disease) is a chronic infectious disease caused by *Mycobacterium leprae*, and the organism can be found in all parts of the body except the central nervous system, while producing skin and nerve lesions only in the cooler areas of the body. Existing since antiquity in an atmosphere of mystery, superstition, and fear, the disease, left untreated, can produce marked disfigurement due to gross deformities of the face, progressive loss of sensation in the hands and feet, and blindness. With our present knowledge and with early detection and treatment of the disease, leprosy can be cured and the stigmata attached to the disease can be avoided.

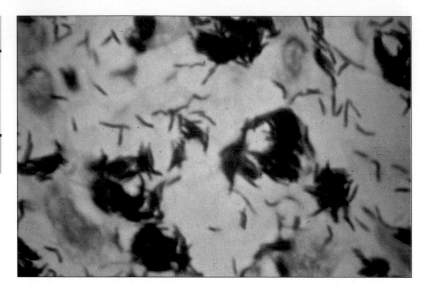

**FIGURE 9-2** Acid-fast stain of *Mycobacterium leprae*. This acid-fast–stained slide shows the great number of *M. leprae* that can be seen in a skin biopsy specimen from a patient with lepromatous leprosy.

## A. Characteristics of *Mycobacterium leprae*: The organism

*M. leprae* first identified by Hansen (1873) as causative agent of leprosy; one of the first microbial pathogens of humans identified

Acid-fast bacillus 0.3–0.4 × 2–7 μm

Considered an obligate intracellular parasite

Will survive for prolonged periods at -80° C and in dried secretions up to 9 days in a hot, humid climate

## B. Characteristics of *Mycobacterium leprae*: Culture and growth

Has not been cultivated in artificial media

Growth in mouse footpad first reported in 1960 by Shepard

Maximum growth in mouse footpad at 27–30° C

Divides on average every 12.5 days during log phase of growth in mouse footpad; it is the slowest growing bacterial pathogen

Has unique ability to oxidize dyhydrophenylaline (DOPA)

Growth also reported in:
 9-banded armadillo
 Nude mouse
 Neonatally thymectomized Lewis rat

## C. Characteristics of *Mycobacterium leprae*: Infectivity

Host specificity: Not confined to humans alone, but also:
 Wild 9-banded armadillos (*Dasypus novencinctus*) caught in Louisiana and Texas
 Chimpanzee (*Pan troglodytes*) and mangabey (*Cercocebus torquatus atys*) from West Africa
Incubation period: Extremely variable, ranging from months to ≥ 2 decades, but usually about 3–5 years; shorter for tuberculoid than lepromatous disease
Seems to have predilection for nerves and for cooler parts of body

**FIGURE 9-3** Characteristics of *Mycobacterium leprae*. The organism is similar in appearance to *M. tuberculosis*, but unlike *M. tuberculosis*, it has not been cultured on artificial media. The method of growing *M. leprae* in the footpads of mice is used as a tool for research and for determining the sensitivity and resistance of the bacterium to drugs. **A,** Organism characteristics. **B,** Culture and growth characteristics. **C,** Infectivity characteristics.

# EPIDEMIOLOGY

### Estimated number of leprosy cases by WHO region, 1995

| WHO region | Estimated cases, *n* | Estimated prevalence per 10,000 population |
|---|---|---|
| Africa | 219,000 | 4.1 |
| Americas | 219,000 | 2.9 |
| Southeast Asia | 1,259,000 | 9.3 |
| Europe | 6000 | 0.1 |
| Eastern Mediterranean | 61,000 | 1.5 |
| Western Pacific | 70,000 | 0.4 |
| **Total** | **1,834,000** | **3.3** |

WHO—World Health Organization.

**FIGURE 9-4** Estimated number of leprosy cases by World Health Organization (WHO) region, 1995. The WHO began a policy of using multidrug therapy for leprosy in 1981, which resulted in a decrease in the prevalence of the disease worldwide. In 1991, the WHO proposed a goal of eliminating leprosy as a public health problem by the year 2000 by reducing the prevalence to < 1/10,000 population. With approximately 600,000 new cases per year, there has been no significant change in the incidence, but prevalence has fallen with 6 months to 2 years of multidrug therapy. The global coverage of multidrug therapy is about 75%. In the United States, there are approximately 7400 cases, and approximately 200 new cases occur per year, with 80% occurring in immigrants. (*Adapted from* WHO [1].)

### Modes of transmission

Respiratory tract
Skin contact

**FIGURE 9-5** Modes of transmission of leprosy. The exact mode of transmission is not known, but the most widely held theory involves the respiratory tract. Untreated lepromatous patients daily discharge from $10^7$ to $10^8$ bacteria from their nares by coughing and sneezing, thereby releasing viable *Mycobacterium leprae* in droplets. The bacteria enters the body via the nasal mucous membrane causing a bacillemia. Transfer via direct skin contact with bacilli discharged from ulcerations in patients might occur but is not likely. Armadillos in Louisiana and Texas have been found to be infected with *M. leprae* and develop a generalized disease, presumably due to their cooler core body temperature; however, it is unknown if transmission occurs from armadillos to humans.

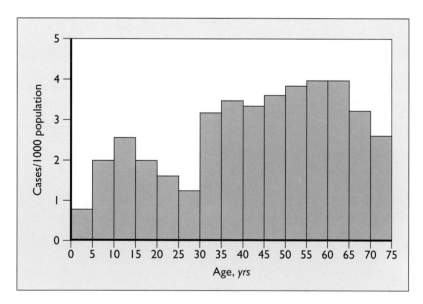

**FIGURE 9-6** Age-specific incidence rates for leprosy in a highly endemic area of India. Leprosy can occur at any age starting at 2 to 2.5 months and extending into the late 80s and 90s. The incidence peaks at 10 to 14 years of age and again at 30 to 60. As people live longer, more cases are occurring in the 60 to 80 age group, especially in more developed countries. Men are affected twice as often as women in most parts of the world. (*Adapted from* Nordeen [2].)

# PATHOGENESIS

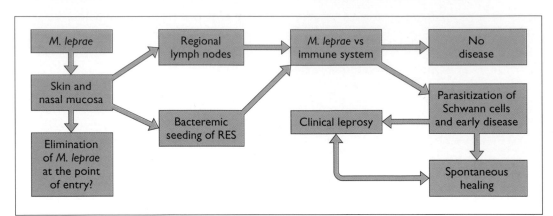

**FIGURE 9-7** Pathogenesis of Hansen's disease. *Mycobacterium leprae* probably enter the body through either a break in the skin or the nasal mucosa. It elicits remarkably little inflammation but, in susceptible individuals, interacts with immunologic factors to determine the type of disease, distribution of lesions, and types of reaction that can occur before or after effective treatment. After an initial inflammatory response to the organisms as seen on biopsy, a granuloma forms from macrophages. (RES—reticuloendothelial system.)

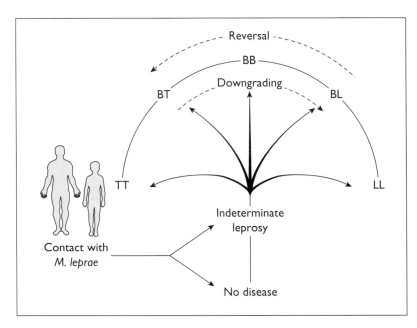

**FIGURE 9-8** Ridley-Jopling classification of Hansen's disease. The classification of leprosy is based on the immunologic status of the patient, the patient's ability to mount a cell-mediated immune response to the bacillus, and the histologic pattern on biopsy. Indeterminate disease falls outside this spectrum. Patients with a high degree of tissue resistance develop tuberculoid (TT) disease, whereas those with no resistance develop lepromatous leprosy (LL). Between these two extremes is the very unstable borderline part of the spectrum, which encompasses borderline tuberculoid (BT), midborderline (BB), and borderline lepromatous (BL) disease, where the great majority of cases occur. Another classification was initiated in 1982 by the World Health Organization for treatment purposes; it defines disease as paucibacillary (negative skin scrapings at any four sites) or multibacillary (positive skin scrapings at any site) and is used worldwide to determine the length of treatment regimens [3].

# CLINICAL ASPECTS

## Diagnostic Testing

### Diagnostic studies in patients with suspected leprosy

1. Physical examination
   a. Examination of skin
   b. Motor and sensory testing
   c. Palpation of peripheral nerves for enlargement and/or tenderness
2. Biopsy of skin for histopathology and determination of MI and BI
3. Skin scrapings for MI and BI determination

BI—bacteriologic index; MI—morphologic index.

**FIGURE 9-9** Diagnostic studies in leprosy. Skin biopsy is performed for histopathologic examination, using hematoxylin-eosin as well as the Fite-Faraco stains. The histopathologic features of leprosy are remarkably heterogeneous and constitute a full spectrum, not a set of discrete steps or categories. Histopathologic classification is based primarily on 1) the pattern of the inflammatory infiltrate (organized into granulomas or disorganized), 2) morphology of the macrophages present (epithelioid vs vacuolated), 3) involvement of cutaneous nerves, and 4) presence and number of *Mycobacterium leprae* in Fite-stained sections. The evaluation of cutaneous nerves is critical and often decisive in establishing the diagnosis, and for this reason a good full-thickness biopsy is very important. *M. leprae* are weakly acid-fast, and a satisfactory search for them requires a Fite (or other modified) acid-fast staining procedure. (*See* Fig. 9-10.)

**Bacteriologic index**

0 = None found per 100 OIF
1+ = 1–10 per 100 OIF
2+ = 1–10 per 10 OIF
3+ = 1–10 per 1 OIF
4+ = 10–100 per 1 OIF
5+ = 100–1000 per 1 OIF
6+ = 1000+ per 1 OIF

OIF—oil immersion field.

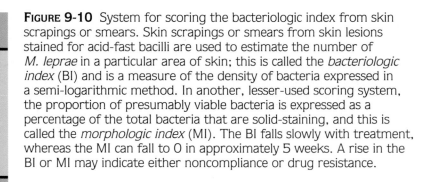

**FIGURE 9-10** System for scoring the bacteriologic index from skin scrapings or smears. Skin scrapings or smears from skin lesions stained for acid-fast bacilli are used to estimate the number of *M. leprae* in a particular area of skin; this is called the *bacteriologic index* (BI) and is a measure of the density of bacteria expressed in a semi-logarithmic method. In another, lesser-used scoring system, the proportion of presumably viable bacteria is expressed as a percentage of the total bacteria that are solid-staining, and this is called the *morphologic index* (MI). The BI falls slowly with treatment, whereas the MI can fall to 0 in approximately 5 weeks. A rise in the BI or MI may indicate either noncompliance or drug resistance.

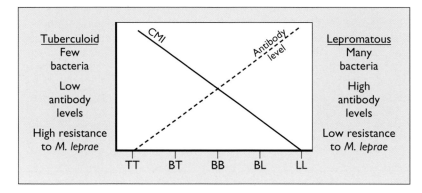

**FIGURE 9-11** Cellular and humoral immune response in Hansen's disease. The cell-mediated immune (CMI) response ranges from high in tuberculoid (TT) leprosy to low or none in lepromatous (LL) leprosy, whereas antibody levels show the opposite trend. (BB—midborderline; BL—borderline lepromatous; BT—borderline tuberculoid.)

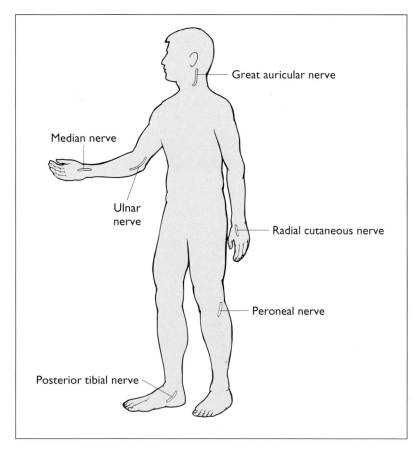

**FIGURE 9-12** Examination of peripheral nerves in leprosy. The larger nerves should be palpated for enlargement or tenderness in a patient with leprosy. Any branch of a peripheral nerve, including the facial branches, can be involved.

# Indeterminate Leprosy

| Indeterminate leprosy: Nature of lesions |
|---|
| 1. One or very few hypopigmented macules |
| 2. Smooth surface |
| 3. Ill-defined margin |
| 4. May have diminished sensation |
| 5. Skin smears usually negative |

**FIGURE 9-13**  Nature of lesions in indeterminate leprosy.

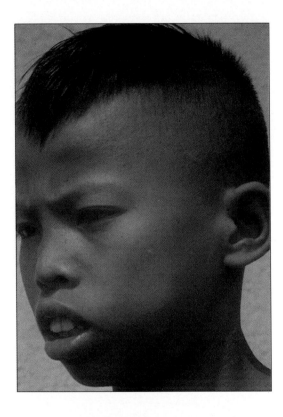

**FIGURE 9-14**  Indeterminate Hansen's disease lesion on the left cheek of a young man. Indeterminate leprosy is the earliest lesion seen in the disease and often is not recognized because of its innocuous appearance. Although most heal spontaneously, the rest, approximately 30%, become determinate and enter the Ridley-Jopling spectrum of the disease. On biopsy, a few acid-fast bacilli may be seen. This type of leprosy is rarely diagnosed in the United States, but when detected, treatment is indicated to prevent progression. (*From* Guinto *et al.* [4]; with permission.)

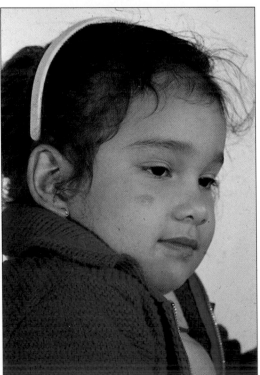

**FIGURE 9-15**  Indeterminate lesion on the right cheek of a young girl. This child, with a family history of leprosy and an erythematous lesion on her right cheek, was diagnosed as having indeterminate leprosy by skin biopsy. For diagnosis, a 2-mm skin biopsy is done on the face, whereas a 4-mm biopsy is recommended for other sites. In the United States, leprosy should be considered in any immigrant, all immunosuppressed individuals, and those with a family history of the disease.

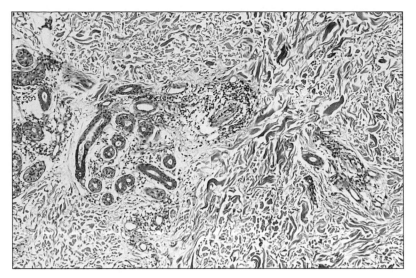

**FIGURE 9-16** Histopathologic features of indeterminate leprosy. The designation "indeterminate" indicates that the diagnosis of leprosy is definitely established but that precise placement on the spectrum is not warranted, usually because the extent of inflammatory infiltrate is insufficient. In routine hematoxylin-eosin–stained sections, the chronic inflammatory infiltrate is nonspecific in character, usually occurring in the mid- and upper dermis. Inflammation is often perivascular but also may be distributed around hair follicles or eccrine glands. Involvement of cutaneous nerves is a valuable indicator also but often is not clearly evident due to the paucity of inflammatory infiltrate. Acid-fast organisms should be unequivocally demonstrated in the biopsy when indeterminate leprosy is diagnosed, though they are often rare. The rarity of bacilli does not mean, however, that the patient necessarily falls into the tuberculoid portion of the spectrum; rather, this lesion is early, and without treatment it may evolve into any portion of the spectrum. In cutaneous lesions of leprosy with more extensive inflammation, which can be classified within the spectrum, the chronic mononuclear cell infiltrates are typically distributed as broad bands or columns, following the course of neurovascular structures in the dermis. Involvement of hair follicles, especially at their bases (*see* Fig. 9-19), and of eccrine glands and arrector pili muscle may eventually destroy these structures, resulting clinically in hair loss, skin dryness, and loss of skin elasticity. (Hematoxylin-eosin stain.)

## Tuberculoid Leprosy

**Tuberculoid leprosy: Nature of lesions**

1. One or few lesions
2. Asymmetrical
3. Large—can cover one extremity or entire trunk
4. Definite edge
5. Rough and scaly
6. Usually anesthetic—an anesthetic "ringworm" lesion

**FIGURE 9-17** Nature of lesions in tuberculoid leprosy.

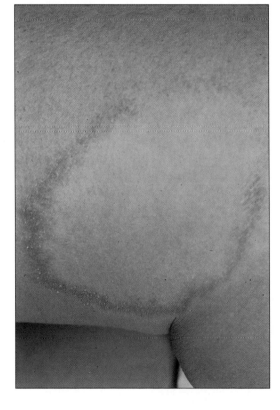

**FIGURE 9-18** Polar tuberculoid leprosy lesion on the thigh. A large, anesthetic, hypopigmented lesion with erythematous borders is seen on the patient's thigh. Many of these lesions will heal without treatment, indicating that the patient possesses a high degree of immunity. With diagnosis, treatment of 6 to 12 months is adequate, with little fear of reactive episodes occurring in this polar form of the disease.

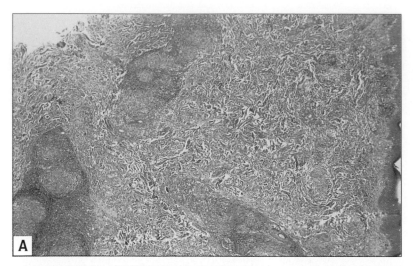

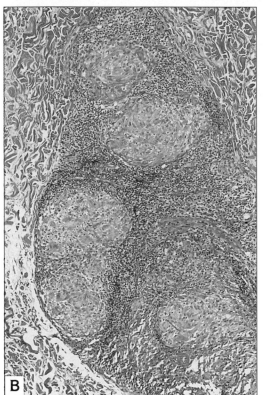

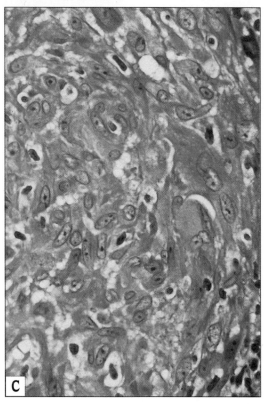

**FIGURE 9-19** Histopathologic features of tuberculoid leprosy. **A**, Polar tuberculoid leprosy is characterized by well-formed, mature epithelioid granulomas. **B**, On higher power, a central core of large, polygonal epithelioid cells is surrounded by a mantle of lymphocytes. The lymphocytic component of the infiltrate may vary from small to large. **C**, Multinucleated giant cells may be present, including Langhans' giant cells, but caseous necrosis is almost never present. Granulomatous inflammation of cutaneous nerves is typically demonstrable if the nerves have not been totally obliterated by the process. The intraneural, perineural, and epineural inflammation results in substantial enlargement of cutaneous nerves. Acid-fast organisms are rare and most often found within nerves; frequently, several serial Fite-stained sections must be examined to demonstrate them. In both tuberculoid and borderline tuberculoid lesions, if the inflammatory infiltrates are located in the upper dermis, they typically extend directly into the basal layer of the epidermis. (*All panels*, hematoxylin-eosin stain.)

# Borderline Tuberculoid Leprosy

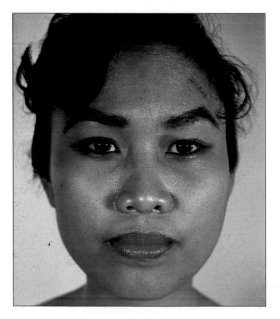

**FIGURE 9-20** Borderline tuberculoid leprosy. A hypopigmented anesthetic skin lesion appears on the left forehead. The healing scar in it is from an excisional biopsy of an enlarged branch of a facial nerve.

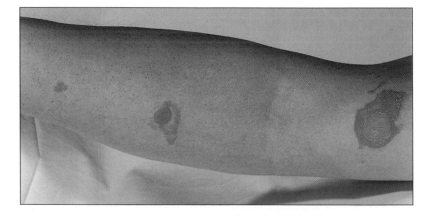

**FIGURE 9-21** Erythematous plaquelike anesthetic lesions of borderline tuberculoid leprosy on the arm. Skin smears were negative. With treatment, this patient could develop a type 1 reaction, causing an ulnar neuropathy with edema of the previous lesions and onset of new lesions. Intervention with corticosteroids will reverse the neuropathy and prevent permanent disability.

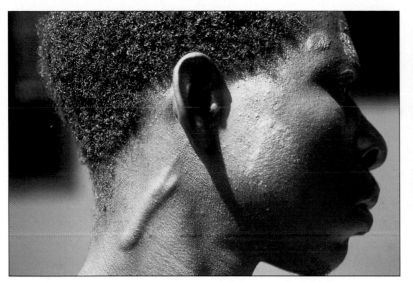

**FIGURE 9-22** Enlarged greater auricular nerve in borderline tuberculoid leprosy. Other branches of the facial nerve are also enlarged in the neck of this patient. Skin lesions can be seen on the cheek and forehead. The nerves may or may not be tender, and any branch of a peripheral nerve may be enlarged and palpable.

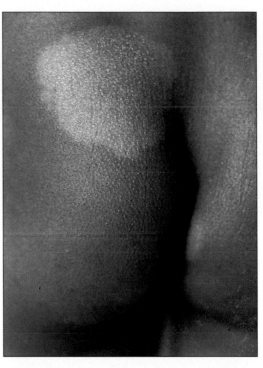

**FIGURE 9-23** Large hypopigmented, circumscribed, anesthetic lesion on the buttocks of a patient with borderline tuberculoid leprosy. This patient with paucibacillary disease and negative skin smears also shows several smaller anesthetic lesions. Treatment with dapsone and rifampin would be necessary for at least 6 months while the patient was monitored for signs of reaction.

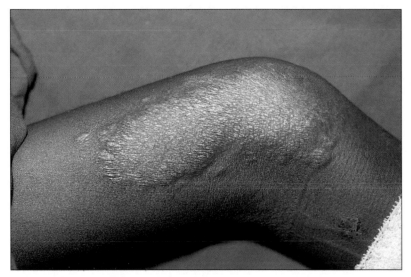

**FIGURE 9-24** A large, infiltrated, well-demarcated, anesthetic scaly lesion of borderline tuberculoid leprosy on a man's knee. Small satellite lesions help to classify this lesion clinically as borderline tuberculoid rather than polar tuberculoid leprosy. Skin scrapings were negative.

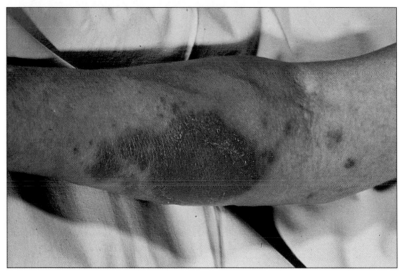

**FIGURE 9-25** A hyperpigmented, anesthetic, lesion with several smaller satellite lesions on the arm of a patient with borderline tuberculoid leprosy.

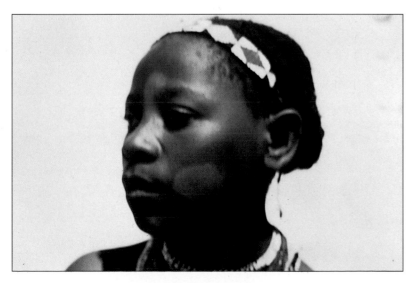

**FIGURE 9-26** Multiple anesthetic, erythematous lesions of borderline tuberculoid leprosy on a woman's face. If only one lesion were present, this presentation could be classified as polar tuberculoid leprosy, but with multiple lesions, borderline tuberculoid leprosy is the clinical and histologic diagnosis.

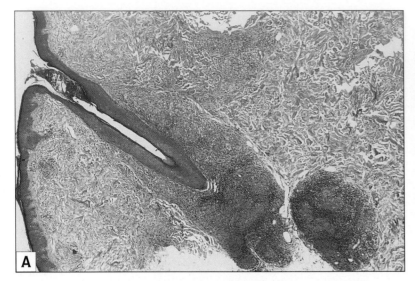

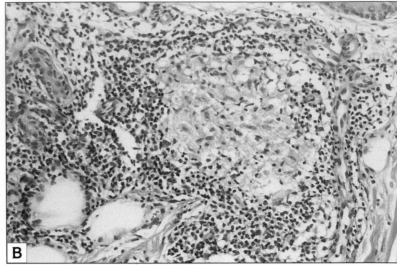

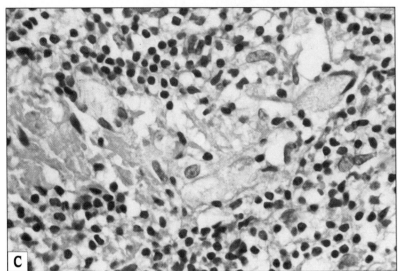

**FIGURE 9-27** Histopathologic features of borderline tuberculoid (BT) leprosy. **A**, BT leprosy is characterized by a granulomatous inflammatory infiltrate that is less well organized than that of polar tuberculoid (TT) lesions. **B**, A substantial portion of the central, epithelioid macrophages may show cytoplasmic vacuolation and they are less tightly knit, giving a "looser" appearance to the granulomas. **C**, Multinucleated giant cells, if present, are less numerous than in TT lesions, and caseous necrosis does not occur in BT lesions. The lymphocytic mantle often comprises a greater proportion of the infiltrate than in polar TT lesions. (*All panels*, hematoxylin-eosin stain.)

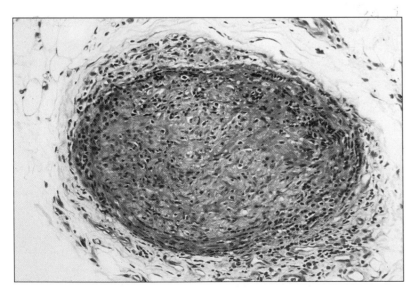

**FIGURE 9-28** Histologic section showing involvement of cutaneous nerves in borderline tuberculoid disease. Inflammation and enlargement of cutaneous nerves are characteristic in borderline tuberculoid leprosy, but nerves may be less extensively enlarged than in tuberculoid lesions. (Hematoxylin-eosin stain.)

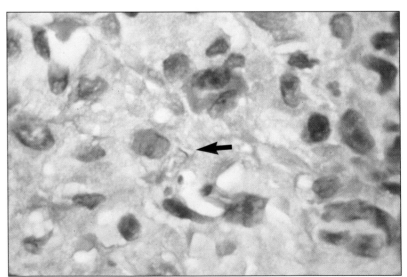

**FIGURE 9-29** Fite stain of cutaneous nerve section showing presence of acid-fast organisms. Acid-fast organisms (*arrow*) are not easily demonstrable but usually can be found, particularly by searching in cells in and around cutaneous nerves. In some lesions, serial sections must be examined.

# Midborderline Leprosy

| Borderline leprosy: Nature of lesions |
| --- |
| 1. Numerous |
| 2. Symmetrical |
| 3. Definite edge |
| 4. Sensation varies |
| 5. Large and small |
| 6. Rough and scaly |

**FIGURE 9-30** Nature of lesions in midborderline leprosy.

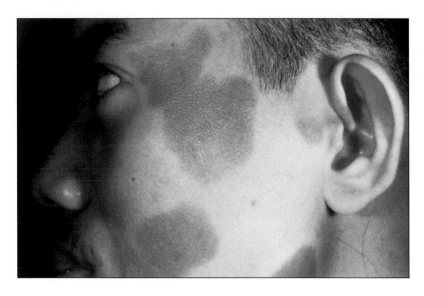

**FIGURE 9-31** Multiple large hyperpigmented lesions of midborderline leprosy on a man's face. Lesion borders range from vague to well demarcated. Other lesions, some anesthetic and some with normal sensation, appear on the trunk and extremities of this patient. Inside the lesions, skin scrapings show a bacteriologic index of 2+ to 3+. Treatment with a three-drug regimen for at least 2 to 3 years is recommended for this multibacillary case.

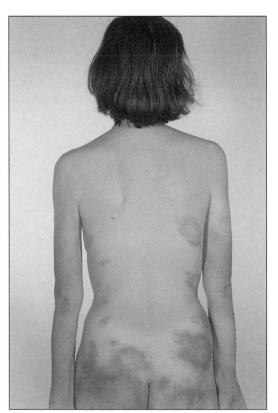

**FIGURE 9-32** Multiple lesions of midborderline leprosy on the back and thighs. The lesions vary in size and have hypesthesia in the center with central clearing of others. Skin smears varied from 1+ to 3+. With many bacteria in an unstable part of the spectrum, this patient is a candidate for a type 1 (reversal) reaction while under treatment.

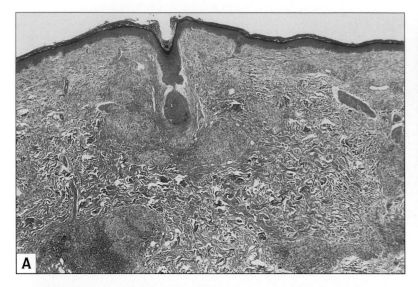

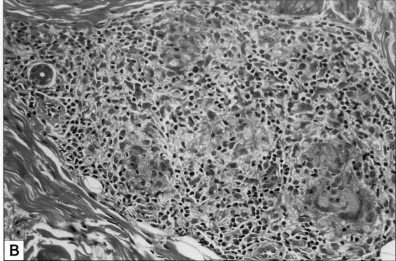

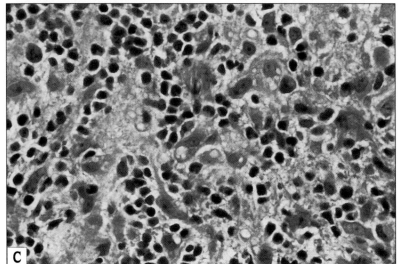

**FIGURE 9-33** Histopathologic feature of midborderline (BB) leprosy. BB lesions display the most dimorphic range of histopathologic features in leprosy. **A** and **B**, Loose, immature granulomas of the borderline tuberculoid type may be seen in one portion of a lesion (*panel 33A*), whereas vacuolated macrophages of borderline lepromatous type predominate in a nearby focus of the same lesion (*panel 33B*). **C**, Most epithelioid-like macrophages show at least some vacuolation. Giant cells are less commonly encountered, and Langhan-type cells are not seen. The quantity of the lymphocytic component is variable. (*All panels*, hematoxylin-eosin stain.)

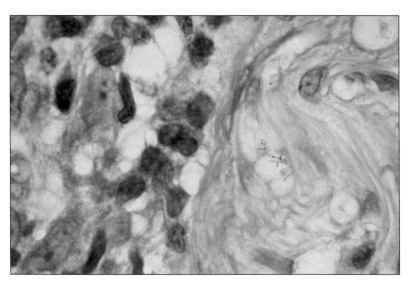

**FIGURE 9-34** Fite stain showing acid-fast organisms in a cutaneous nerve section in midborderline leprosy. Acid-fast organisms usually are more readily demonstrated in some portions of the midborderline lesion but may be scarce in other areas. If scarce in histiocytes, they are likely to be demonstrated in cutaneous nerves, as seen here.

# Borderline Lepromatous Leprosy

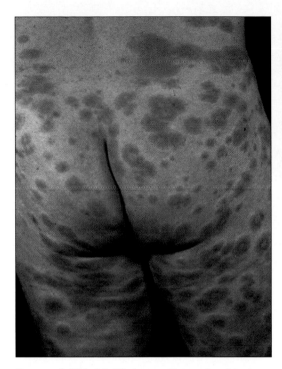

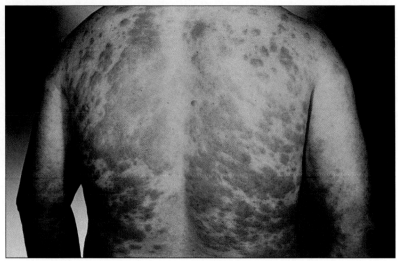

**FIGURE 9-36** Widespread erythematous lesions of borderline lepromatous leprosy on a patient's back. Widespread erythematous lesions can occur over the entire body, with relative sparing of the midline of the back, which is a warmer area where *M. leprae* do not thrive. This patient had no sensory loss in the lesions but had loss of sensation to pain and temperature in his distal extremities, thus being at risk for ulcerations, especially on the plantar surfaces of his feet. Skin lesions clear with treatment, but long-standing sensory loss is permanent. Skin scrapings were 3+ to 4+ anywhere on this patient's body. Borderline lepromatous patients are at risk for both type I (reversal) and type 2 (erythema nodosum leprosum) reactions.

**FIGURE 9-35** Multiple medium-sized lesions of borderline lepromatous leprosy covering a patient's buttocks and thighs. Multiple medium-sized lesions with central clearing with skin scrapings of 3+ to 4+ covered almost the entire body of this man.

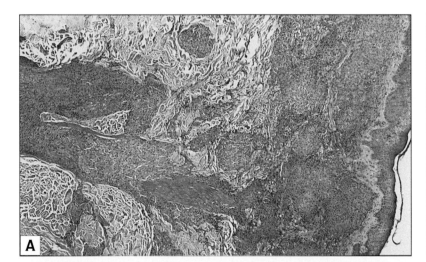

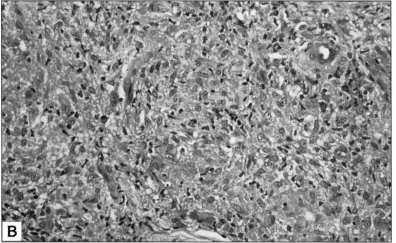

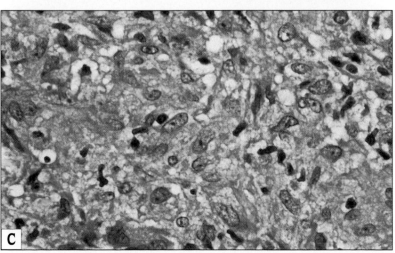

**FIGURE 9-37** Histopathologic features of borderline lepromatous leprosy. **A** and **B**, Borderline lepromatous lesions typically reveal poorly organized or disorganized chronic inflammatory infiltrates appearing as broad bands (*panel 37A*) or sheets (*panel 37B*) of cells following a neurovascular distribution. **C**, The cytoplasm of histiocytes is mildly to extensively vacuolated; epithelioid cells are scarce if present at all. (*All panels*, hematoxylin-eosin stain.)

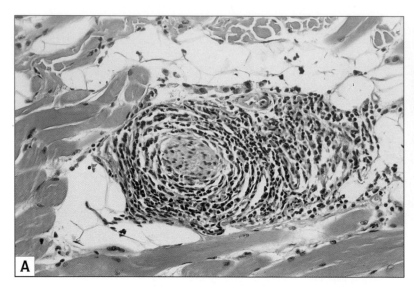

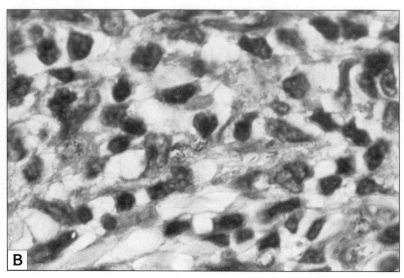

**FIGURE 9-38** Histopathologic sections showing cutaneous nerve involvement in borderline lepromatous leprosy. **A,** The inflammatory involvement of cutaneous nerves is often accompanied by laminar, concentric thickening of the perineurium and epineurium, resulting in an "onion skin" appearance. (Hematoxylin-eosin stain.) **B,** On Fite staining, *M. leprae* are present in moderate to large numbers in histiocytes and in both the intraneural and epineural components of the nerves.

# Lepromatous Leprosy

| Lepromatous leprosy: Nature of lesions |
|---|
| 1. Many |
| 2. Small |
| 3. Symmetrical |
| 4. Vague edge |
| 5. Surface smooth |
| 6. Sensation variable |
| 7. Tend to coalesce |

**FIGURE 9-39** Nature of lesions in lepromatous leprosy.

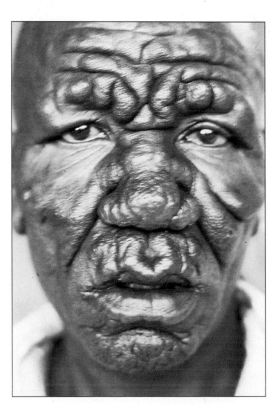

**FIGURE 9-40** Lepromatous leprosy causing leonine facies. Far-advanced, untreated, polar lepromatous leprosy can result in the leonine facies shown in this patient. He has madarosis (loss of eyebrows), partial collapse of the nose, and nasal congestion, with a heavy bacterial load of 6+ anywhere on his body. Also, he has a loss of sensation in his distal extremities. Without treatment, this patient, with a high morphologic index indicating many solid-staining *M. leprae*, is considered a reservoir of infection. Treatment with multidrug therapy for 2 to 3 years is indicated. These patients are at risk for a type 2 reaction, called *erythema nodosum leprosum*.

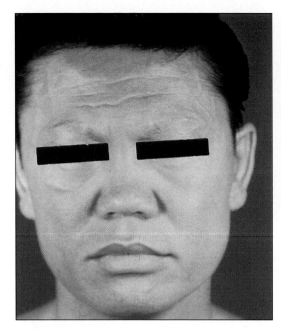

**FIGURE 9-41** Lepromatous leprosy presenting with madarosis and diffuse infiltration of the skin without any specific skin lesions. Skin scrapings show a bacteriologic index of 6+ with an morphologic index ranging from 1% to 4%.

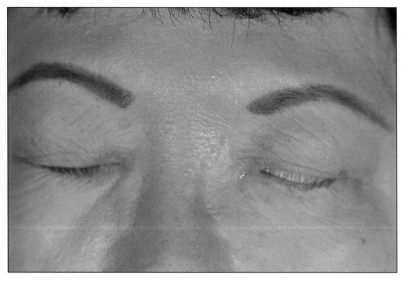

**FIGURE 9-42** Loss of eyebrows (madarosis) and lagophthalmos in lepromatous leprosy. What is seen on this patient are eyebrow pencil markings. The left eye does not close completely (lagophthalmos). Loss of eyebrows is primarily a finding in advanced lepromatous disease, but lagophthalmos can occur in association with any stage of Hansen's disease.

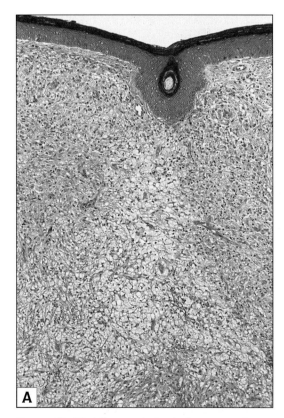

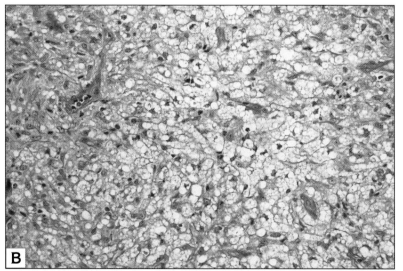

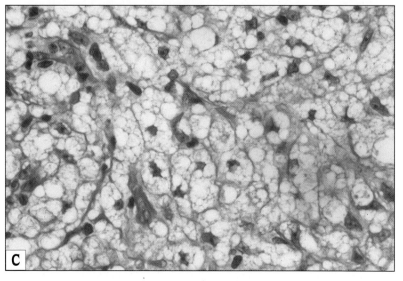

**FIGURE 9-43** Histopathologic features of lepromatous leprosy. **A,** Lepromatous lesions present with the picture of a completely anergic response to large numbers of acid-fast organisms. **B** and **C,** Little or no organization is apparent (*panel 43B*), and a small lymphocytic component is scattered randomly among the sheets of vacuolated macrophages in the dermis (*panel 43C*). (*All panels,* hematoxylin-eosin stain.)

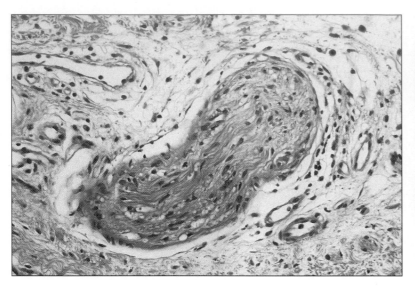

**FIGURE 9-44** Histologic section showing cutaneous nerve involvement in lepromatous leprosy. Cutaneous nerves may be extensively infiltrated by both *M. leprae* and mononuclear cells, but show little perineural thickening. (Hematoxylin-eosin stain.)

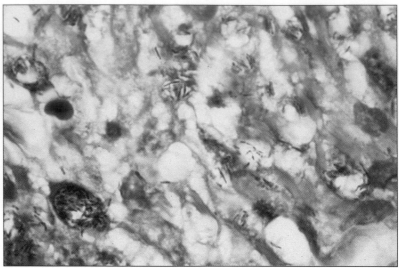

**FIGURE 9-45** Fite-stained section showing globi of acid-fast organisms in lepromatous leprosy. Acid-fast organisms are numerous within histiocytes and cutaneous nerves, and they may be clustered in microcolonies termed *globi*.

### Indications of nerve damage in leprosy

Nerve pain or tenderness
  Ulnar      Median
  Peroneal    Posterior tibial
  Facial
Loss of sensation or weakness in hand, foot, or eye

**FIGURE 9-46** Indications of nerve damage in leprosy. Leprosy is the leading cause of disabling neuropathy in the world. Therefore, when there is any indication of acute nerve damage, intervention with corticosteroids should be an emergency procedure. Involvement of the ulnar and median nerve can cause a clawed hand; the peroneal nerve, a footdrop; the posterior tibial nerve, clawed toes; facial nerve, various facial deformities. Neuropathy may be the first presentation of the disease, which can cause a diagnostic problem for the neurologist or family physician.

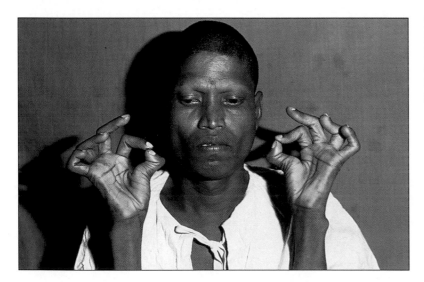

**FIGURE 9-47** Bilateral median and ulnar nerve paralysis. Although this patient was classified as having borderline lepromatous leprosy, the loss of eyebrows suggests lepromatous leprosy. In any event, treatment for borderline lepromatous and lepromatous leprosy is the same. In this case, these hands can be helped by surgery.

# TREATMENT OF LEPROSY

### A. Current US recommendations for treatment of leprosy: Paucibacillary disease

Dapsone 100 mg/day + rifampin 600 mg/day × 6 mos
*then*
Dapsone monotherapy × 3 yrs (indeterminate and tuberculoid) or 5 yrs (borderline tuberculoid)

### B. Current US recommendations for treatment of leprosy: Multibacillary disease

Dapsone 100 mg/day + rifampin 600 mg/day for 3 yrs
*then*
Dapsone monotherapy × 10 yrs (midborderline) or life (borderline lepromatous and lepromatous)
Clofazimine 50 mg/day × 3 yrs—add if mouse footpad study is not done or unsuccessful

**FIGURE 9-48** Current US recommendations for treatment of leprosy. The current US regimens have been used for many years with no evidence of relapse to date, but these regimens remain rather long, ranging from 3 to 5 years in paucibacillary leprosy to life for multibacillary disease (borderline lepromatous and lepromatous disease). **A**, Recommendations for paucibacillary leprosy. **B**, Recommendations for multibacillary leprosy.

### A. Multidrug treatment regimen recommendations by WHO: Paucibacillary disease

Rifampin 600 mg once monthly, supervised
*plus*
Dapsone 100 mg/day, unsupervised
Both given for 6 mos, then discontinued

WHO—World Health Organization.

### B. Multidrug treatment regimen recommendations by WHO: Multibacillary disease

Rifampin 600 mg once monthly, supervised
*plus*
Clofazimine 300 mg once monthly, supervised, and 50 mg/day, unsupervised
*plus*
Dapsone 100 mg/day, unsupervised
All medications continued for 2 yrs, then discontinued

WHO—World Health Organization.

**FIGURE 9-49** Multidrug treatment regimen recommendations for leprosy by the World Health Organization (WHO). The WHO introduced multidrug therapy in 1981 to counter the widespread occurrence of secondary dapsone resistance (in up to 19% of patients on dapsone monotherapy) and emerging instances of primary dapsone resistance in newly diagnosed untreated cases. Over a 9-year period of follow-up of multidrug regimens, the cumulative risk of relapse after stopping treatment was 1.09% for paucibacillary disease and 0.74% for multibacillary disease, which is much lower than the relapse rate after stopping any form of monotherapy. **A**, Recommendations for paucibacillary leprosy. **B**, Recommendations for multibacillary leprosy. (*Adapted from* WHO [5].)

### A. Investigational multidrug regimens in the United States: Paucibacillary disease

Dapsone 100 mg/day
*plus*
Rifampin 600 mg/day (or monthly)
Continue for 1 yr, then discontinue

**FIGURE 9-50** Investigational multidrug regimens in the United States. In the United States, certain short-term drug regimens containing rifampin are considered experimental for the treatment of leprosy, and their use remains investigational here. **A**, Recommendations for paucibacillary leprosy. (*continued*)

**B. Investigational multidrug regimens in the United States: Multibacillary disease**

**For proven dapsone-sensitive disease**
  Dapsone 100 mg/day
    *plus*
  Rifampin 600 mg/day

  Dapsone 100 mg/day
    *plus*
  Rifampin 600 mg/day
    *plus*
  Clofazimine 50 mg/day

The standard WHO multibacillary disease regimen

All medications given for 2 yrs, then discontinued

WHO—World Health Organization.

**FIGURE 9-50** (*continued*) **B.** Recommendations for multibacillary leprosy. The dapsone–rifampin regimen is used only in patients whose disease is shown to be fully sensitive to dapsone with a mouse footpad study. For all other cases, triple therapy with dapsone–rifampin–clofazimine is recommended. (Information about using these regimens can be obtained from the Clinical Branch, Gillis W. Long Hansen's Disease Center, Carville, LA.)

# REACTIONAL STATES

**Clinical features of reactional states in Hansen's disease**

| Type 1 (reversal reaction) | Type 2 (erythema nodosum leprosum) |
|---|---|
| Occurs in borderline tuberculoid, midborderline, and borderline lepromatous leprosy | Occurs in borderline lepromatous and lepromatous leprosy |
| Skin inflammation in existing lesions | New nodules in normal-appearing skin |
| Asymmetrical skin and nerve involvement | Diffuse skin and nerve involvement |
| Nerve pain may be acute and nerve damage rapid | Nerve pain chronic and nerve damage slow |

**FIGURE 9-51** Clinical features of reactional states in Hansen's disease. Type 1 (reversal) reactions can occur across the full spectrum of disease except technically at polar tuberculoid and polar lepromatous leprosy. Type 2 (erythema nodosum leprosum) reactions occur in borderline lepromatous and lepromatous disease only. Some experts call the Lucio phenomenon, which is rare and more severe, a third type of reaction. Any type of reaction can occur during and after treatment, and most are considered medical emergencies. Intervention with corticosteroids to reverse the reaction and prevent deformities is indicated. A fourth type of reaction, called *downgrading*, may occasionally occur in patients who have just started treatment or are not on effective therapy. This type of reaction is improved by antileprosy treatment, and corticosteroids may be utilized if a neuropathy is present.

**Precipitating factors in reactional status**

Physical or mental stress
Pregnancy
Surgical procedures
Injuries
Intercurrent infections
Antibacterial treatment

**FIGURE 9-52** Precipitating factors in reactional states. All patients should be counseled that reactions may occur, that their disease is not worsening during a reaction, and that prompt treatment can relieve symptoms and prevent deformity.

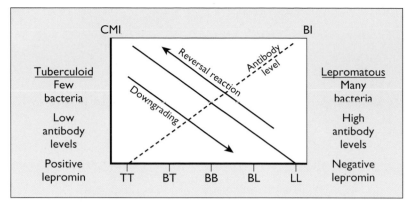

**FIGURE 9-53** Reactional states in the Hansen's disease spectrum. Immunity is high in tuberculoid (TT) and low or absent in lepromatous (LL) leprosy. LL has many bacteria, high antibody levels and a negative lepromin skin test as opposed to TT. The etiology, pathogenesis, and epidemiology of reactions are not fully understood [6]. (BB—midborderline; BI—bacteriologic index; BL—borderline lepromatous; BT—borderline tuberculoid; CMI—cell-mediated immunity.)

**Diagnosis of reaction**

New erythematous skin lesions
Painful or tender nerves
Pain and/or swelling of hands and feet
Acute febrile illness

**FIGURE 9-54** Diagnosis of reaction. Differentiation between reaction and reactivation of disease can be difficult clinically, and a skin biopsy may be helpful. All of the findings listed in the figure can occur in type 1 or type 2 reactions. The emergency treatment of reactional states is the same in either type—continue antileprotic medications and start corticosteroids.

# Type 1 (Reversal) Reactions

**Clinical features of reversal reactions**

May be present at time of diagnosis and usually occurs within first 6 months of treatment
Nerve damage may occur rapidly if neuritis is present
Reversal reaction with acute neuritis is a medical emergency

**FIGURE 9-55** Clinical features of type 1 (reversal) reaction. The patient must be informed that reactions can occur while under adequate treatment and that these are not an indication that their disease is worsening. Instead, their immunologic status is improving, which is the cause of the reaction.

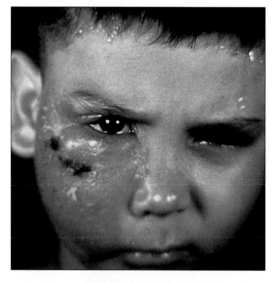

**FIGURE 9-56** Reversal reaction in borderline tuberculoid leprosy. After treatment this boy developed a type 1 reaction over a previous facial lesion and was left with a permanent partial paralysis.

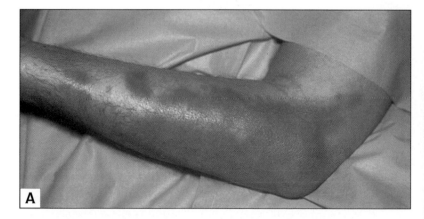

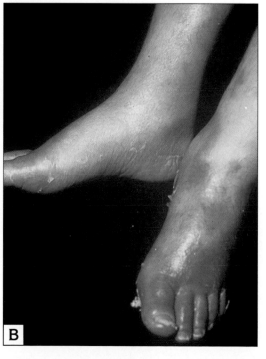

**FIGURE 9-57** Reversal reaction in borderline lepromatous leprosy. After 1 year of multidrug treatment, this patient developed a severe type 1 reaction with erythema and edema of previous lesions, onset of new lesions, edema of all extremities, and severe pain in his hands and feet. **A.** Erythematous lesions on the patient's arms. **B.** Edema and erythema in the patient's feet. Skin scrapings were 3+ to 4+, making him at great risk for neuropathy. However, he responded to treatment with prednisone without any sequelae.

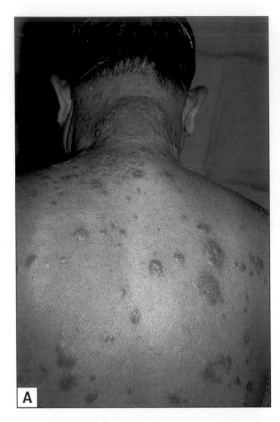

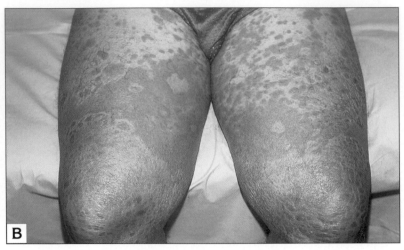

**FIGURE 9-58** Reversal reaction in borderline lepromatous leprosy. This man aged 62 years had a skin rash for years before the diagnosis of leprosy was made from a biopsy. After treatment with dapsone, rifampin, and clofazimine, he developed severe edema of his extremities and was diagnosed as being in congestive heart failure, but he also developed new erythematous lesions all over his body. He actually was having a type 1 reaction. He was treated with prednisone with good results but was left with loss of protective sensation in his feet. **A**, A large plaquelike lesion seen on the patient's posterior neck. **B**, Erythematous lesions on the legs.

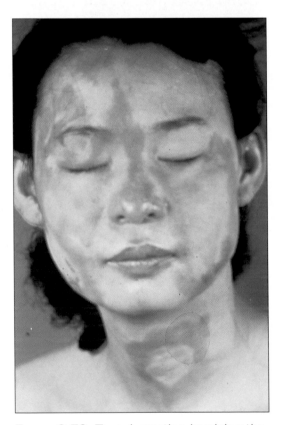

**FIGURE 9-59** Type 1 reaction involving the face in borderline leprosy.

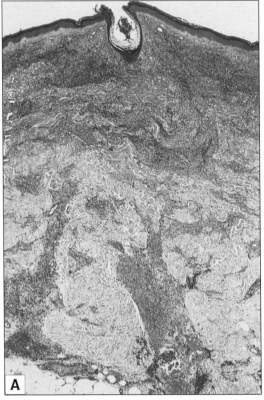

**FIGURE 9-60** Histopathologic features of type 1 reactions. Reversal reactions occur in patients in the borderline portions of the leprosy spectrum (borderline lepromatous–midborderline–borderline tuberculoid). The increased inflammation that is clinically characteristic of these lesions, however, is not matched by distinctive histologic features, and the diagnosis cannot be unequivocally confirmed histologically. **A**, Such nonspecific features as edema in the upper dermis may be seen, and an increase in lymphocytes or in the number of multinucleated giant cells may be demonstrable if a previous biopsy of the same or a similar lesion is available for comparison. (*continued*)

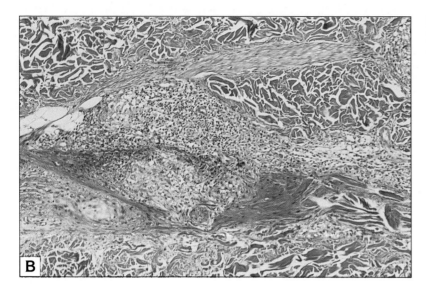

FIGURE **9-60** (*continued*) **B**, The biopsy appears to reveal an intensification of the inflammation within a cutaneous nerve. (*Both panels*, hematoxylin-eosin stain.)

| Treatment of type 1 reversal reactions | |
| --- | --- |
| **Mild** | **Severe** |
| Symptomatic treatment | Prednisone, 40–80 mg/day as single dose × 5–7 days, then taper to elimination over 2–6 mos |
| | Clofazimine, 300 mg/day × 6 wks, and then at reduced dose × 6–12 mos (in selected cases) |
| *Continue antibacterial treatment at full doses* | |

FIGURE **9-61** Treatment of type 1 reversal reactions. The dosage of prednisone may need to be higher than 40 to 60 mg in some severe cases to control reactions, particularly in patients taking rifampin. Rifampin, being a potent inducer of the hepatic P450 enzyme system, causes important drug interactions with other drugs, such as corticosteroids, and thus will decrease the effectiveness of prednisone. At times, the dosage of prednisone is increased to 100 to 120 mg/day, whereas rifampin is given only once monthly [7].

# Type 2 Reactions

| A. Erythema nodosum leprosum: Definition |
| --- |
| Immune complex disorder |
| Tumor necrosis factor levels increase during erythema nodosum leprosum |
| Neutrophil infiltration |
| Occurs in borderline lepromatous and lepromatous disease |

| B. Erythema nodosum leprosum: Clinical features |
| --- |
| Usually 1–3 years after beginning treatment |
| Involves skin, nerves, eyes, other organs |
| May present as febrile illness |
| Nerve damage usually slow |

FIGURE **9-62** Erythema nodosum leprosum, or type 2 reaction, is a systemic disease, and patients frequently are hospitalized in an intensive care unit with fever and ulcerating nodules for treatment of a septicemia before the correct diagnosis is made. After a single injection of a corticosteroid, dramatic improvement can be noted in the patient's condition in several hours. **A**, Definition. **B**, Clinical features.

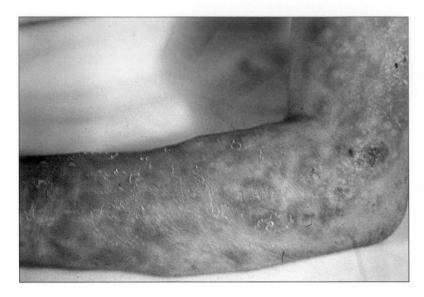

**FIGURE 9-63** Erythema nodosum leprosum lesions on the arm. This patient has erythematous nodules over most of his body, including his arms, where some have ulcerated. Erythema nodosum leprosum can present as severe systemic disease with high fever, malaise, and many nodules that ulcerate. It may be associated with hepatosplenomegaly, arthralgias, and generalized lymphadenopathy and can occur in borderline lepromatous and lepromatous leprosy before or after treatment.

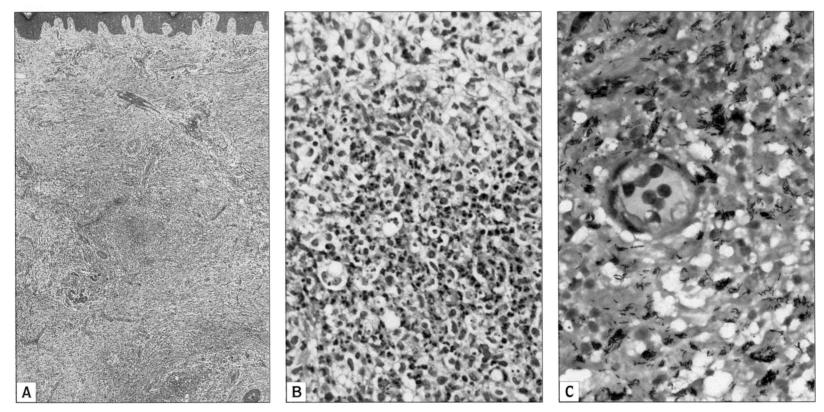

**FIGURE 9-64** Histopathologic features of type 2 reaction. Erythema nodosum leprosum (ENL) occurs in patients in the lepromatous portion of the leprosy spectrum (lepromatous–borderline lepromatous). **A**, ENL is characterized histologically by the presence of an acute inflammatory infiltrate superimposed on a chronic lepromatous background. **B** and **C**, Focal collections of neutrophils and eosinophils (*panel 64B*) are intermingled with vacuolated, heavily infected macrophages (*panel 64C*). Superficial ulceration may also be present. (*continued*)

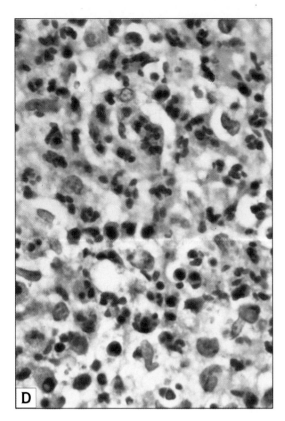

**FIGURE 9-64** (*continued*) **D**, Even a small focus of acute inflammation with polymorphonuclear leukocytes (PMNs) should arouse strong suspicion of ENL, because PMNs are not seen in nonreacting leprosy lesions. The acute inflammation characteristic of this reaction is very transient, however, and PMNs may not be found if the ENL lesion is more than 24 hours old when the biopsy is performed. Similarly, PMNs are seldom found if the patient has been treated with corticosteroids or thalidomide prior to biopsy. Thus, although histopathologic findings can confirm the clinical diagnosis of ENL, absence of the characteristic acute inflammatory infiltrate may be due to treatment or to the poor selection of the biopsy site and cannot be taken as proof of the absence of this reaction. (*Panels 64A, 64B, and 64D,* hematoxylin-eosin stain; *panel 64C,* Fite stain.)

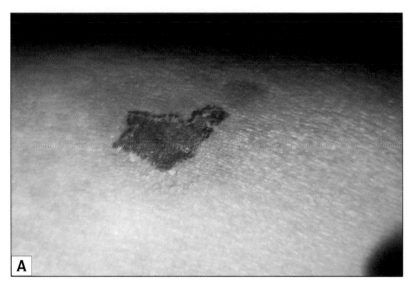

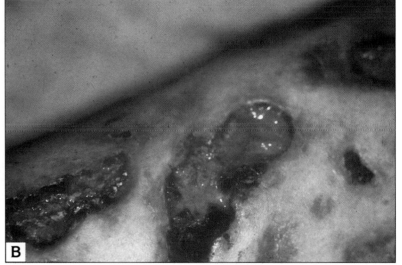

**FIGURE 9-65** Lucio's phenomenon. This rare type of reaction occurs in untreated lepromatous leprosy cases, usually in Mexico, where it was first described by Lucio and Alvarado in 1852. It presents as a diffuse skin infiltration of the entire body and is known as *lepra bonito*—the beautiful leprosy. **A**, This figure shows the very early lesion, a hemorrhagic infarct, which later ulcerates by a necrotizing vasculitis to form deep ulcerations with the appearance of third-degree burns. **B**, Several days later, the reaction has progressed, with deep ulcerations that can involve the entire skin despite treatment with corticosteroids. Standard therapy for Hansen's disease plus corticosteroids is the best treatment, but this patient died of a gram-negative septicemia secondary to severe immunosuppression with high doses of prednisone [8].

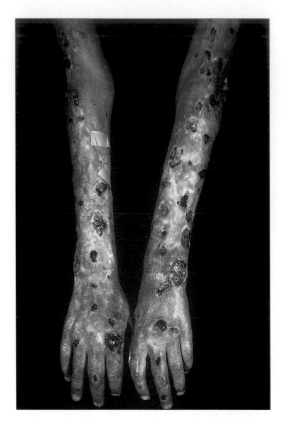

**Figure 9-66** Lucio phenomenon with extensive ulceration involving the arms. This uncommon form of reaction is probably related to erythema nodosum leprosum but is much more severe. The ulcerations are caused by a necrotizing vasculitis. The lesions can ultimately involve most of the skin and not infrequently result in death. Standard therapy for Hansen's disease plus corticosteroids is the best therapy now available but is not always effective. Otherwise, care is given as for a third-degree burn.

| Treatment of type 2 reaction | |
| --- | --- |
| **Mild** | **Severe** |
| Symptomatic treatment | Thalidomide 400 mg/day tapered to 100 mg/day |
| | Prednisone 40–80 mg/day |
| | Clofazimine 100–300 mg/day |
| *Continue antibacterial treatment at full dose* | |

**Figure 9-67** Treatment of type 2 reactions. Treatment with prednisone is effective in about 24 hours, thalidomide in 2 to 3 days, and clofazimine in 2 to 3 months. At present in the United States, thalidomide cannot be used in fertile women, except with hospitalization, monthly pregnancy tests, and an effective birth control method.

# COMPLICATIONS OF LEPROSY

| Association of HIV infection and leprosy |
| --- |
| Association of the two diseases |
|   Malawi—No |
|   Ethiopia—No |
|   Uganda—No |
|   Tanzania—Yes (relative risk 2.2 for multibacillary disease) |
| Use gloves for skin smears |

**Figure 9-68** Association of HIV infection and leprosy. In countries where leprosy and HIV infection are endemic, leprosy has not been found to be more common in patients with both diseases, except in one study in Tanzania that showed that the relative risk of developing multibacillary leprosy in a patient who was HIV positive was 2.2. A more recent study in Uganda showed no relationship between leprosy and HIV and recommended that dually infected patients be followed to better understand the immunology of leprosy. Universal precautions should be used when testing patients to prevent transmission of HIV, hepatitis B virus, and other blood-borne infections [9].

## Complications of leprosy due to bacterial invasion

1. Neurologic
   Sensory nerve loss ± enlarged and/or
      tender nerves
   Motor nerve loss with paralysis (ulnar,
      median, radial, peroneal, posterior
      tibial, facial) and deformities
2. Ear, nose, and throat
   Megalobule of ears
   Leonine facies
   Rhinitis with nasal septal perforation
      and nasal collapse
   Laryngitis with hoarseness
3. Bone and joint
   Loss of anterior nasal spine
   Destruction of alveolar process with
      loss of upper central incisors
   Tibial periostitis
   Primary lepromatous osteomyelitis
      with phalangeal involvement

4. Testes
   Destruction of Leydig cells leading to
      testicular atrophy and sterility
5. Eye
   Madarosis
   Punctate keratitis
   Pannus formation
   Corneal nodules
6. Connective tissue
   Dactylitis
   Tenosynovitis

**FIGURE 9-69** Complications of leprosy due to bacterial invasion. Most if not all complications due to invasion of the bacterium occur in borderline lepromatous and lepromatous leprosy. It is difficult to separate complications from reactions because they overlap most of the time. These complications can be prevented with early diagnosis and treatment, and most occur only in longstanding, untreated cases.

## Complications of Hansen's disease due to reactional states

1. Neurologic
   Sensory loss ± enlarged tender nerves
   Motor nerve loss with paralysis and deformities
2. Bone and joint
   Arthritis
   Arthralgia
   Acute tibial osteitis
   Absorption and fracture
3. Testes
   Acute orchitis

4. Eye
   Acute iridocyclitis
   Acute scleritis and episcleritis
   Lagophthalmos due to involvement of CN VII
   Corneal anesthesia with ulcerations due to CN V
   Glaucoma
   Cataract
   Blindness
5. Kidney
   Acute glomerulonephritis of all types (also
      involves liver, spleen, and adrenals)
   Secondary amyloidosis

CN—cranial nerve.

**FIGURE 9-70** Complications of Hansen's disease due to reaction.

**FIGURE 9-71** Complications causing hand and foot problems.

## Complications of leprosy causing hand and foot problems

1. Anesthesia
   Ulcers from trauma
   Burns
   Cuts
   Puncture wounds
   Blisters
   Acute cellulitis and osteomyelitis leading to amputation
   Absorption of bones
   Fractures without pain
2. Paralysis of muscles
   Clawing of fingers
   Clawing of toes
   Foot drop
   Various muscle imbalances producing deformities

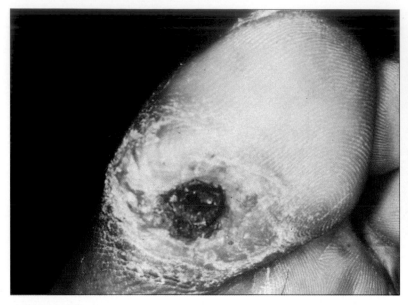

**FIGURE 9-72** Toe ulcer in an insensate foot. This patient who had lepromatous leprosy walked unknowingly with a rock in his shoe, which caused an ulcer in his insensate foot.

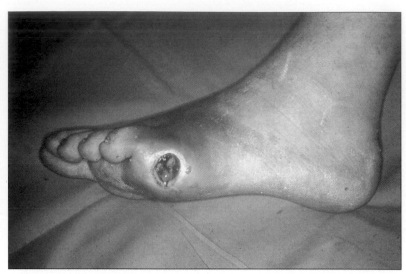

**FIGURE 9-73** Infected foot ulcer. Wearing a tight shoe on an insensate foot produced this ulcer. It was followed by an acute cellulitis, which, without proper immobilization of the foot and systemic antibiotics, would place this patient at great risk for osteomyelitis and possible amputation of part of the foot.

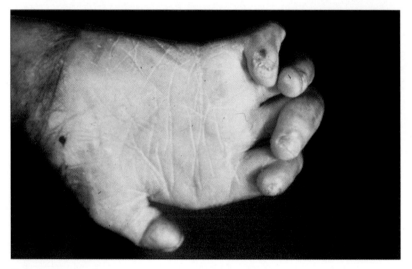

**FIGURE 9-74** Clawed hand in lepromatous leprosy. This clawed hand is a result of ulnar and median nerve paralysis and is also anesthetic. Reconstructive surgery can produce excellent cosmetic and good functional results.

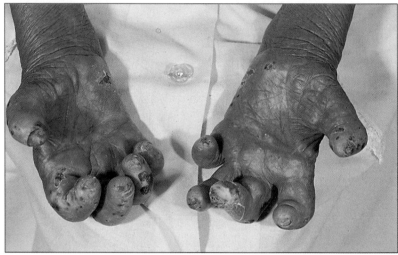

**FIGURE 9-75** Absorption and shortening of digits. In an insensate hand, repetitive stress and recurrent infections bring about gradual absorption of the bone, causing shortening of the fingers and resulting in a mitten hand.

**FIGURE 9-76** Lepromatous infiltration of ear. Complication can be prevented with early diagnosis and treatment of the disease and prompt treatment of reactions.

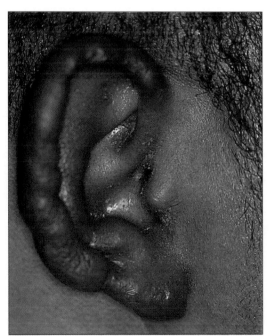

# PROSPECTS FOR ADVANCES

## Prospects for leprosy treatment and control

1. Newer multidrug short-term regimens
2. Clinical study of experimental drugs such as:
   Clarithromycin
   Minocycline
   Sparfloxacin
   Ofloxacin
   Fusidic acid
   Dihydrofolate reductase inhibitors
3. Vaccination studies
   BCG
   Other vaccines in trials (*eg*, heat-killed *M. leprae*/BCG)
4. Prophylaxis studies using BCG, dapsone, and rifampin
5. Diagnostic problems
   Studies of serum phenolic glycolipid–1 antibody levels
   Use of polymerase chain reaction in complicated cases
6. Radiorespirometric assays *in vitro* for screening of drugs for antileprosy activity
7. Continuous monitoring for multidrug resistance *M. leprae*
8. Continued leprosy research
9. Improved reaction therapy

BCG—bacille Calmette-Guérin.

**FIGURE 9-77** Prospects for leprosy treatment and control. Many short-term multidrug studies are now being conducted in various parts of the world. The bacille Calmette-Guérin vaccine seems to induce some protection against leprosy, but this effect varies between countries. Diagnostic studies using phenolic glycolipid–1 have been inconclusive, whereas polymerase chain reaction from biopsy specimens can detect small numbers of bacteria. With the World Health Organization's goal of eliminating leprosy as a public health problem by the year 2000, funding for research in leprosy may soon become inadequate. Corticosteroids and thalidomide are excellent drugs for control of reactions, but both have potentially severe side effects, necessitating the search for new agents [10–12].

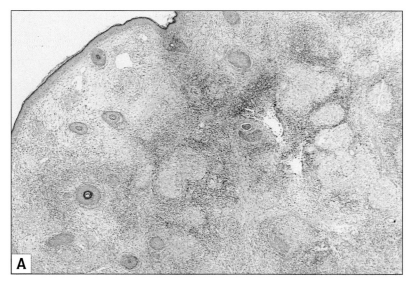

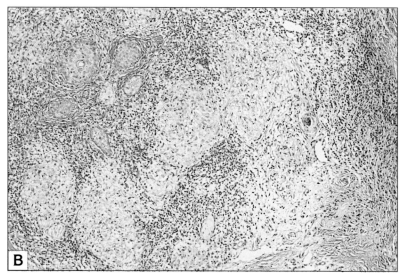

**FIGURE 9-78** Polymerase chain reaction (PCR) technique used for confirming diagnosis of leprosy in nonspecific cases. PCR can be used to identify *Mycobacterium leprae* in tissues using primers and probes for a 360-basepair fragment of an 18-kDa protein gene of the organism. The technique is most useful in determining the identity of the organisms when clinical and/or histopathologic features present inconsistencies. **A–C**, In one representative case, the clinical lesion had not responded to treatment, and although granulomas without identifiable organisms predominated in some parts of the lesion (*panels 78A and 78B*), other areas did contain moderate numbers of acid-fast bacilli (*panel 78C*). (*continued*)

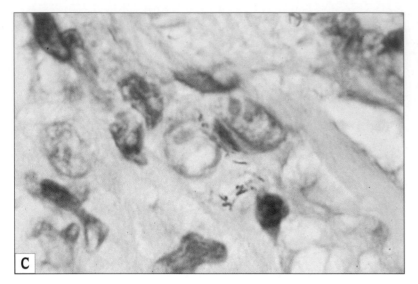

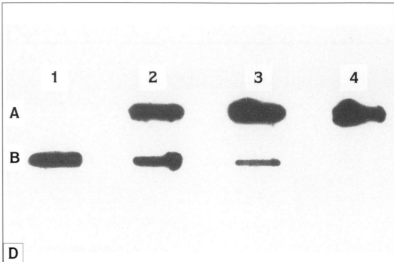

**FIGURE 9-78** (*continued*) **D**, Results of PCR amplification and slot-blot hybridization: negative control (*A1*), replicate tests of the biopsy sample showing positive bands for the *M. leprae* gene (*A2–4*), and positive controls (*B1–4*). Positive controls represent the PCR product from 330, 33, 3, and 0.3 bacilli, respectively. Although PCR theoretically can identify very rare organisms, in practice the results indicate that if *M. leprae* cannot be found by standard histologic examination in specimens highly suspect for leprosy, then only approximately 50% of these specimens will yield a positive PCR result [13]. (*Panels 78A and 78B*, hematoxylin-eosin stain; *panel 78C*, Fite stain.) (Panel 78D *courtesy of* T. Gillis, MD.)

# REFERENCES

1. Progress toward elimination of leprosy as a public health problem. *Wkly Epidemiol Rec* 1995, 25:177–182.

2. Nordeen SK: The epidemiology of leprosy. *In* Hastings RC (ed.): *Leprosy.* New York: Churchill Livingstone; 1985:29–45.

3. Ridley DS, Jopling WH: Classification of leprosy according to immunity—a five group system. *Int J Lepr* 1996, 34:255–273.

4. Guinto RS, *et al.*: *An Atlas of Leprosy*, rev. ed. Tokyo: Sasakawa Memorial Health Foundation; 1984:4.

5. Chemotherapy of leprosy: Report of a WHO study group. *WHO Tech Rep Ser* 1994, 847.

6. Scollard DM, Smith T, Bhoopat L, *et al.*: Epidemiological characteristics of leprosy reactions. *Int J Lepr* 1994, 62:559–567.

7. Bochering SM, Baciewics AM, Self TH: Update on rifampin drug interactions: II. *Arch Intern Med* 1992, 152:711–716.

8. Rea TH, Ridley DS: Lucio phenomenon: A comparative histologic study. *Int J Lepr* 1979, 47:161–166.

9. Kawuma HJS, Bwire R, Adatu-Engwam F: Leprosy and infection with the human immunodeficiency virus in Uganda: A case-control study. *Int J Lepr* 1992, 62:521–526.

10. Convit J, Sampan C, Zunigam M, *et al.*: Immunoprophylactic trial with combined *Mycobacterium leprae*/BCG vaccine against leprosy: Preliminary results. *Lancet* 1992, 339:446–450.

11. Smith PG: The Serodiagnosis of leprosy. *Lepr Rev* 1992, 63:97–100.

12. Brennan PJ: The microbiology of *Mycobacterium leprae* Pt II. Reflections on major developments and those responsible for them. *Int J Lepr* 1994, 62:594–598.

13. Williams DL, Gillis TP, Fiallo P, *et al.*: Detection of *Mycobacterium leprae* and the potential for monitoring antileprosy drug therapy directly from skin biopsies by PCR. *Mol Cell Probes* 1992, 6:401–410.

# SELECTED BIBLIOGRAPHY

Bryceson A, Pfaltzgraff RE: *Leprosy*, 3rd ed. London: Churchill Livingstone; 1990.

Clements BH: Leprosy. *In* Sanders CV, Nesbitt LT Jr (eds.): *The Skin and Infection.* Baltimore: Williams & Wilkins; 1995:147–156.

Hastings RE (ed.): *Leprosy*, 2nd ed. New York: Churchill Livingstone; 1994.

Jacobson RR: Leprosy. *In* Ropel RE (ed.): *Conn's Current Therapy*, 41st ed. Philadelphia: W.B. Saunders; 1995: 87–91.

Jamet P, Bo Boohong JI, Merchanx Chemotherapy Study Group: Relapse after long-term follow up of multibacillary patients treated by WHO multidrug regimen. *Int J Lepr* 1995, 63:195–201.

# CHAPTER 10

# Viral Hemorrhagic Fevers

C.J. Peters
S.R. Zaki
P.E. Rollin

# TAXONOMY

| Viruses associated with the hemorrhagic fever syndromes |
| --- |

| Arenaviridae | Bunyaviridae | Flaviviridae |
| --- | --- | --- |
| Junín | *Nairovirus* | Mosquito-borne |
| Machupo |   Crimean-Congo hemorrhagic fever |   Yellow fever |
| Guanarito | *Phlebovirus* |   Dengue viruses 1–4 |
| Sabiá |   Rift Valley fever | Tick-borne |
| Lassa | *Hantavirus* |   Kyasanur Forest disease |
| |   Hantaan, Puumala, Seoul, others |   Omsk hemorrhagic fever |
| |   Sin Nombre, Black Creek Canal, | **Filoviridae** |
| |     Bayou, others |   Marburg |
| | |   Ebola (four subtypes) |

**FIGURE 10-1** Viruses associated with the hemorrhagic fever syndromes. Several viruses, belonging to four different virus families, have been implicated as causing the hemorrhagic fever syndrome in a significant proportion of their human infections. The causative viruses are all RNA viruses with a lipid envelope and are all zoonotic. The oldest and best known is yellow fever virus, and the most recently discovered is a tick-borne flavivirus isolated in the Middle East in 1995; this latter virus is related to the virus causing Kyasanur Forest disease.

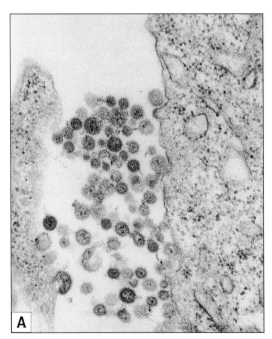

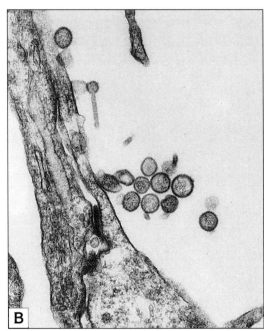

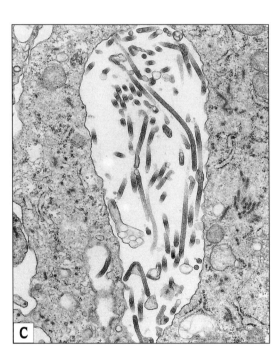

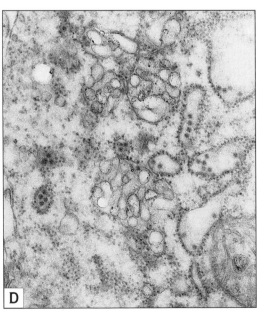

**FIGURE 10-2** Electron micrographs of viruses from the four families causing hemorrhagic fever syndrome. Each of the virus families differs in its genomic structure, replication strategy, and morphology. The characteristic ultrastructural morphology of representative family members is shown: **A**, Arenaviridae, Machupo virus. **B**, Bunyaviridae, Sin Nombre virus, the agent responsible for the 1993 Four-Corners outbreak in the southwestern United States. **C**, Filoviridae, Ebola virus isolate, from the 1995 Kikwit, Zaire, outbreak. **D**, Flaviviridae, yellow fever virus. (Panel 2A *courtesy of* S.G. Whitfield, MS; panels 2B–2D *courtesy of* C.S. Goldsmith, MS.)

## A. Epidemiologic features of the hemorrhagic fever viruses and their diseases: Arenaviridae

| Virus | Disease | Incubation, d | Geography | Vector/reservoir | Human infection |
|---|---|---|---|---|---|
| Junín | Argentine HF | 7–14 | Argentine pampas | Small field rodent, *Calomys musculinus* | Infects mostly agricultural workers<br>Aerosol transmission to humans |
| Machupo | Bolivian HF | 7–14 | Bolivia, Beni province | Small field rodent, *C. callosus* | Rural residents and farmers main target; rodent can invade towns to cause epidemics<br>Aerosol transmission to humans |
| Guanarito | Venezuelan HF | — | Venezuela, Portuguesa state | Chronic infection of field rodent *Zygodontomys brevicauda* | Occurs in newly developed area in Venezuela with small farms |
| Sabiá | ? | — | Rural area near Sao Paulo, Brazil (?) | Presumably chronic infection of unidentified rodents | Single infection observed in nature: little definitive information on potential |
| Lassa | Lassa fever | 5–16 | West Africa | Chronic infection of rodents of genus *Mastomys* | Reservoir rodent is common in Africa, and the disease is a major cause of severe febrile illness in West Africa<br>Spread to humans by aerosols and by capturing the rodent for consumption, as well as person-to-person transmission<br>Rare nosocomial spread<br>Lassa fever is most commonly exported HF |

HF—hemorrhagic fever.

## B. Epidemiologic features of the hemorrhagic fever viruses and their diseases: Bunyaviridae

| Virus | Disease | Incubation, d | Geography | Vector/reservoir | Human infection |
|---|---|---|---|---|---|
| Rift Valley fever | Rift Valley fever | 2–5 | Sub-Saharan Africa | Vertical infection of floodwater *Aedes* mosquitoes<br>Epidemics occur from horizontal transmission by many different mosquito species between domestic animals, especially sheep and cattle | Humans acquire by mosquito bite; contact with blood or offal of infected sheep, cattle, or goats; and aerosols generated from infected domestic animals<br>No interhuman transmission observed |
| Crimean-Congo HF | Crimean-Congo HF | 3–12 | Africa<br>Middle East<br>Balkans<br>Southern USSR<br>Western China | Tick–mammal–tick infection<br>Vertical infection in ticks<br>*Hyalomma* ticks may be the natural reservoir, but other genera may become infected and transmit | Tick bite; squashing ticks; and exposure to aerosols or fomites from slaughtered cattle and sheep (domestic animals do not show illness but may become infected when transported to market or held in pens for slaughter)<br>Many nosocomial epidemics observed |
| Hantaan, Puumala, Seoul, others | HFRS | 9–35 | Worldwide, depending on rodent reservoir | Horizontal infection in a single rodent genus or species typical of the virus | Aerosols from infected rodents<br>Some infections acquired from secondary aerosols or droplets from rodent excreta and secreta or from rodent bites<br>Interhuman transmission never documented |
| Sin Nombre, Black Creek Canal, Bayou, others | Hantavirus pulmonary syndrome | 7–30(?) | Americas | As for hantaviruses causing HFRS | As for hantaviruses causing HFRS |

HF—hemorrhagic fever; HFRS—hemorrhagic fever with renal syndrome.

**FIGURE 10-3** Epidemiologic features of the hemorrhagic fever viruses and their diseases. The different viruses cause similar disease syndromes with individual variations in epidemiology, pathogenesis, and some aspects of the clinical presentation. Infection is usually acquired from an arthropod or rodent vector, and thus most of the viruses are a risk in rural settings (with the exception of the Seoul or dengue viruses, which have urban vectors, or yellow fever virus, which may have urban and rural vectors). There is interhuman or nosocomial infection in several of the diseases. **A,** Arenaviridae. **B,** Bunyaviridae. (*continued*)

**C. Epidemiologic features of the hemorrhagic fever viruses and their diseases: Filoviridae and Flaviviridae**

| Virus | Disease | Incubation, d | Geography | Vector/reservoir | Human infection |
|---|---|---|---|---|---|
| **Filoviridae** | | | | | |
| Marburg Ebola (four subtypes) | Filovirus HF | 3–16 | Africa Philippines (?) | Unknown | Infection of index case occurs by unknown route; later spread among human or nonhuman primates by close contact with case<br>Aerosol transmission observed in some monkey infections |
| **Flaviviridae** | | | | | |
| Yellow fever | Yellow fever | 3–6 | Africa South America | Mosquito–monkey–mosquito maintenance, with occasional human infection<br>Formerly large epidemics among humans with *Aedes aegypti* as vector | Mosquito infection of unvaccinated humans entering forest and encountering infected sylvatic vector<br>Epidemics in African savannas by specific *Aedes* mosquito vectors<br>Most dangerous situation is interhuman transmission by *A. aegypti*<br>Fully developed cases are no longer viremic, and direct interhuman transmission not believed a problem; virus is highly infectious (including aerosols) in laboratory |
| Dengue viruses 1-4 | Dengue HF, dengue shock syndrome | 3–15 | Tropics and subtropics worldwide | Maintained by *A. aegypti*–human–*A. aegypti* transmission with frequent geographic transport of virus | Actually four different viruses with homotypic immunity but heterotypic priming for severe disease<br>Dengue HF is an uncommon complication of heterotypic infection |
| Kyasanur Forest disease | Kyasanur Forest disease | 3–8 | Limited area of Mysore state, India | Tick–vertebrate–tick | In rural areas, virus activity often signaled by monkey deaths |
| Omsk HF | Omsk HF | 3–8 | Western Siberia | Poorly understood cycle involving ticks, voles, muskrats, and possibly water-borne transmission | Muskrat trappers classically involved |
| Unnamed | ? | ? | Middle East (?) Africa (?) | Unknown; probably involves tick–domestic livestock–tick cycle, as in genetically related tick-borne flaviviruses | Transmitted by unknown route to humans working in livestock-related occupations |

HF—hemorrhagic fever.

**Figure 10-3** (*continued*) **C**, Filoviridae and Flaviviridae.

## Clinical characteristics of the hemorrhagic fever syndromes

| Disease | Duration* | Case:infection ratio | Case mortality | Characteristic features |
|---|---|---|---|---|
| **Arenaviridae** | | | | |
| South American HF (Junín, Machupo, Guanarito, Sabiá viruses) | 10–14 | Most (> 1/2) result in disease | 15%–30% | Typical cases have hypotension, shock, obvious bleeding, and neurologic symptoms, such as dysarthria and intention tremor. Some have virtually pure neurologic syndrome. |
| Lassa fever | 10–14 | Mild infections probably common | ~ 15% | Severe prostration and shock; not associated with such florid hemorrhagic or neurologic manifestations as in South American HF, except in severe cases. Less thrombocytopenia. Deafness in 20%. |
| **Bunyaviridae** | | | | |
| Rift Valley fever | 3–7 | ~ 1% | ~ 50% | Severe disease associated with bleeding, shock, anuria, icterus. Encephalitis and retinal vasculitis also occur, but without overlap with HF syndrome. |
| Crimean-Congo HF | 7–10 | 20%–100% | 15%–30% | Most severe bleeding and ecchymoses of all HFs. |
| Hemorrhagic fever with renal syndrome | 5–14 | > 3/4 Hantaan 1/20 Puumala | 5%–15% Hantaan < 1% Puumala | Febrile prodrome followed by shock and renal failure. Bleeding during febrile, shock, and renal failure. Puumala infections have similar course but much milder. |
| Hantavirus pulmonary syndrome | 5–10 | Very high | 40%–50% | Febrile prodrome followed by acute pulmonary edema and shock. |
| **Filoviridae** | | | | |
| Marburg or Ebola HF | 7–9 | Probably high | 25%–90% | Most severe of HF. Marked weight loss and prostration. Maculopapular rash common. Patients have had late sequelae (hepatitis, uveitis, orchitis) often with virus isolation from biopsy or aspiration. |
| **Flaviviridae** | | | | |
| Yellow fever | 7–10 | 80%–95% | 20% | Acute febrile period with defervescence accompanied in severe cases by jaundice, renal failure. |
| Dengue HF/dengue shock syndrome | 4–7 | 0.007% of nonimmune and 1% of heterologous immune | Probably < 1% | High fever for 3–5 days with shock lasting 1–2 days. Dengue shock syndrome is most dangerous manifestation of dengue and is due to acute vascular leak. Attack rates, mortality vary with epidemic virus strain and surveillance. |
| Kyasanur Forest disease/Omsk HF | 10–12 | Variable | 0.5%–9% | Typical biphasic disease with febrile or hemorrhagic period often followed by central nervous system involvement. Similar to tick-borne encephalitis except hemorrhagic manifestations not characteristic of first phase of tick-borne encephalitis. |

*Typical time to death or improvement in days.

HF—hemorrhagic fever.

**Figure 10-4** Clinical characteristics of the hemorrhagic fever syndromes. Viral hemorrhagic fever is characterized clinically by its disproportionate effect on the vascular system. Typical manifestations are related to a loss of vascular regulation (vasodilatation, hypotension), vascular damage (leakage of protein into the urine, edema in soft tissues of the face and other loose connective tissues, and petechial hemorrhage in the skin and internal organs), and a severe systemic derangement that presents as fever, myalgia, and asthenia but which proceeds to a state of prostration. Frank hemorrhage is common with most of the viruses (though not universal) and usually originates from mucosal surfaces. Patients with severe cases of hemorrhagic fever generally develop shock, diffuse bleeding, and central nervous system dysfunction.

# GEOGRAPHIC DISTRIBUTION AND EPIDEMIOLOGY

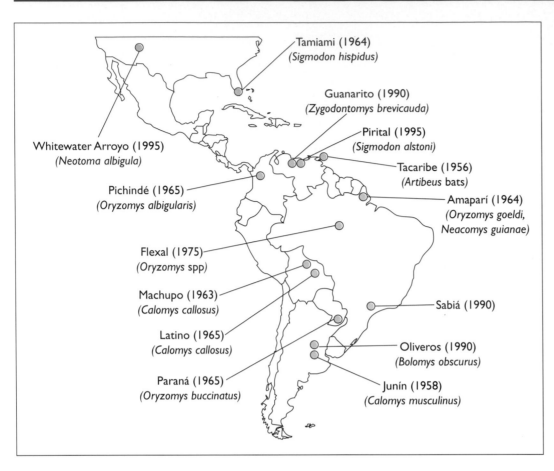

**FIGURE 10-5** Geographic distribution of arenaviruses in the Americas. The arenaviruses are widely distributed chronic infections of rodents that spread virus to humans, largely through aerosols of excreta and secreta. The best known arenavirus is lymphocytic choriomeningitis virus, from the common house mouse (*Mus musculus*); it is found in Europe, where the rodent originated, and elsewhere through the introduction of the reservoir rodent. In the Americas, the known distributions of arenaviruses causing hemorrhagic fever appear to be focal, and in virtually all cases, each arenavirus has had a single rodent host. The American or Tacaribe complex arenaviruses and their rodent reservoirs are shown on the map. Pathogenic arenaviruses (shown in *orange*) are found in Argentina (Junín virus), Bolivia (Machupo virus), Venezuela (Guanarito virus), and Brazil (Sabìa virus), with numerous arenaviruses of unknown significance for human disease found elsewhere in the Americas as well. (*Courtesy of* A. Sanchez, PhD.)

Tamiami (1964)
(*Sigmodon hispidus*)

Guanarito (1990)
(*Zygodontomys brevicauda*)

Pirital (1995)
(*Sigmodon alstoni*)

Whitewater Arroyo (1995)
(*Neotoma albigula*)

Tacaribe (1956)
(*Artibeus* bats)

Pichindé (1965)
(*Oryzomys albigularis*)

Amaparí (1964)
(*Oryzomys goeldi,
Neacomys guianae*)

Flexal (1975)
(*Oryzomys* spp)

Machupo (1963)
(*Calomys callosus*)

Sabiá (1990)

Latino (1965)
(*Calomys callosus*)

Oliveros (1990)
(*Bolomys obscurus*)

Paraná (1965)
(*Oryzomys buccinatus*)

Junín (1958)
(*Calomys musculinus*)

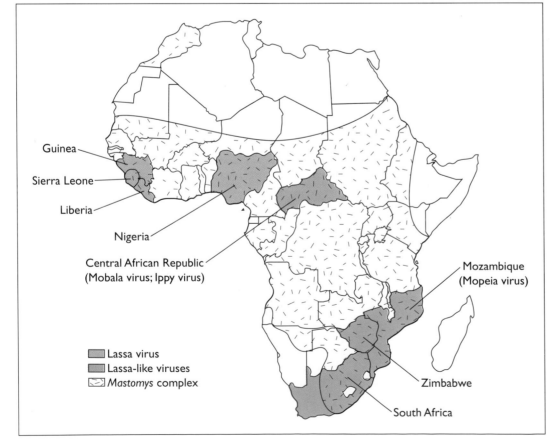

**FIGURE 10-6** Geographic distribution of arenaviruses in Africa. Lassa fever is a major infectious disease in the west African countries of Sierra Leone, Liberia, Nigeria, and probably Guinea, but it presumably also occurs elsewhere. The distribution of the potential reservoirs (rodents of the genus *Mastomys*) is extensive, but the genetic match between human pathogenic Lassa virus and the different rodent genotypes is unknown. Related African arenaviruses of *Mastomys* and other rodents are less well studied, may be less pathogenic for humans, and are found in several other countries. (*Courtesy of* A. Sanchez, PhD.)

Guinea

Sierra Leone

Liberia

Nigeria

Central African Republic
(Mobala virus; Ippy virus)

Mozambique
(Mopeia virus)

Zimbabwe

South Africa

Lassa virus
Lassa-like viruses
*Mastomys* complex

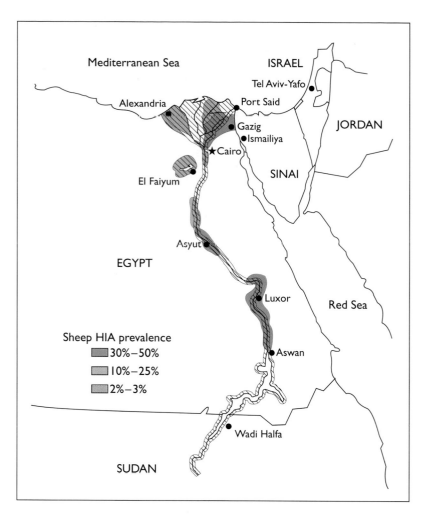

**FIGURE 10-7** Geographic distribution of Rift Valley fever in Egypt between 1977 and 1979. Rift Valley fever (RVF) virus, a bunyavirus of the genus *Phlebovirus*, was discovered in the 1930s during an epidemic in the Rift Valley in Kenya, but actually it is distributed throughout sub-Saharan Africa. The disease is endemic most years, but during times of heavy rainfall, RVF virus may be transmitted more intensively, and when herds of sheep and cattle are present, large epizootics may occur. The virus is not endemic in Egypt, but importation of the virus has caused epidemics during 1977 to 1979 and 1993 to 1995. RVF virus carries a potential for introduction into receptive areas with high mosquito populations and domestic livestock worldwide. This figure shows the extent of the 1977 to 1979 RVF epidemic in Egypt, as measured by the prevalence of antibodies in sheep, which is proportional to human seroprevalence. This figure emphasizes the importance of domestic animals as amplifiers of infection, surveillance tools, and targets for control of human disease through animal vaccination. An estimated 1 million human infections occurred after the introduction of the virus in 1977; 20,000 cases with 700 deaths were reported officially. (HIA—hemagglutination inhibitory antibody.)

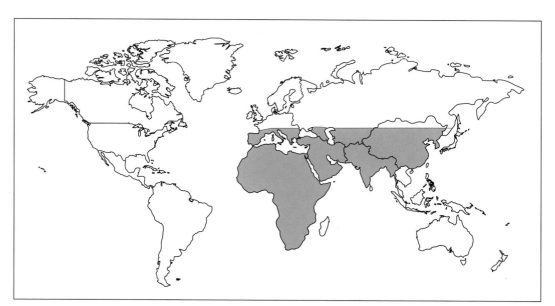

**FIGURE 10-8** World distribution of *Hyalomma* ticks, vectors of Crimean-Congo hemorrhagic fever. Crimean-Congo hemorrhagic fever virus is also a member of the family Bunyaviridae, genus *Nairovirus*. It is found over much of the range of the *Hyalomma* ticks. The disease, which is certainly underdiagnosed, has been particularly prominent in Africa, the Middle East, central Asia, and the Balkans. This map shows the distribution of the tick reservoir and therefore the maximum extent of the virus' natural range. Crimean-Congo hemorrhagic fever virus may spread outside this area by export of domestic animals bearing infected ticks. Humans may become infected by tick bite, crushing an infected tick, or exposure to the blood of viremic livestock. Acutely infected cattle and sheep do not become sick, in contrast to Rift Valley fever, but they have virus in the blood that poses a risk to slaughterhouse workers and others. (*Courtesy of* R. Swanepoel, DVM, PhD.)

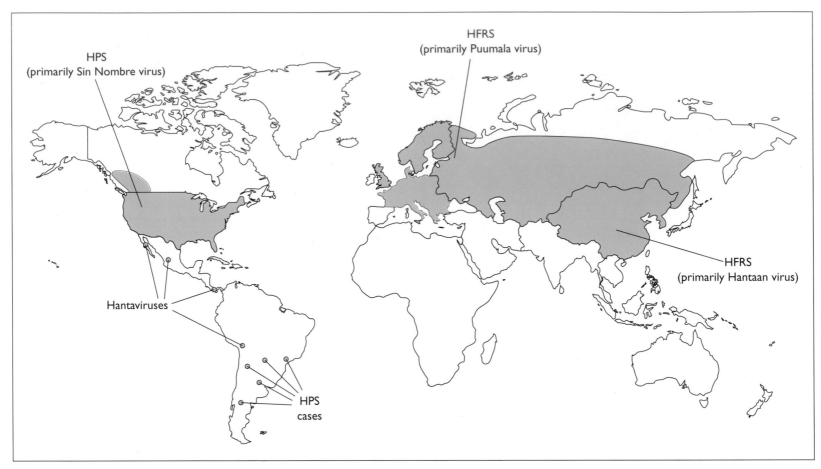

**FIGURE 10-9** World distribution of *Hantavirus*-induced hemorrhagic fever syndromes. Hantaviruses are the most important cause of hemorrhagic fever worldwide. This map shows the major distribution of hemorrhagic fever with renal syndrome (HFRS) and is based on a combination of rodent reservoir distribution and reported cases. The main virus responsible for HFRS in Asia is Hantaan virus, which chronically infects the striped field mouse (*Apodemus agrarius*). In Europe the major virus is Puumala virus, which causes milder disease and is associated with the bank vole, *Clethrionomys glareolus*. Both viruses, as well as Dobrava virus from *A. flavicollis* are active in the Balkans. Several other rodent species carry viruses implicated in hantavirus pulmonary syndrome (HPS), including Bayou and Black Creek Canal viruses in the southern United States. The rodents in the Americas (family Muridae, subfamily Sigmodontinae) that have been associated with viruses causing HPS as of 1996 are not found in Europe and Asia, suggesting that true HPS may be a New World disease. Seoul virus, a hantavirus not shown on this map, was first isolated in Seoul, Korea. It is carried by the common sewer rat, gray rat, or Norway rat (*Rattus norvegicus*) and has a wide distribution. Seoul virus has been implicated as a cause of HFRS in Asia and rarely in the Americas. (*Courtesy of* K. Wagoner, PhD.)

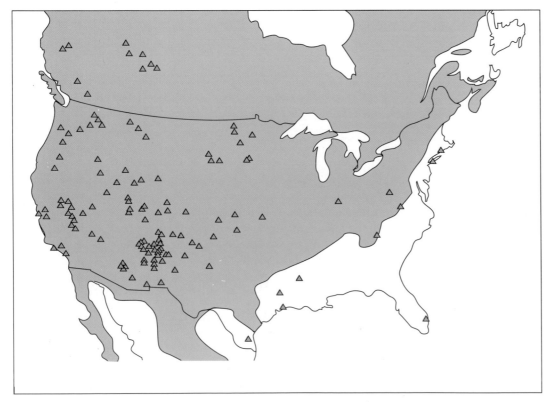

**FIGURE 10-10** Distribution of *Peromyscus maniculatus* and cases of hantavirus pulmonary syndrome (HPS) in North America, as of 1996. In the Americas, HPS is the major manifestation of infection with hantaviruses. Most HPS in North America is caused by Sin Nombre virus, which is carried by the deer mouse (*P. maniculatus*). The map compares the distribution of HPS cases (*orange triangles*) and the range of this mouse (*green shading*). HPS on the east coast outside the range of the deer mouse has been caused by a virus closely related to Sin Nombre virus that is carried by the white-footed mouse (*P. leucopus*). In the southeast, Bayou virus (rice rat, *Oryzomys palustris*) and Black Creek Canal virus (cotton rat, *Sigmodon hispidus*) have been implicated as causes of HPS.

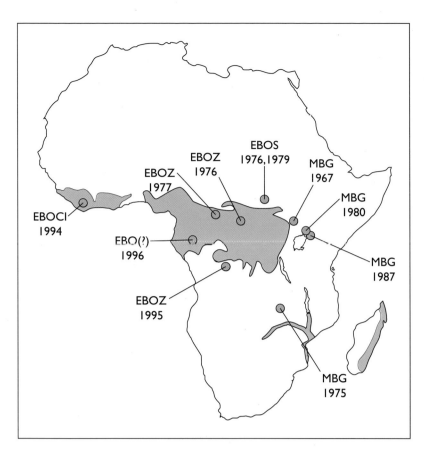

**FIGURE 10-11** Distribution of filovirus infection in Africa. The filoviruses are rare agents but pose a threat because of their unknown transmission cycle and high mortality rate when they do infect humans. Almost all filovirus infections have been in tropical or subtropical Africa. Ebola virus (EBO) appearances are distributed throughout central Africa, either within or adjacent to tropical forests. The four subtypes of Ebola virus, each of which is a distinct virus, are named for the geographic area in which they were first found (CI—Cote d'Ivoire; S—Sudan; Z—Zaire) and the date of the outbreak. The 1996 Gabon outbreak virus has not been characterized. There are two periods when outbreaks have been recognized, 1976 to 1979 and 1994 to 1996. In addition, a less pathogenic subtype (Ebola, Reston) has been found in monkeys imported from the Philippines. Marburg virus (MBG) has been recognized primarily around Mount Elgon in Kenya and Uganda, but one case did occur in a traveler in the savanna regions of Zimbabwe. For each index cases, the source of infection (a human or nonhuman primate) has never been ascertained, but the subsequent transmission is between humans in a setting of close contact or use of improperly sterilized needles and syringes. (*Green shading* indicates tropical rain forest.)

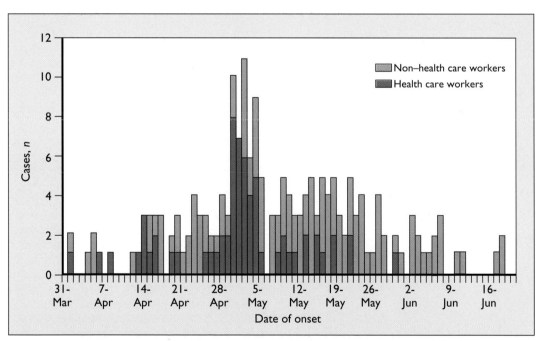

**FIGURE 10-12** Suspected Ebola hemorrhagic fever cases by occupation in Zaire in 1995. Filoviruses are readily transmissible to close contacts and have resulted in serious epidemics in Africa. Ebola outbreaks in 1976 and 1995 have each resulted in > 300 cases with a mortality of 77% to 90%. Underequipped hospitals lacking proper barrier nursing equipment and sterilization of needles and syringes have been important amplifiers of infection, although disease also occurs frequently in family contacts (16% in the 1995 Kikwit epidemic). This figure shows the progress of the 1995 Ebola epidemic in the town of Kikwit, Zaire. Total cases are shown in *yellow*, and cases among health care workers in *red*. Health care workers comprised 30% of the casualties, but transmission to medical staff virtually ceased when gowns, gloves, and respiratory protection were provided and coupled with proper training; this occurred in mid-May (see *arrow*), and only a single death in the staff occurred in late May.

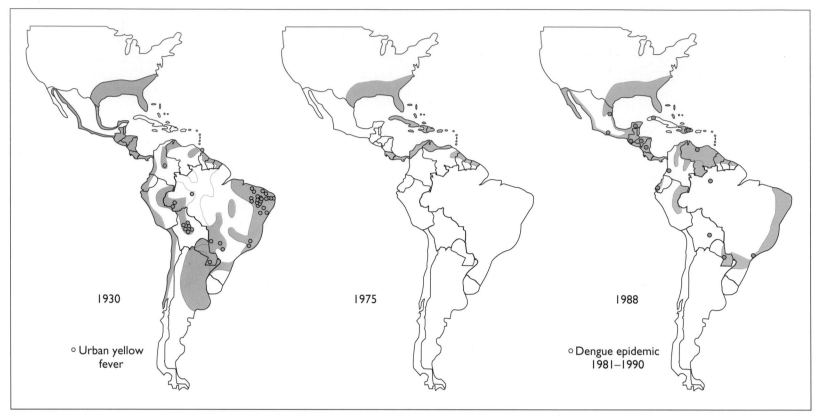

**FIGURE 10-13** Changing distribution of *Aedes aegypti* mosquito in the Americas between 1930 and 1988. Flaviviruses that cause hemorrhagic fever are either mosquito- or tick-borne. The agents associated with mosquitoes, yellow fever and dengue viruses, share an urban vector in the mosquito *A. aegypti*. This mosquito colonized the New World from Africa in post-Colombian times and was responsible for transmission of urban yellow fever in the Americas until its virtual eradication in the 1960s. This map shows the distribution of *A. aegypti* (*green areas*) in three time periods. In the *left panel*, historical locations of urban yellow fever epidemics are shown by *orange dots*. By 1975, the large scale eradication of *A. aegypti* was accomplished in cooperating nations through the intensive control of breeding sites and application of DDT. By 1988, there has been a reinvasion of the mosquito vector and the transmission of epidemic dengue viruses by *A. aegypti*. The high level of dengue virus circulation in South America, Mexico, and the Caribbean suggests that this mosquito could once again transmit yellow fever in the great and small cities of South America.

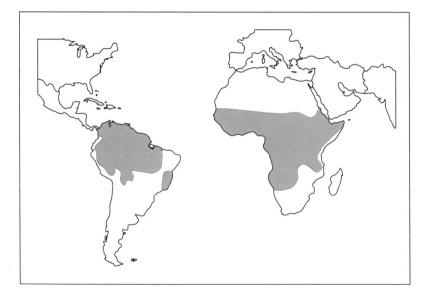

**FIGURE 10-14** Distribution of jungle yellow fever in South America and Africa. The yellow fever virus circulates primarily in forested areas in a cycle involving monkeys and mosquitoes other than *Aedes aegypti*. Note the overlap in South America between jungle yellow fever and the areas with extensive *A. aegypti* infestation (*see* Fig. 10-13); this overlap increases the likelihood that urban yellow fever transmitted by *A. aegypti* will occur in the near future. Urban yellow fever occurs in some towns and cities of Africa from time to time. Timely information on changes in disease distribution and yellow fever vaccine requirements can be obtained from Health Information for Travelers, Centers for Disease Control and Prevention, Atlanta, GA 30333 (fax 404-332-4565 requesting document no. 220022#; telephone 404-332-4559; or http://www.cdc.gov).

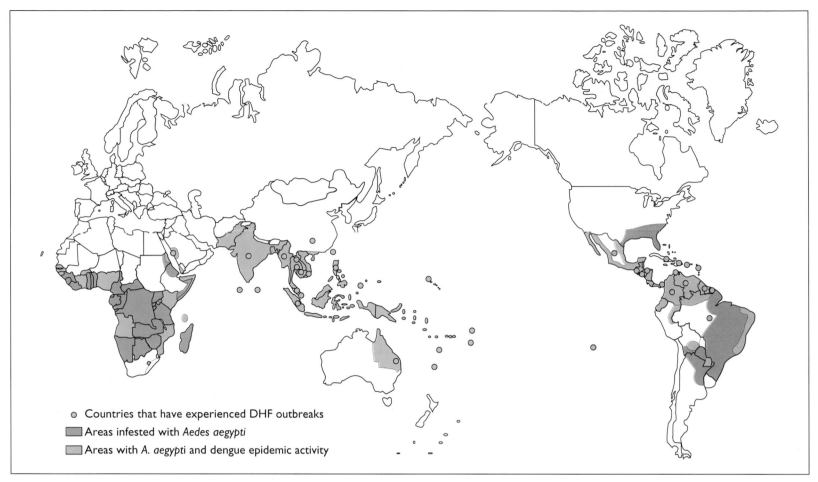

o Countries that have experienced DHF outbreaks

▨ Areas infested with *Aedes aegypti*

▨ Areas with *A. aegypti* and dengue epidemic activity

**FIGURE 10-15** Distribution of dengue in 1996. The high level of transmission of dengue viruses by large *Aedes aegypti* mosquito populations has resulted in the emergence of dengue hemorrhagic fever (DHF) in the Americas as well as in Asia. Dengue hemorrhagic fever occurs in most of the areas shown as epidemic for dengue. There are four distinct dengue viruses. They do not cross-protect, but rather infection with one of the viruses may provide the background to immunologically enhance infection after exposure to another dengue virus (*see* Fig. 10-52). The increase in regions where multiple dengue viruses are transmitted and the worldwide movement of dengue viruses have resulted in increasingly large areas of Asia, South America, and the Caribbean suffering with dengue hemorrhagic fever. It was first recognized in southeast Asia in the 1950s. (*Asterisks* indicate countries that have experienced dengue hemorrhagic fever outbreaks.) (*Courtesy of* Centers for Disease Control and Prevention.)

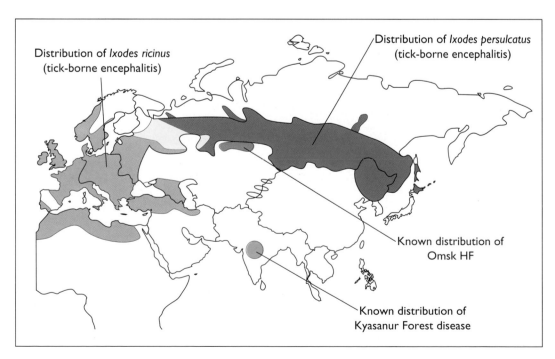

Distribution of *Ixodes ricinus*
(tick-borne encephalitis)

Distribution of *Ixodes persulcatus*
(tick-borne encephalitis)

Known distribution of
Omsk HF

Known distribution of
Kyasanur Forest disease

**FIGURE 10-16** Distribution of tick-borne flaviviruses in Eurasia. The tick-borne flaviviruses comprise a large group of viruses with a wide distribution. Tick-borne encephalitis occurs across Europe into Asia, corresponding to the distribution of *Ixodes ricinus* in the western areas and *I. persulcatus* in the eastern areas. The tick-borne hemorrhagic fever (HF) agents cause hemorrhagic disease sometimes followed by an encephalitic phase. They occur focally in specific areas of the world.

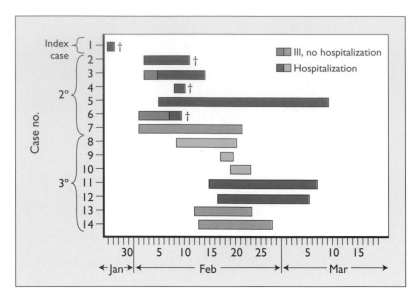

**FIGURE 10-17** Nosocomial transmission of Crimean-Congo hemorrhagic fever (HF) in Rawalpindi, Pakistan, in 1976. Nosocomial transmission of HF is not common, but dissemination in hospitals or among family members has been described occasionally for most HFs. Hantaviruses and the flaviviruses are regarded as posing no risk for medical personnel. Filoviruses occur rarely but they have been responsible for the largest hospital outbreaks (*eg*, Ebola, *see* Fig. 10-11), and their 25% to 90% mortality is dramatic. The commonest cause of nosocomial outbreaks is Crimean-Congo HF virus, which resulted in a hospital epidemic in Rawalpindi, Pakistan, in 1976. An infected shepherd was thought to have an intractable bleeding ulcer and underwent surgery, with disastrous results for the surgeon and operating room staff. As is usually the case, tertiary cases were fewer in number and milder. (*Daggers* indicate death.) (*Adapted from* Burney *et al.* [1].)

# VECTORS

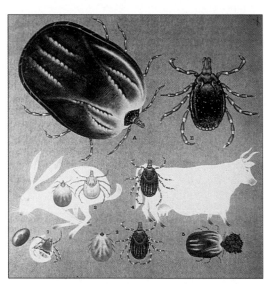

**FIGURE 10-18** Life cycle of *Hyalomma marginatum*, vector of Crimean-Congo hemorrhagic fever. Because these viruses all involve one or more intermediates in their transmission, the habits and dynamics of the vectors are important in understanding the risks of acquiring the diseases. For example, the tick species essential to the natural cycle of Crimean-Congo hemorrhagic fever virus belongs to the genus *Hyalomma* (*see also* Fig. 10-8). Humans are only occasionally attacked and may recognize the specific tick vector. One of the most important vectors is *Hyalomma marginatum* (*left*—female; *right*—male). After hatching (*1*), the tick feeds on small mammals such as hares in its immature stages (*2*, feeding; *3*, developing into nymph) and later prefers larger animals such as domestic livestock (*4*, feeding; *5*, oviposition). Ticks may be infected transovarially or from feeding on infected hosts; the virus survives the maturation of the tick through larval, nymphal, and adult stages. (*Courtesy of* the National Institute of Virology, Sandringham, South Africa.)

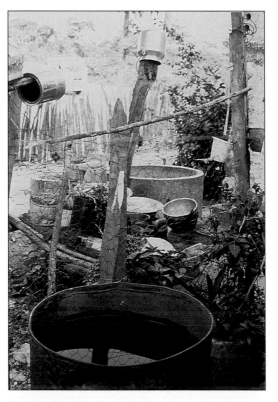

**FIGURE 10-19** Outdoor water containers providing breeding sites for mosquitoes. Vector control through elimination of breeding sites can sometimes be a practical objective. The pictured containers in a Caribbean backyard are excellent for breeding by *Aedes aegypti*, which will reproduce only in relatively clean, still water. At the turn of the century, William Gorgas acted to eliminate or cover these types of sites and thus rendered Havana and the Panama Canal zone free of yellow fever. Failure of community mobilization, appearance of insecticide resistance, difficulties in removing nonbiodegradable breeding sites (such as discarded tires), and the need for water jars in houses without piped water are all cited as obstacles to repeating Gorgas accomplishments, and so dengue and dengue hemorrhagic fever are worldwide problems in the tropics and subtropics today. (*Courtesy of* G. Clark, PhD.)

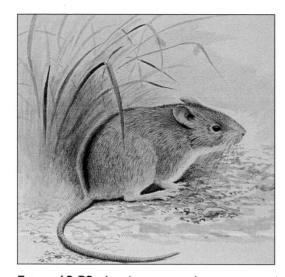

**FIGURE 10-20** *Apodemus agrarius* mouse, vector of Hantaan virus in Asia. A history of specific contact with rodents may be diagnostically significant with rodent-borne viruses, but it has low sensitivity and specificity in part because rodent reservoirs may be relatively common and the viruses are usually transmitted by aerosols. Knowledge of the presence and population density of the rodent is sufficient to suspect infection. This handsome creature is *A. agrarius*, the striped field mouse and vector of Hantaan virus over much of Asia and parts of Europe. (*From* Bjarvall and Ullstrom [2]; with permission.)

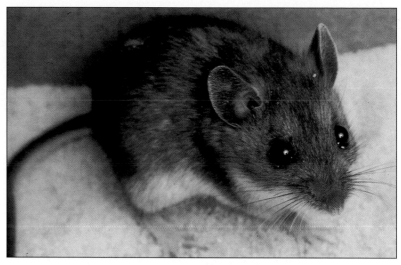

**FIGURE 10-21** The deer mouse, *Peromyscus maniculatus*, vector of Sin Nombre virus. Sin Nombre and its variants cause hantavirus pulmonary syndrome and are associated with the deer mouse (*P. maniculatus*) and the white-footed mouse (*P. leucopus*). The geographic range of the deer mouse is shown in Figure 10-10. (*Courtesy of* L. Lien Yang, MS.)

# CLINICAL SYNDROME OF HEMORRHAGIC FEVER

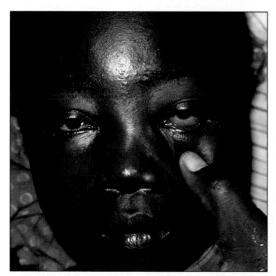

**FIGURE 10-22** Conjunctival suffusion in hemorrhagic fever. One of the early signs of abnormal vascular regulation is conjunctival suffusion, seen here in a patient with Lassa fever. This suffusion may be both bulbar and palpebral. Erythema of the oropharyngeal mucous membranes also may be noted. (*Courtesy of* M. Monson, MD.)

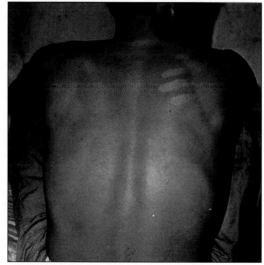

**FIGURE 10-23** Acute erythema with blanching in Bolivian hemorrhagic fever. There is often a diffuse erythematous suffusion over the face, anterior thorax (often on the upper part or V-area around the neck), and posterior thorax, which blanches to pressure. These cutaneous or mucous membrane signs usually do not appear in hantavirus pulmonary syndrome, perhaps reflecting the compartmentalization of the pathologic process within the thorax or a different spectrum of mediators. (*Courtesy of* K. Johnson, MD.)

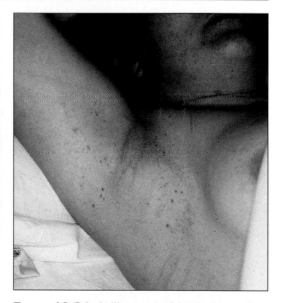

**FIGURE 10-24** Axillary petechiae in Argentine hemorrhagic fever. Infection with most of the hemorrhagic fever viruses leads to thrombocytopenia in addition to the underlying vascular lesions. The resulting petechiae are the most frequent sign of hemorrhagic manifestations, if they are carefully sought. The axilla is the commonest site for diagnostically significant petechiae. In Lassa fever, thrombocytopenia and petechiae are less severe, and bleeding manifestations are less common; functional platelet defects may be important. Patients with hantavirus pulmonary syndrome virtually always develop thrombocytopenia; severe cases may develop hemorrhage often associated with disseminated intravascular coagulation. (*Courtesy of* J. Maiztegui, MD.)

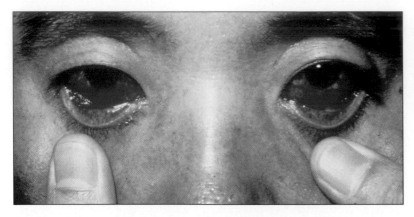

**FIGURE 10-25** Subconjunctival hemorrhage in hemorrhagic fever with renal syndrome. The presence of subconjunctival hemorrhages is common in all hemorrhagic fevers and has been emphasized in clinical descriptions of hemorrhagic fever with renal syndrome, as seen in this patient. (*Courtesy of* H.W. Lee, MD.)

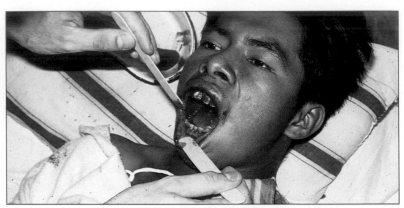

**FIGURE 10-26** Gingival hemorrhage in Bolivian hemorrhagic fever. Gingival hemorrhages occur commonly in hemorrhagic fever, as seen in this patient with Bolivian hemorrhagic fever. Severe hemorrhage is usually manifest by bleeding from mucosal surfaces (particularly the oropharynx, gastrointestinal tract, and female genital tract) or by ecchymoses. (*Courtesy of* K. Johnson, MD.)

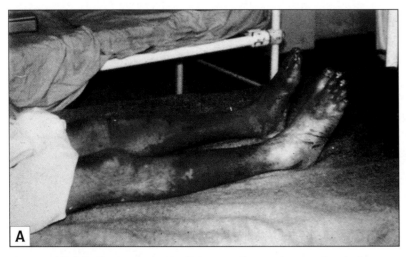

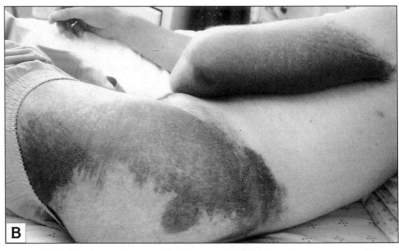

**FIGURE 10-27** Ecchymoses in Crimean-Congo hemorrhagic fever. **A** and **B**, Although there has never been a valid study to compare hemorrhages in Crimean-Congo hemorrhagic fever to those in other diseases, the hemorrhages and ecchymoses in it are often dramatic. (Panel 27A *courtesy of* D.I.H. Simpson, MD; panel 27B *courtesy of* R. Swanepoel, DVM, PhD.)

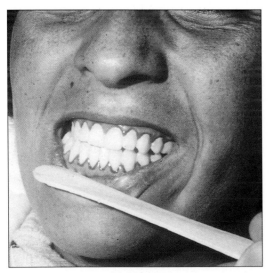

**FIGURE 10-28** Periodontal erythema in Argentine hemorrhagic fever. Pharyngitis and enanthems are commonly described but are not usually specific for any disease, with the exception of a periodontal dilatation of the vascular bed, which is believed to be indicative of Argentine hemorrhagic fever. (*Courtesy of* D. Enria, MD.)

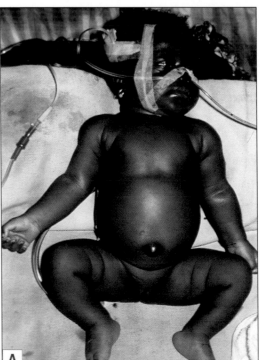

**FIGURE 10-29** Facial edema. **A**, In the more severe cases of hemorrhagic fever, vascular leakage leads to puffy eyes, cervical edema, and serous effusions, as seen in this child with Lassa fever. Such extensive and diffuse findings imply a poor prognosis. (*continued*)

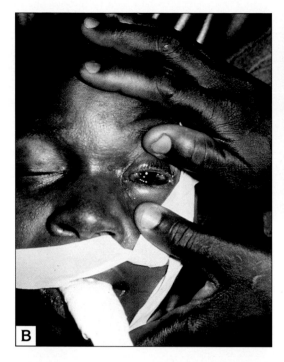

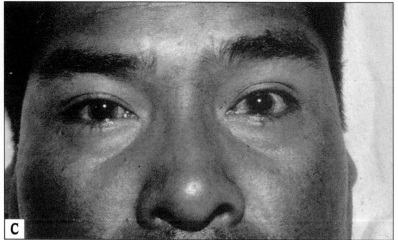

**FIGURE 10-29** (*continued*) **B,** Periorbital edema, chemosis, and subconjunctival hemorrhage are seen in another patient with Lassa fever. **C,** A man with Argentine hemorrhagic fever shows periorbital edema, flushing, and conjunctival injection. (Panels 29A and 29B *courtesy of* M. Monson, MD; panel 29C *courtesy of* H.W. Lee, MD; panel 29A *from* Monson *et al.* [3]; with permission.)

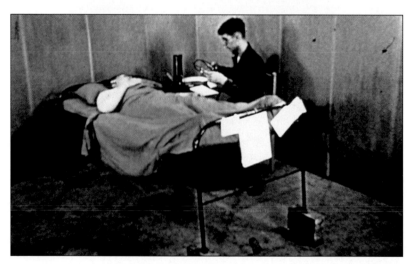

**FIGURE 10-30** Hypotension and shock in hemorrhagic fever with renal syndrome. Combating the hypotension and, in more severe cases, shock is difficult because of the presence of increased vascular permeability. Fluid infusions may be followed by pulmonary edema. In the cases in which hemodynamic measurements have been made, cardiac output has been decreased and systemic vascular resistance increased. As shown in this figure, during the Korean war, shock in hemorrhagic fever with renal syndrome (which typically lasts a few hours to 2 days) was managed by infusion of human serum albumin, use of the Trendelenburg position to permit reversal of the central volume, and administration of pressors. This figure is adapted from a US Army training film from the period.

# PATHOGENESIS OF SPECIFIC HEMORRHAGIC FEVERS

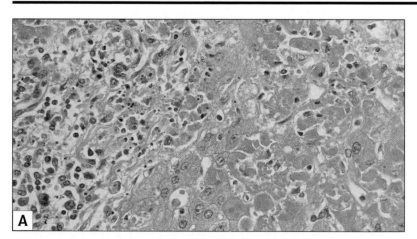

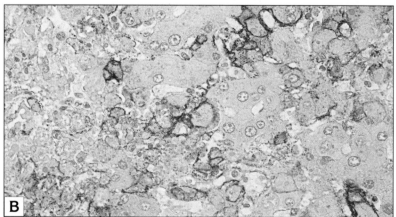

**FIGURE 10-31 A,** Hepatocellular necrosis as seen in fatal Lassa fever. There is no single histologic lesion that links the various hemorrhagic fevers, underscoring the difficulty in understanding the severe disease process on a purely light-microscopic basis. **B,** Using immunohistochemistry, abundant Lassa viral antigens (red) are observed in cytoplasm of sinusoidal macrophages of liver as well as within hepatocytes. Pathogenesis of arenaviral and other hemorrhagic fevers is thought to involve infection of the endothelium, macrophages, and other cells to varying degrees. There also is evidence for secretion of physiologically active mediators, including cytokines and lipid molecules. The degree to which actual viral damage of the infected cell, immunopathology, and other more subtle effects interact to produce disease is under study.

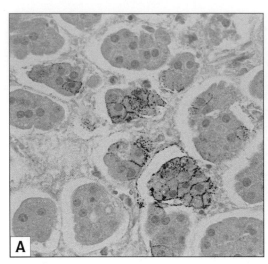
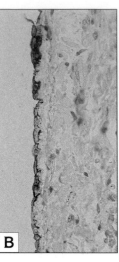

**Figure 10-32  A**, Photomicrograph showing viral antigens in morphologically unremarkable adrenocortical cells in a case of Lassa hemorrhagic fever. **B**, Photomicrograph showing immunohistochemical staining of viral antigens in serosal cells on surface of liver of a case of Bolivian hemorrhagic fever. Extensive infection of macrophages and mesothelial cells lining several serosal surfaces is characteristic of arenavirus infections and helps explain serous effusions seen in these patients. The arenavirus hemorrhagic fevers are notorious for causing more extensive infection than morphologic lesions would suggest. In some disease models, arenavirus-infected cells have a major functional deficit that is not detected by measurements of other cellular activities or by morphologic changes.

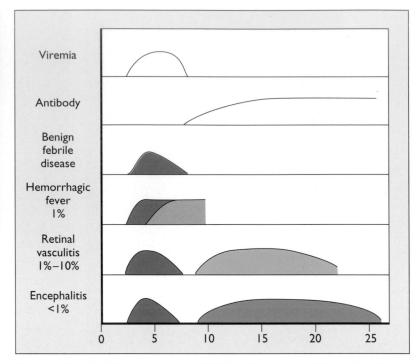

**Figure 10-33**  Clinical course of Rift Valley fever. Rift Valley fever is unusual in that most infected persons have only a self-limited febrile illness, but a small proportion develop hemorrhagic fever, viral encephalitis, or retinal vasculitis. Both the retinal vasculitis and encephalitis have their onset after viremia and acute illness have ceased. The encephalitis is a typical necrotizing viral lesion; the pathogenesis of the retinal lesion is not known. There is no known propensity for patients with one of these syndromes to develop another.

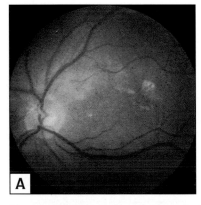
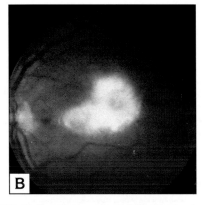

**Figure 10-34**  Retinal lesions in Rift Valley fever. **A** and **B**, Retinal lesions develop in 1% to 10% of patients with Rift Valley fever and are helpful in recognizing virus epidemics. These retinal photographs show the different characteristics, which consist of hemorrhage, infarct, and inflammation. The prognosis for recovery follows from the type of lesion encountered. Most described retinopathy is macular, but it is not known if this is because patients with macular lesions seek medical attention more commonly. (*Courtesy of* J. Meegan, PhD; panel 34B *from* Siam *et al.* [4]; with permission.)

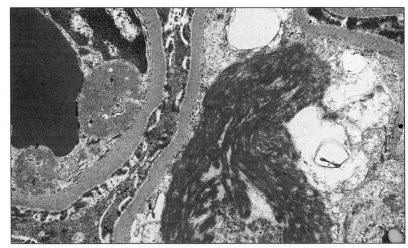

**Figure 10-35**  Electron micrograph of glomerulus with fibrin in Rift Valley fever. Nonhuman primates infected with Rift Valley fever virus develop a disease similar to human hemorrhagic fever, which has allowed some inferences as to the pathogenesis of the disease. Disseminated intravascular coagulation (DIC) occurs in rhesus monkeys, perhaps as a result of direct viral damage to the endothelium by this highly cytopathic virus. The renal glomerulus pictured here shows extensive fibrin deposition. DIC does not occur in all hemorrhagic fevers but is thought to play a role in Crimean-Congo hemorrhagic fever and perhaps filovirus infections. It occurs regularly in the early stages of Hantaan infection and may occur in severe cases of hantavirus pulmonary syndrome. It is doubtful if there is any significant participation in arenavirus or flavivirus infections. (*Courtesy of* J. White, PhD; *from* Peters *et al.* [5]; with permission.)

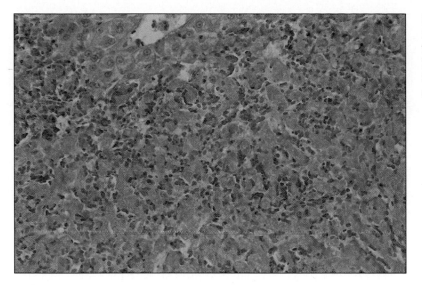

**FIGURE 10-36** Histologic section of liver showing midzonal necrosis in Rift Valley fever. Hemorrhagic fever from Rift Valley fever virus results in extensive midzonal liver necrosis. This distribution of hepatic lesions, illustrated here by tissue from a fatally infected rhesus monkey, is also found in yellow fever. (*Courtesy of* T. Slone, DVM.)

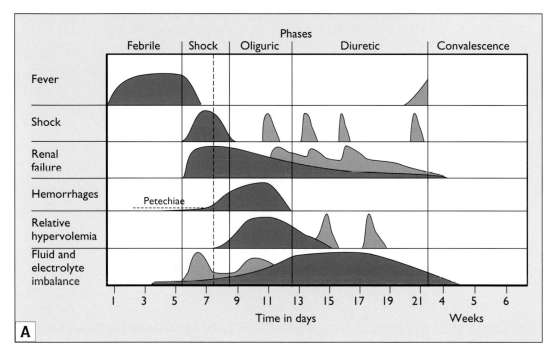

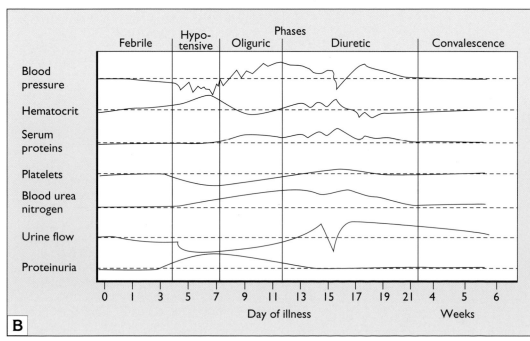

**FIGURE 10-37** Clinical and laboratory course in hemorrhagic fever with renal syndrome, based on the Korean War experience. **A** and **B**, The lesions in hemorrhagic fever are generally diffuse, and no one organ is singled out by the process. Hemorrhagic fever with renal syndrome (HFRS) is an exception because the systemic findings are accompanied by impressive damage to three target organs. The disease unrolls in a series of events that begins with fever, followed by shock, and culminating with renal failure. Recovery is marked by heavy diuresis and an inability to concentrate urine that may persist for weeks. These figures describe the course of events in moderate or severe HFRS caused by a virus such as Hantaan virus, which was responsible for HFRS during the Korean war. Milder cases of Hantaan infection and many cases of HFRS due to one of the other serotypes that cause less severe disease may skip one or more of the stages. In such a situation, the renal failure may be ascribed to transient hypotension, antibiotics administered during the febrile stage, or otherwise misdiagnosed. (*Adapted from* Sheedy *et al.* [6].)

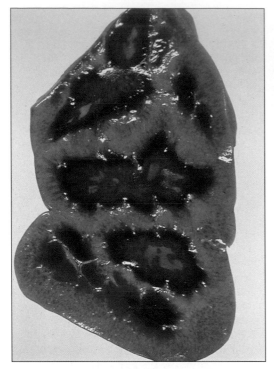

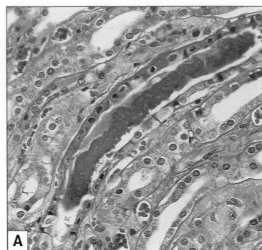

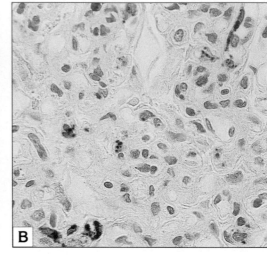

**FIGURE 10-39** Renal histopathologic changes in a patient with hemorrhagic fever with renal syndrome. **A**, This figure shows interstitial edema and tubular lesions, including dilatation, degeneration, and sloughing of tubular epithelium. **B**, Immunohistochemical stain reveals the presence of Hantaan antigen in endothelial cells of this glomerulus.

**FIGURE 10-38** Gross autopsy view of kidney in hemorrhagic fever with renal syndrome. The renal medulla is the site of hemorrhage and congestion. The renal involvement can be detected by magnetic resonance imaging, computed tomography scan, and radioisotope renography. (*Courtesy of* J.S. Lee, MD.)

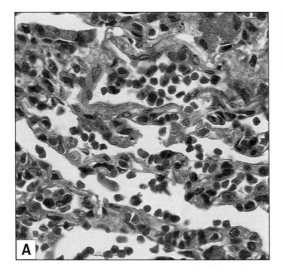

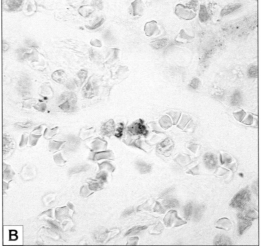

**FIGURE 10-40** Interstitial pneumonitis in a fatal case of hemorrhagic fever with renal syndrome (HFRS). **A**, Histologic features somewhat similar to those seen in hantavirus pulmonary syndrome (HPS) can be seen in lungs of severe cases of HFRS. **B**, However, immunohistochemical staining for hantaviral antigens shows only focal staining of pulmonary endothelial cells and macrophages. Compare the pattern and distribution to that seen in HPS in Figure 10-45.

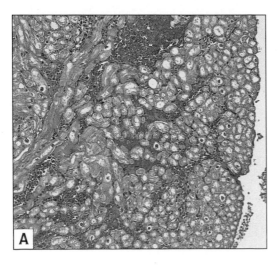

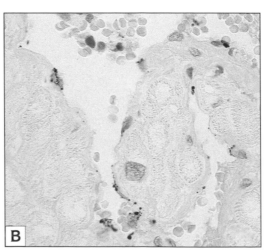

**FIGURE 10-41** Right atrial lesion of hemorrhagic fever with renal syndrome (HFRS). Three gross lesions are characteristic of HFRS: 1) medullary hemorrhage of the kidney (Fig. 10-38), 2) anterior pituitary necrosis (not shown), and 3) hemorrhage of the right atrium of the heart (shown here). Hemodynamic measurements have shown functional changes in association with these findings. **A** and **B**, Congestion and hemorrhage (*panel 41A*) are seen in juxtaposition to Hantaan virus antigens in endothelial cells lining the endocardium (*panel 41B*).

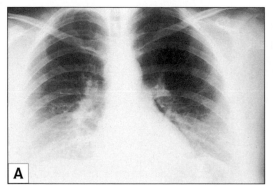
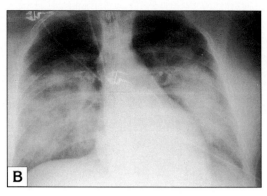

onset follows a febrile prodrome of 1 to 10 days' duration (typically 3–5 days). The chest radiograph occasionally may be normal very early in the pulmonary phase of HPS, but it soon progresses to the more typical pattern of bilateral interstitial or alveolar pulmonary edema. The findings differ from those of adult respiratory distress syndrome in that indications of interstitial edema (Kerley B lines, peribronchial cuffing) are more common and the distribution is more central. These radiographs represent typical films in an HPS patient on presentation (*panel 42A*) and 3 days later (*panel 42B*). (*Courtesy of L. Ketai, MD.*)

**FIGURE 10-42** Chest radiographs showing progression of pulmonary edema in hantavirus pulmonary syndrome (HPS). **A** and **B**, In HPS, the lung is the target organ, with a distinctive bilateral pulmonary edema due to increased vascular permeability. The abrupt

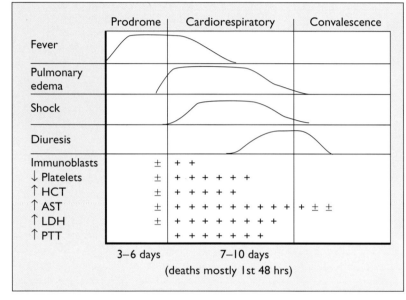

**FIGURE 10-43** Clinical course of hantavirus pulmonary syndrome (HPS). The course of HPS differs from that for hemorrhagic fever with renal syndrome, seen in Figure 10-38. Both show a febrile prodrome that leads to hypotension and end-organ failure. In both diseases, the onset of the immune response precedes severe organ failure, which is thought to be immunopathologic in nature. In the case of HPS, the hypotension does not result in shock until the onset of respiratory failure, but this may reflect the severe physiologic impact of the lung edema. (AST—aspartate aminotransferase; HCT—hematocrit; LDH—lactate dehydrogenase; PTT—partial thromboplastin time.)

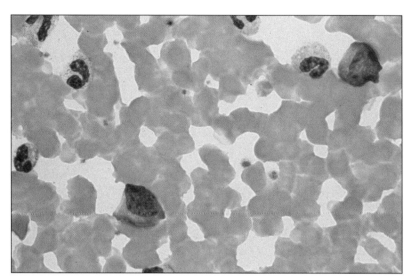

**FIGURE 10-44** Atypical lymphocytes in hantavirus pulmonary syndrome (HPS). In HPS and hemorrhagic fever with renal syndrome, the atypical lymphocytes are predominantly CD8+, DR+ immunoblasts. Other peripheral blood features of diagnostic importance in HPS are 1) thrombocytopenia, which is almost always present and is an early and useful diagnostic finding; 2) hemoconcentration, which reflects the increased permeability of the pulmonary capillaries to protein; 3) normal or elevated total leukocyte count; and 4) left shift.

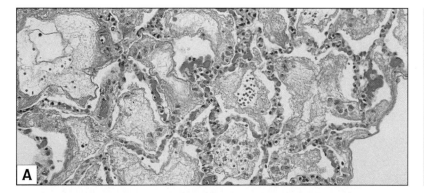
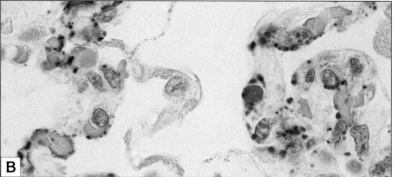

**FIGURE 10-45** Microscopic features of hantavirus pulmonary syndrome. **A**, Interstitial pneumonitis and interalveolar edema. **B**, Immunohistochemical stain showing hantaviral antigens predominantly within endothelial cells of the pulmonary microvasculature. The acute pulmonary edema of hantavirus pulmonary syndrome correlates with the abundant hantaviral antigen selectively found in pulmonary capillary endothelium as well as the presence of CD4+ and CD8+ lymphoblasts and activated macrophages. Protein-rich fluid floods into the interstitium and alveoli, without any morphologic lesion in the blood-gas barrier at the light-microscopic level. The pathogenesis differs from that of the neutrophil-mediated lesion of classic adult respiratory distress syndrome, just as the hantavirus pulmonary syndrome differs in its detailed clinical, pathologic, and radiologic picture.

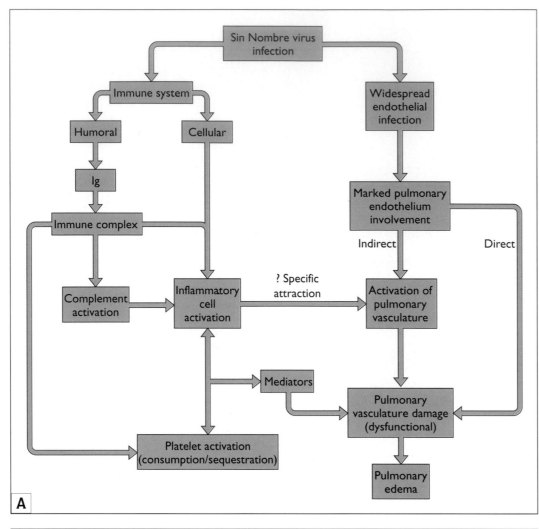

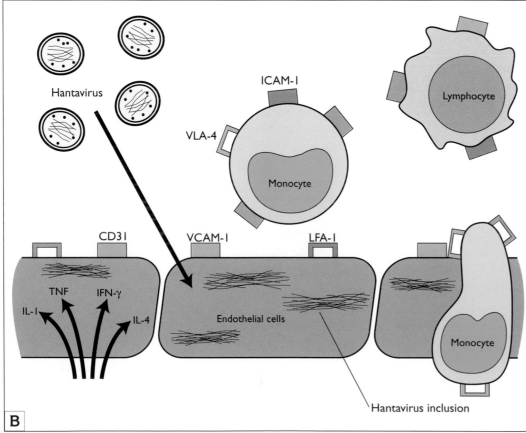

**FIGURE 10-46** Hypothesized pathogenesis of hantavirus pulmonary syndrome (HPS). Pulmonary edema and functional derangement of vascular endothelium are central in the pathogenesis of HPS. **A**, Some possible mechanisms by which immunologic and pharmacologic mediators of inflammation may interact to induce the shock syndrome in HPS. **B**, Preliminary data suggest that the mechanism of inflammatory cell recruitment of the lungs of HPS patients is consistent with specific attraction and adherence of a selective population of inflammatory cells to a specialized activated endothelium [8]. (ICAM—intercellular adhesion molecule; IFN-γ—interferon-γ; IL—interleukin; LFA-1—leukocyte function–associated antigen 1; TNF—tumor necrosis factor; VCAM-1—vascular cellular adhesion molecule; VLA-4—very late antigen-4.) (Panel 46A *adapted from* Zaki *et al.* [7]; panel 46B *courtesy of* N. Zaki.)

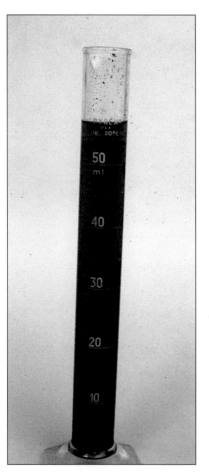

**FIGURE 10-47** Viral antigens in lung tissue in a fatal case of viral hemorrhagic fever. The finding of viral antigens in capillary endothelia is not a unique feature of hantavirus pulmonary syndrome (HPS) and can be seen in a number of viral hemorrhagic fevers. In this figure, Ebola virus antigens are seen in infected endothelium, but, in contrast to HPS, they also can be seen in macrophages, fibroblasts, and other parenchymal cells of this lung section. In such cases, the organ dysfunction and the vasculopathy appear to be a consequence of a direct cytolytic injury and the elaboration of soluble mediators of inflammation.

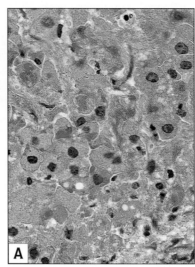
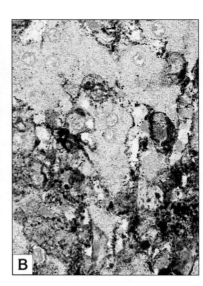

**FIGURE 10-48** Photomicrograph demonstrating Ebola virus in liver. **A**, Hepatocellular necrosis and typical intracytoplasmic viral inclusions are seen in liver of a patient with Ebola virus hemorrhagic fever. At the electron microscope level, inclusions are seen to consist of viral nucleocapsids (not shown). **B**, The staining of inclusions and massive load in hepatocytes, Kuppfer cells, and sinusoidal lining cells is illustrated in an immunohistochemical preparation.

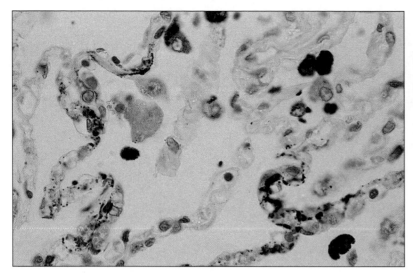

**FIGURE 10-49** Black vomit in yellow fever. The classic hemorrhagic fever is yellow fever, and one of the most characteristic clinical manifestations is the occurrence of black vomit, which was mistakenly regarded in the early literature as having some degree of specificity for the disease. As quoted by Ashbel Smith in his account of the yellow fever epidemic in Galveston, Texas, in 1839: "But the efforts of the citizens even then were paralyzed, by the absurd denial of a few who feared their pecuniary interests would be damaged by a knowledge of the existence of yellow fever among us, aided by the *gross ignorance* of others, who in their pointless hostility to the name of yellow fever, declared the recent Epidemic to be the Plague— They were, however, most signally rebuked by the disease stamping almost every fatal case with its *unequivocal seal* of *black vomit*" (author's italics) [8]. (*Courtesy of* J.W. LeDuc, PhD, and F. Pinheiro, MD.)

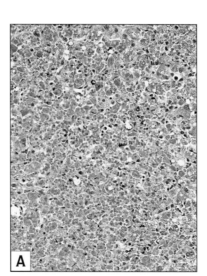
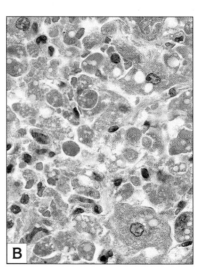

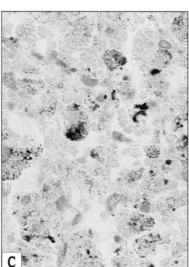

**FIGURE 10-50** Liver histology in a case of yellow fever. **A**, Yellow fever virus infection of the liver results in a characteristic acidophilic midzonal necrosis. **B**, However, this pattern and the acidophilic hepatocytes (Councilman-like body) can be seen in a number of other viral hemorrhagic fevers (HFs). **C**, Immunohistochemical staining is helpful in confirming the diagnosis and demonstrates infection of both hepatocytes and Kuppfer cells. The initial infection in experimental yellow fever is in the Kuppfer cell, but later hepatocytes become involved. The distribution, like that of Rift Valley fever, is midzonal. Extensive liver damage is a feature of most but not all fatal yellow fever cases. Other HFs may also have sufficient liver involvement for jaundice to appear, particularly Rift Valley fever, Crimean-Congo HF, and the filoviruses.

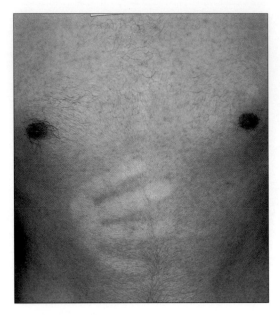

**FIGURE 10-51** Maculopapular rash of dengue. Dengue viruses have been implicated as causing hemorrhagic fever either as primary infections or, more commonly, when sequential infections with different dengue viruses occur in highly endemic areas. Dengue virus infection often produces a characteristic macular rash during the first day or two of fever and may also be accompanied by a maculopapular rash occurring around day 5 of disease. The latter rash corresponds to the time of defervescence or remission and may be present in dengue hemorrhagic fever patients in addition to a petechial rash. (*Courtesy of* C. Hoch, MD.)

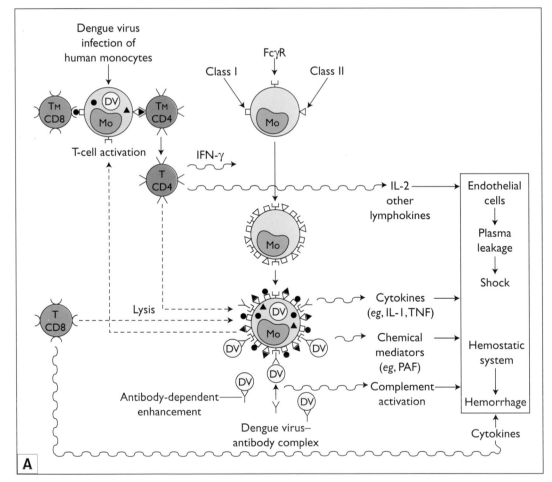

**FIGURE 10-52** Pathogenesis of dengue hemorrhagic fever and shock syndrome. **A,** Dengue virus is remarkable for infecting macrophages almost exclusively in its pathogenesis. The virus enters the cell through viral receptors or the Fc receptor, and this latter property is responsible for the occurrence of hemorrhagic fever in a small number of secondary dengue infections. Secondary dengue hemorrhagic fever (DHF)/dengue shock syndrome (DSS) occurs in persons previously infected with one dengue virus type who are infected with a heterologous dengue virus. The heterotypic antibody is not protective, but cross-reacting antibodies attach to the virus and enhance macrophage infection through Fc receptor–mediated endocytosis (as depicted in the bottom part of *panel 52A*). The secondary antibody response to the new infecting dengue virus plus the enhanced virus output lead to formation of phlogistic immune complexes. The resulting activated complement components may cause damage directly and also through interactions with the coagulation system. The cellular immune system is also important. (DV—dengue virus; IL—interleukin; PAF—platelet activating factor; TNF—tumor necrosis factor.) (*continued*)

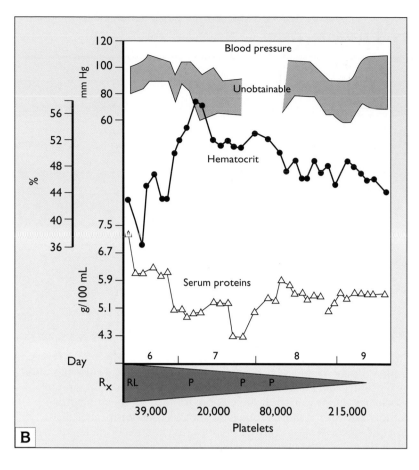

**B**

**FIGURE 10-52** (*continued*) Memory T cells (TM) that recognize cross-reacting epitopes on the new dengue virus species are activated and secrete interferon-γ (IFN-γ), tumor necrosis factor (TNF), and other cytokines, as well as proliferate. IFN-γ upregulates the Fc receptors on the macrophages, which further increases the antibody-dependent enhancement of infection of the dengue target cell. The T cells also interact with macrophages, including the potential for lysis of infected macrophages by cross-reactive CD8+ T cells known to be present. The result of this extensive release of cytokines and other mediators is the abrupt onset of a shock state due to enhanced vascular permeability. This is referred to as DSS and may also be accompanied by a hemorrhagic state, DHF. The dissociation of the two findings in some patients leads to the use of both appellations, allowing the more commonly dangerous DSS to be conceptualized separately. **B**, The clinical course of DSS. At the time of defervescence the vascular leak leads to a rising hematocrit just as serum proteins leave the vascular system. The resulting falling blood pressure can usually be treated effectively with infusions of crystalloid or, at times, colloid until the condition reverses. (P—plasma; RL—Ringer's lactate.) (Panel 52A *adapted from* Kurane and Ennis [9]; panel 52B *adapted from* Halstead [10].)

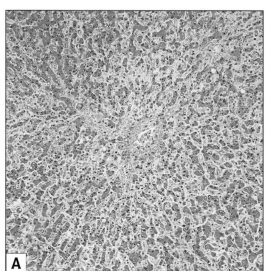

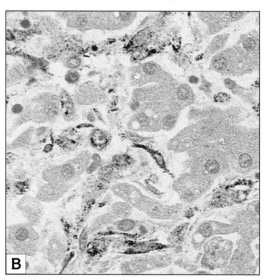

**FIGURE 10-53** Liver histology in dengue hemorrhagic fever. **A**, In this liver section from a fatal case of dengue hemorrhagic fever there is hepatic necrosis with a centrolobular distribution. **B**, When the same sample is stained for dengue antigens, selective localization to the Fc-bearing Kuppfer cells is seen with minor involvement of the endothelial cells.

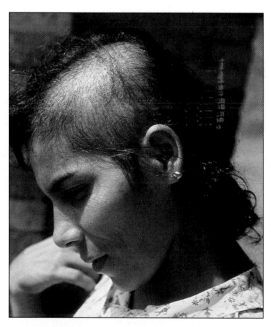

**FIGURE 10-54** Alopecia in a woman recovering from Bolivian hemorrhagic fever. Recovery from hemorrhagic fever is usually complete, but convalescence is prolonged. This young woman shows alopecia after Bolivian hemorrhagic fever, a finding that has been noted particularly in the South American hemorrhagic fever but that may occur after any severe febrile illness. (*Courtesy of* K. Johnson, MD.)

# PREVENTION AND TREATMENT

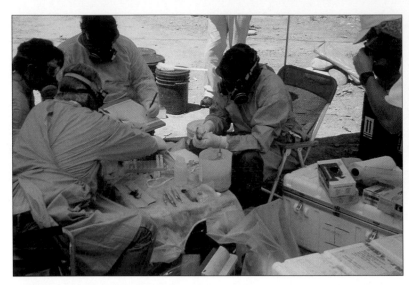

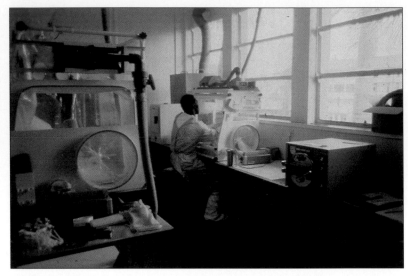

**FIGURE 10-55** Rodent collection in the US southwest. When investigating the reservoirs of hazardous rodent-borne viruses, workers should take extensive precautions, as seen with this team of ecologists and mammalogists working in the southwestern United States. Respiratory protection against small-particle aerosols is provided by fitted respirators, and eye protection is worn. Materials are present for weighing, measuring, obtaining blood samples, and removing tissue samples. In the background, the red buckets are used for copious cleansing of instruments between uses, so that virus isolation and polymerase chain reaction tests on samples are not contaminated by carryover between animals.

**FIGURE 10-56** Hazardous materials laboratory in Kenya. In the United States, many of the hemorrhagic fever viruses are classified as biosafety level 4 agents, and work on them must be done in specialized laboratories. It is possible to have quite satisfactory containment for limited studies of such viruses with carefully thought-out execution but less elaborate construction. This African laboratory is made negative pressure with respect to the rest of its building by blowers that exhaust through HEPA filters (seen behind the virologist). Work on hazardous samples is conducted in flexible plastic film isolators, shown in use by the virologist in the background. These isolators are kept at a slight negative pressure to the room and exhausted through HEPA filters.

## A. Prevention and treatment of viral hemorrhagic fevers: Arenaviridae

| Disease | Prevention | Treatment |
|---|---|---|
| Argentine hemorrhagic fever | Safe, effective vaccine used for high-risk residents of endemic area | Infusion of convalescent plasma during first 8 days of illness reduces mortality from 15%–30% to < 1% |
| Bolivian hemorrhagic fever | Elimination of specific reservoir rodents from towns is practical and effective. Sporadic cases due to exposure outside towns; person-to-person contact cannot be prevented | Ribavirin likely effective and should be used in this and other arenavirus diseases unless alternative therapy available |
| Lassa fever | None; intensive village-based rodent control may reduce risk | Ribavirin effective in reducing mortality; use in higher risk patients, *eg*, if aspartate aminotransferase > 150 |

**FIGURE 10-57** Prevention and treatment of hemorrhagic fevers. Viral illnesses are often thought to be refractory to medical intervention, but there are several approaches to prevent or treat the hemorrhagic fevers (HFs). The process begins with surveillance in the endemic zones to define patterns of transmission and risks of infection. Recognition of disease in travelers is important, as well. Various preventive approaches are different for each disease, such as vector eradication (*Aedes aegypti* for dengue or urban yellow fever; rodents for urban Bolivian HF), avoidance of the vector (tick-borne diseases; rodent-borne disease to the extent practical), elimination of the virus from a critical host (Rift Valley fever virus vaccine for domestic animals), or vaccines (vaccines for jungle yellow fever, Argentine HF). (*continued*)

### B. Prevention and treatment of viral hemorrhagic fevers: Bunyaviridae

| Disease | Prevention | Treatment |
|---------|-----------|-----------|
| Rift Valley fever | Vaccination of domestic livestock prevents epizootics/epidemics but not sporadic, endemic infections of humans<br>Human vaccine safe and effective but limited supply | Ribavirin should be tried in HF patients based on studies in experimental animals |
| Crimean-Congo HF | Tick avoidance<br>No slaughter of acutely infected animals (these cattle are healthy but viremic and therefore a threat)<br>Barrier nursing of suspected patients | Ribavirin should be used based on *in vitro* sensitivity and on uncontrolled South African experience |
| HF with renal syndrome | Rodent control and avoidance impractical in most cases<br>Investigational vaccines deserve further development | Early diagnosis and supportive care life-saving<br>Ribavirin has positive effect during initial 4 days of illness and should be used in Hantaan infection if available |
| Hantavirus pulmonary syndrome | Rodent avoidance may be useful<br>Care should be taken before entering or cleaning closed buildings with rodent infestations | Early diagnosis and supportive care potentially life-saving<br>Avoidance of hypoxia and excessive hydration coupled with careful management of shock |

HF—hemorrhagic fever.

### C. Prevention and treatment of viral hemorrhagic fevers: Filoviridae and flaviviridae

| Disease | Prevention | Treatment |
|---------|-----------|-----------|
| Ebola or Marburg HF | Barrier nursing and needle sterilization in African hospitals<br>Avoid close contact with suspected patients<br>Careful evaluation of sick nonhuman primates | None other than supportive, which may be of limited utility |
| Yellow fever | Vaccine is probably safest and most effective in the world<br>Control of *Aedes aegypti* would eliminate urban transmission, but sylvan transmission remains | None other than supportive |
| Dengue HF | Reduction of dengue transmission by *A. aegypti* control<br>Currently investigational vaccines will probably be available soon; possibly useful in travelers but unlikely to prevent hyperendemic dengue transmission that leads to dengue HF | Supportive care effective and greatly reduces mortality |
| Tick-borne HF (Kyasanur, Omsk HF) | Avoidance of ticks | Supportive care |

HF—hemorrhagic fever.

**FIGURE 10-57** (*continued*) Failure of prevention can be rescued by use of passive antibodies, antiviral drugs, or supportive therapy. Supportive therapy should include the reasonable measures that would be employed in any very sick patient with a fragile vascular bed and also be directed toward specific defects, such as the renal lesion of hemorrhagic fever with renal syndrome, careful fluid and oxygenation management of hantavirus pulmonary syndrome patients, and adequate volume replacement in dengue HF. **A**, Arenaviridae. **B**, Bunyaviridae. **C**, Filoviridae and Flaviviridae.

# REFERENCES

1. Burney MI, Ghafoor A, Saleen M, *et al.*: Nosocomial outbreak of viral hemorrhagic fever caused by Crimean hemorrhagic fever-Congo virus in Pakistan, January 1976. *Am J Trop Med Hyg* 1980, 29:941–947.

2. Bjarvall A, Ullstrom S: *The Mammals of Britain and Europe.* London: Croom Helm; 1986.

3. Monson MH, Cole AK, Frame JD, *et al.*: Pediatric Lassa fever: A review of 33 Liberian cases. *Am J Trop Med Hyg* 1987, 36:408–415.

4. Siam AL, Meegan JM, Gharbawai KF: Rift Valley fever ocular manifestation: Observations during the 1977 epidemic in the Arab Republic of Egypt. *Br J Ophthalmol* 1980, 64:366–374.

5. Peters CJ, Jones D, Trotter R, *et al.*: Experimental Rift Valley fever in rhesus macaques. *Arch Virol* 1988, 99:31–44.

6. Sheedy JA, Froeb HF, Batson HA, *et al.*: The clinical course of epidemic hemorrhagic fever. *Am J Med* 1954, 16:619.

7. Zaki SR, Greer PW, Coffield LM, *et al.*: Hantavirus pulmonary syndrome: Pathogenesis of an emerging infectious disease. *Am J Pathol* 1995, 146:552–579.

8. Smith A: *Yellow Fever in Galveston, Republic of Texas, 1839: An Account of the Great Epidemic.* Austin, TX: University of Texas Press; 1951 [reprint].

9. Kurane I, Ellis FA: Immunity and immunopathology in dengue virus infections. *Semin Immunol* 1992, 4:121.

10. Halstead SB: Dengue. *In* Warren KS, Malmoud AAF (eds): *Tropical and Geographic Medicine*, 2nd ed. New York: McGraw Hill; 1990:675–684.

# SELECTED BIBLIOGRAPHY

Monath TP, Heinz FX: Flaviviruses. *In* Fields BN, Knipe DM, Howley PM, *et al.* (eds.): *Fields Virology*, 3rd ed. Philadelphia: Lippincott-Raven; 1996:961–1034.

Peters CJ: Arenaviruses. *In* Richman DD, Whitley RJ, Hayden FG (eds.): *Clinical Virology* 1996, in press.

Peters CJ: Pathogenesis of viral hemorrhagic fevers. *In* Nathanson N, Ahmed R, Gonzalez-Scarano F, *et al.* (eds.): *Viral Pathogenesis*. Philadelphia: Lippincott-Raven; 1996.

Peters CJ, LeDuc JW: Bunyaviridae: Bunyaviruses, phleboviruses, and related viruses. *In* Belshe R (ed.): *Textbook of Human Virology*, 2nd ed. St. Louis: Mosby Year Book; 1991:571–614.

Peters CJ, Sanchez A, Rollin P, *et al.*: Filoviruses. *In* Fields BN, Knipe DM, Howley PM, *et al.* (eds.): *Fields Virology*, 3rd ed. Philadelphia: Lippincott-Raven; 1996:1161–1176.

# CHAPTER 11

## Systemic Fungal Infections

### Carol A. Kauffman

**Major systemic mycoses seen in the United States**

| Endemic mycoses | Opportunistic mycoses |
|---|---|
| Blastomycosis | Candidiasis |
| Histoplasmosis | Aspergillosis |
| Coccidioidomycosis | Cryptococcosis |
| Sporotrichosis | Mucormycosis (zygomycosis) |

**FIGURE 11-1** Major systemic mycoses seen in the United States.

**Diagnosis of endemic fungal infections**

| Fungal disease | Skin tests | Serology | Culture of fluid or tissue | Histopathology |
|---|---|---|---|---|
| Blastomycosis | NA | Not readily available; EIA most helpful; CF, ID rarely useful | Definitive; may take 4 wks to grow | Definitive; quick; distinctive appearance |
| Histoplasmosis | Rarely helpful in endemic areas | Very helpful; CF, ID available; antigen test (RIA) helpful in some patients | Definitive; may take 6 wks to grow | Definitive; quick; distinctive appearance |
| Coccidioidomycosis | Rarely helpful in endemic areas | Very helpful; CF, ID available | Definitive; grows in days to weeks; dangerous to laboratory workers | Definitive; quick; distinctive appearance |
| Sporotrichosis | NA | Not readily available; LA of some use; EIA perhaps best | Definitive; grows in several weeks | Organisms not often seen; appearance not diagnostic |

CF—complement fixation; EIA—enzyme immunoassay; ID—immunodiffusion; LA—latex agglutination; NA—not available; RIA—radioimmunoassay.

**FIGURE 11-2** Laboratory and other tests useful in the diagnosis of endemic fungal infections.

**Diagnosis of invasive opportunistic fungal infections**

| Fungal disease | Skin tests | Serology | Culture of fluid or tissue | Histopathology |
|---|---|---|---|---|
| Aspergillosis | Not helpful | Not helpful | Easily grown; must differentiate from laboratory contaminant, colonizer | Definitive; quick; proves tissue invasion |
| Mucormycosis | NA | NA | Easily grown; must differentiate from laboratory contaminant | Definitive; quick; proves tissue invasion |
| Candidiasis | Not helpful | Not helpful | Easily grown; must differentiate from colonization | Definitive; quick; proves tissue invasion for certain sites |
| Cryptococcosis | NA | Antigen test (LA) very specific and sensitive | Definitive; easily grown | Definitive; rarely used for CNS disease; muci-carmine stain specific |

CNS—central nervous system; LA—latex agglutination; NA—not available.

**FIGURE 11-3** Laboratory and other tests useful in the diagnosis of opportunistic fungal infections.

## Treatment regimens for the endemic mycoses

| Fungal disease | Preferred regimen | Second-line regimens | Comment |
|---|---|---|---|
| Blastomycosis | Itraconazole | Ketoconazole Fluconazole | Amphotericin B for life-threatening infection |
| Histoplasmosis | Itraconazole | Ketoconazole Fluconazole | Amphotericin B for life-threatening infection |
| Sporotrichosis | Itraconazole | SSKI Fluconazole | Amphotericin B for life-threatening infection |
| Coccidioidomycosis | Itraconazole or fluconazole | Ketoconazole | Amphotericin B for life-threatening infection |
| Meningitis | Fluconazole | Amphotericin B Itraconazole | — |

SSKI—saturated solution of potassium iodide.

**FIGURE 11-4** Treatment regimens for the endemic mycoses.

## Treatment regimens for opportunistic fungal infections

| Fungal disease | Preferred regimen | Second-line regimens | Comment |
|---|---|---|---|
| Cryptococcosis | Amphotericin B + flucytosine followed by fluconazole | Fluconazole + flucytosine Amphotericin B + flucytosine followed by itraconazole | Probably effective regimens for both AIDS and non-AIDS patients |
| Candidiasis | | | |
| Disseminated | Amphotericin B or fluconazole | — | Amphotericin B better for some non-*albicans* species |
| Urinary tract | Fluconazole | Amphotericin B bladder wash | — |
| Oral | Clotrimazole or fluconazole | Ketoconazole Itraconazole | Use clotrimazole first, fluconazole if refractory |
| Esophagitis | Fluconazole | Ketoconazole | — |
| Vaginitis | Fluconazole or local creams, suppositories | Ketoconazole | — |
| Aspergillosis | Amphotericin B | Itraconazole | Amphotericin B for life-threatening infections |
| Mucormycosis | Amphotericin B | — | Surgical debridement crucial |

**FIGURE 11-5** Treatment regimens for the opportunistic fungal infections.

# BLASTOMYCOSIS

## Major disease manifestations of blastomycosis

Systemic
  Fever
  Night sweats
  Fatigue
  Weight loss
Pulmonary
  Cough
  Dyspnea
  Sputum production

Cutaneous
  Indolent, verrucous, nonpainful, nodular or plaquelike lesions, often with central ulcerations
  Acute nodular, pustular, or ulcerated lesions
Other organ involvement
  Osteoarticular (swelling, pain, drainage)
  Genitourinary (frequency, urgency, swelling)

**FIGURE 11-6** Major disease manifestations of blastomycosis.

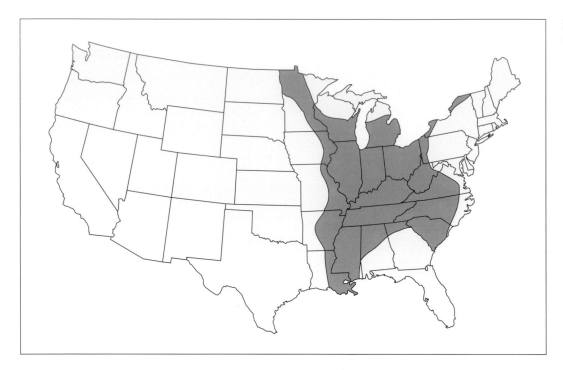

**FIGURE 11-7** Geographic distribution of *Blastomyces dermatitidis* in the United States.

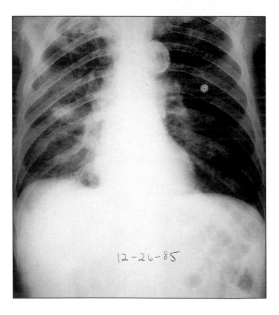

**FIGURE 11-8** Large verrucous skin lesion of blastomycosis on the lateral aspect of the knee. The patient, a man aged 72 years, ran a sawmill in southern Michigan. This lesion was nontender and had been present for at least 6 months. Biopsy revealed large, thick-walled, broad-based budding yeasts typical of *Blastomyces dermatitidis*.

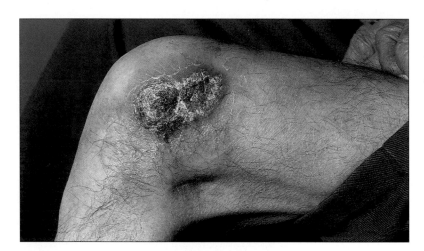

**FIGURE 11-9** Chest radiograph showing multiple nodular lesions and cavitary infiltrate in the right upper lobe in a patient with blastomycosis. Sputum cytology in this patient (*see* Fig. 11-8) showed large, broad-based budding yeasts, and cultures yielded *Blastomyces dermatitidis*.

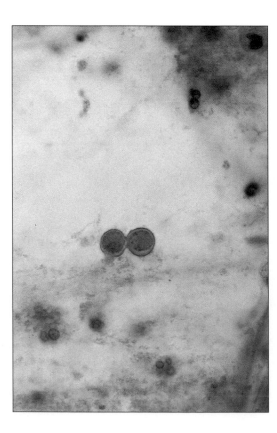

**FIGURE 11-10** Papanicolaou-stained sputum smear in blastomycosis. Sputum was obtained from the patient in Figure 11-9 and stained with Papanicolaou stain. The appearance of this organism is diagnostic for blastomycosis. The organisms are large (8–20 μm) and thick-walled, and the daughter bud is attached to the mother cell by a broad base.

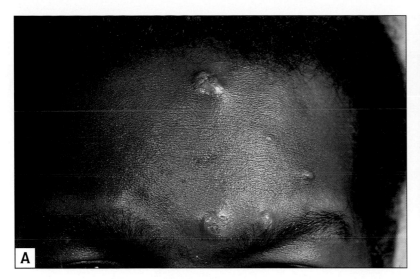

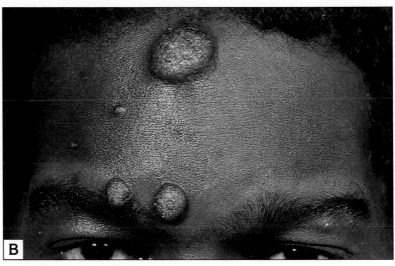

**FIGURE 11-11** Multiple nodular skin lesions in blastomycosis. **A**, Nodular lesions within the first week of development. This man aged 40 years had fever, chills, and shortness of breath and developed more than 100 nodular skin lesions within the course of 2

weeks. **B**, At 2 weeks, the patient shows enlargement of all preexisting lesions and development of several new lesions. (Panel 11A *from* Kauffman [1]; with permission.)

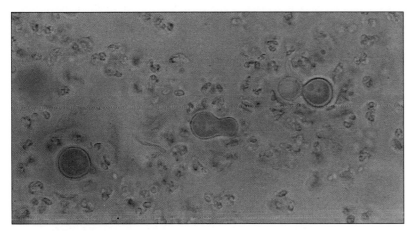

**FIGURE 11-12** Lactophenol cotton blue preparation from a smear of a nodular skin lesion of blastomycosis. Examination of the purulent material obtained from the patient shown in Figure 11-11 showed multiple thick-walled, broad-based, budding yeasts in the midst of surrounding inflammatory cells. Culture yielded *Blastomyces dermatitidis*.

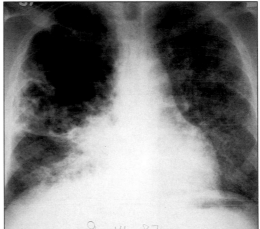

**FIGURE 11-13** Chest radiograph in blastomycosis showing extensive alveolar infiltrates throughout both lung fields. In the same patient (*see* Fig. 11-11), sputum potassium hydroxide preparation showed many yeasts typical of *Blastomyces dermatitidis*, and the organism grew on culture.

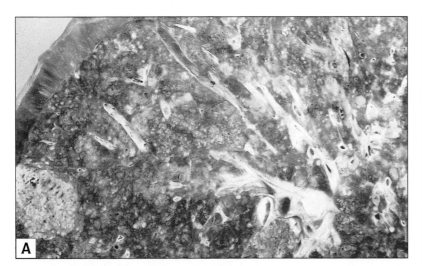

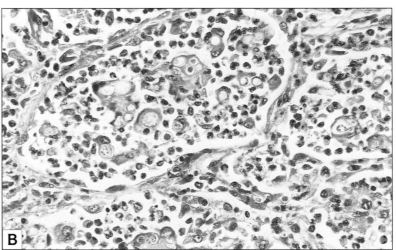

**FIGURE 11-14** Lung tissue examination in blastomycosis. **A**, Gross necropsy specimen of the lung taken from the patient shown in Figure 11-11 shows multiple nodular lesions of varying sizes throughout the lung. **B**, Histopathologic examination with hematoxylin-eosin stain demonstrates overwhelming blastomycosis in

the lungs. Multiple thick-walled yeasts, some of which are budding, are seen within inflammatory cells in the lung parenchyma. Despite amphotericin B treatment, this patient died of overwhelming blastomycosis with involvement of nearly every organ.

# SPOROTRICHOSIS

### Major disease manifestations of sporotrichosis

Systemic
  Uncommon unless disseminated; then fever,
    fatigue, weight loss
Cutaneous
  Nodular, ulcerating, frequently painful lesions
  Drainage of serosanguinous or purulent material
  Regional lymphadenitis
Pulmonary
  Cough
  Purulent sputum
  Hemoptysis
  Dyspnea
Osteoarticular
  Swollen, painful joints
  Drainage
  Tenosynovitis, bursitis

**FIGURE 11-15**  Major disease manifestations of sporotrichosis.

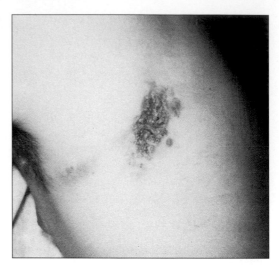

**FIGURE 11-16**  Nodular, ulcerating skin lesions of sporotrichosis. A man aged 27 years was involved in a motor vehicle accident in Michigan, in which he scraped his back on the dirt. Several weeks later, several lesions developed. The posterior lesion drained serous material, the anterior lesion became nodular, and both were painful. The lesions gradually enlarged over the course of the month. Culture yielded *Sporothrix schenckii*. (*From* Kauffman [2]; with permission.)

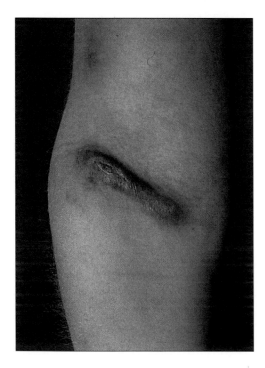

**FIGURE 11-17**
Multiple nodular cutaneous lesions of sporotrichosis. Multiple cutaneous lesions arose in a young woman several weeks after she walked through a recently harvested corn field. These lesions were slightly tender, gradually increased in size over the course of 4 weeks, and were present on both arms and legs. Biopsy revealed granulomatous inflammation but no organisms. *Sporothrix schenckii* was found on culture of the biopsy specimen.

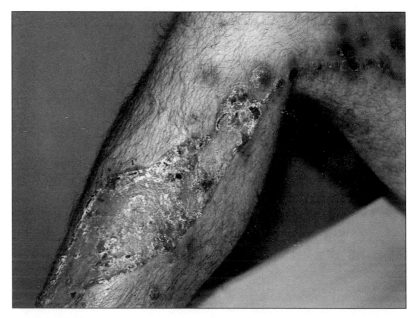

**FIGURE 11-18**  Multiple ulcerating and nodular lesions of cutaneous sporotrichosis on the lower leg. Multiple cutaneous lesions developed after a dirt bike accident in a man aged 22 years. The lesion on the lower leg had been skin-grafted several weeks previously, and then new lesions arose at the borders of the graft. Culture of the material removed at operation yielded *Sporothrix schenckii*, and the patient ultimately responded to oral azole therapy.

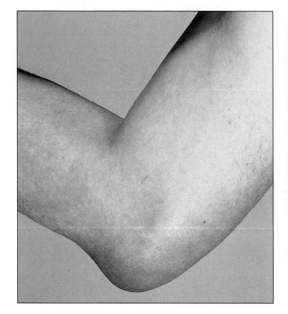

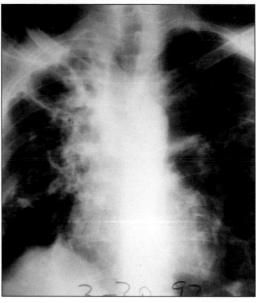

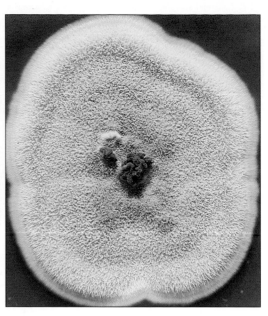

**FIGURE 11-19** Swollen olecranon bursa in osteoarticular sporotrichosis. The elbow was red, warm, tender to touch, and had limitation of movement. Aspirated bursal fluid revealed many neutrophils but no organisms; culture yielded *Sporothrix schenckii*. The patient, a man aged 45 years with chronic alcohol abuse, ultimately developed osteomyelitis in the ulna and severe limitation of joint movement.

**FIGURE 11-20** Chest radiograph from a patient with pulmonary and osteoarticular sporotrichosis. The radiograph shows bilateral cavitation due to sporotrichosis. The patient also had chronic obstructive pulmonary disease. Extensive bilateral infiltrates with upper lobe cavitary lesions are noted.

**FIGURE 11-21** Typical appearance of *Sporothrix schenckii* growing *in vitro* at 25° C on malt extract agar.

# HISTOPLASMOSIS

| Major disease manifestations of histoplasmosis | |
|---|---|
| Systemic<br>  Fever<br>  Night sweats<br>  Fatigue<br>  Weight loss<br>Pulmonary<br>  Cough<br>  Dyspnea<br>  Sputum production<br>    (in chronic cavitary disease)<br>  Hemoptysis<br>    (in chronic cavitary disease) | Reticuloendothelial system<br>  Hepatosplenomegaly<br>  Lymphadenopathy<br>  Pancytopenia<br>Other organ involvement<br>  Adrenal glands (hypotension,<br>    fatigue, electrolyte disturbances)<br>  Mucous membranes<br>    (painful ulcers)<br>  Skin (ulcers, pustules, nodules)<br>  Central nervous system<br>    (headache, confusion) |

**FIGURE 11-22** Major disease manifestations of histoplasmosis.

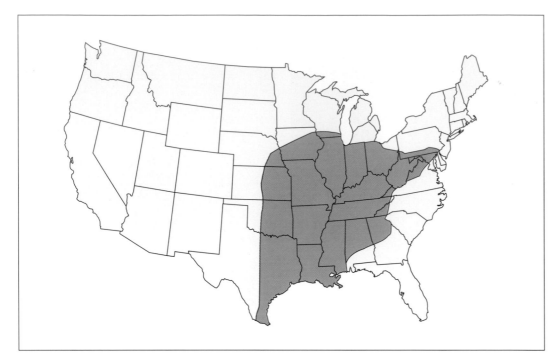

**FIGURE 11-23** Geographic distribution of *Histoplasma capsulatum* in the United States.

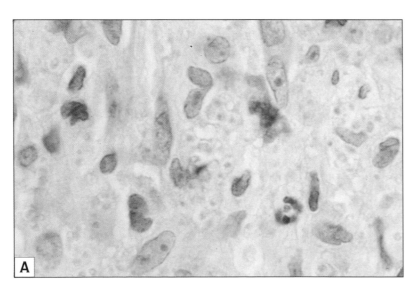

**FIGURE 11-24** Ulcerated skin lesion in histoplasmosis. A farmer aged 72 years from southern Ohio developed multiple coin-shaped ulcerative lesions on his thigh. He had fevers, night sweats, weight loss, pulmonary infiltrates, hepatosplenomegaly, and anemia. Serologic test for *Histoplasma capsulatum* was positive, and culture of bone marrow yielded the organism.

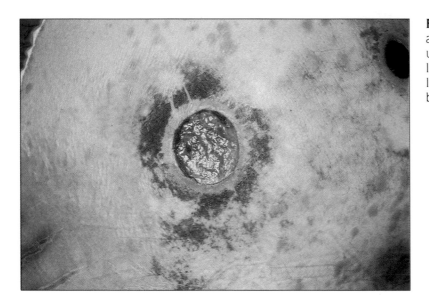

**A**

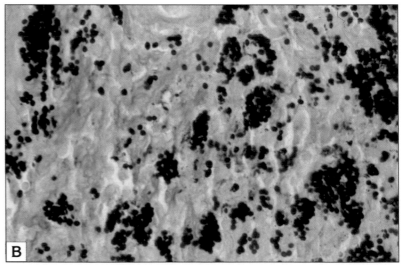

**B**

**FIGURE 11-25** Biopsy of the skin lesion in histoplasmosis. **A**, In the patient shown in Figure 11-24, hematoxylin-eosin staining shows many small round structures that are surrounded by a clear zone throughout the dermis, the typical appearance of

*Histoplasma capsulatum*. **B**, Methenamine silver stain of the same skin lesion shows a profusion of small budding yeasts, approximately 2 to 4 μm in diameter, that are characteristic of *H. capsulatum*.

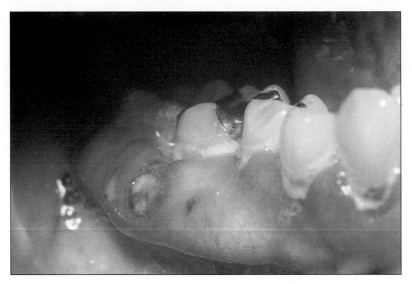

**FIGURE 11-26** Oropharyngeal ulcer of disseminated histoplasmosis. An ulcerated lesion is seen on the gum below the molar teeth in a man aged 65 years who complained of sore mouth, weight loss, and night sweats. Biopsy of this lesion showed small budding yeasts with a morphology typical of *Histoplasma capsulatum*, and the organism grew in culture. (*Courtesy of* J. Galgiani, MD; *from* Kauffman [3]; with permission.)

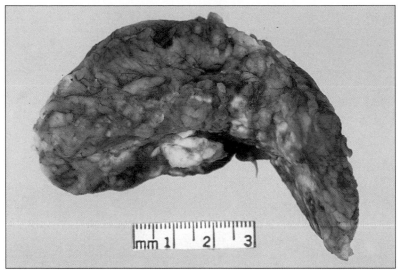

**FIGURE 11-27** Gross necropsy specimen showing adrenal involvement in histoplasmosis. The patient presented with fever, hypotension, and confusion and had a prior history of night sweats, fatigue, fevers, and weight loss. At autopsy, progressive disseminated histoplasmosis involving the adrenals, liver, spleen, lungs, and lymph nodes was found. (*From* Kauffman and Terpenning [4]; with permission.)

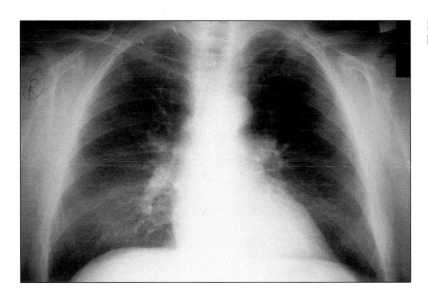

**FIGURE 11-28** Chest radiograph in progressive disseminated histoplasmosis showing diffuse infiltrates bilaterally.

# COCCIDIOIDOMYCOSIS

| Major disease manifestations of coccidioidomycosis | |
|---|---|
| Systemic | Pulmonary |
|   Fever |   Cough |
|   Night sweats |   Dyspnea |
|   Fatigue |   Sputum production |
|   Weight loss | Other organ involvement |
|   Arthralgias (in acute disease) |   Skin (cellulitis, ulcers, nodules, plaques) |
|   Erythema nodosum |   Osteoarticular (swelling, pain, drainage) |
|    (in acute disease) |   Central nervous system (headache, confusion) |

**FIGURE 11-29** Major disease manifestations of coccidioidomycosis.

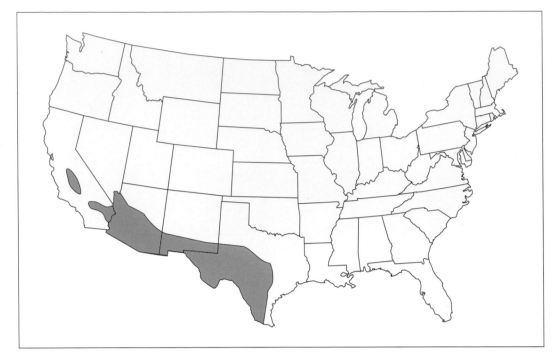

**FIGURE 11-30** Geographic distribution of *Coccidioides immitis* in the United States.

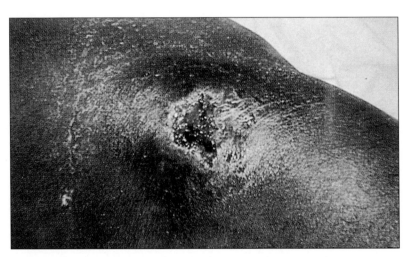

**FIGURE 11-31** Draining sinus tract from a patient aged 37 years with disseminated coccidioidomycosis. This lesion was slightly tender, drained purulent material, and had not healed over the course of 3 months. Culture yielded *Coccidioides immitis*, and the patient responded to therapy with ketoconazole. (*From* Kauffman and Terpenning [4]; with permission.)

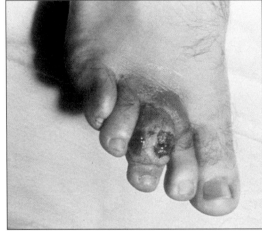

**FIGURE 11-32** Painful, swollen, draining lesion on the toe of a patient with disseminated coccidioidomycosis. Further investigation showed destruction of the digit and involvement of the metatarsal head. Culture yielded *Coccidioides immitis*. (*Courtesy of* N. Ampel, MD.)

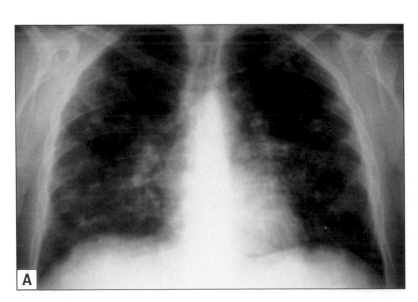

**FIGURE 11-33** Pulmonary coccidioidomycosis. **A**, A chest radiograph of a man aged 40 years with HIV infection. The patient was from Michigan but had previously lived in Phoenix. He had fevers, weight loss, fatigue, dyspnea, and cough. Radiograph shows extensive bilateral nodular infiltrates. Culture of bronchoalveolar lavage fluid yielded *Coccidioides immitis*. (*continued*)

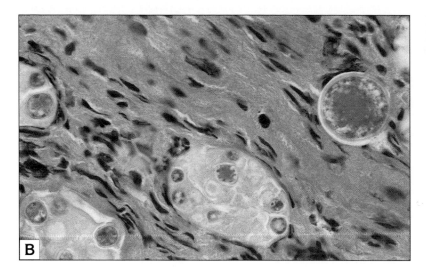

**FIGURE 11-33** (*continued*) **B**, A lung biopsy specimen shows numerous large spherules (50–80 μm) with endospores typical of *Coccidioides immitis*. (Hematoxylin-eosin stain.)

# CRYPTOCOCCOSIS

| Major disease manifestations of cryptococcosis |
| --- |
| Systemic |
|   Fever |
|   Night sweats |
|   Fatigue |
|   Weight loss |
| Central nervous system |
|   Headache |
|   Stiff neck |
|   Visual changes |
|   Nausea and vomiting |
|   Confusion |
|   Personality changes |
|   Cranial nerve palsies |
|   Seizures |
| Pulmonary |
|   Cough |
|   Dyspnea |
| Other organ involvement |
|   Skin (pustules, ulcers, cellulitis) |
|   Osteoarticular (pain, swelling, drainage) |
|   Prostatitis (frequency, urgency) |

**FIGURE 11-34** Major disease manifestations of cryptococcosis.

| Risk factors for cryptococcosis | |
| --- | --- |
| **Predisposing conditions** | **Contributing factors** |
| Hematologic malignancy, especially lymphomas | Corticosteroids |
| Transplantation | Cytotoxic chemotherapy |
| Collagen vascular disease | |
| AIDS | |

**FIGURE 11-35** Risk factors for cryptococcosis.

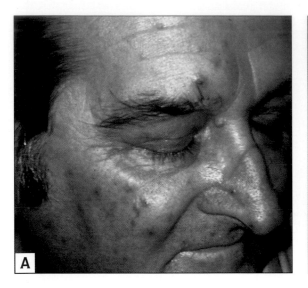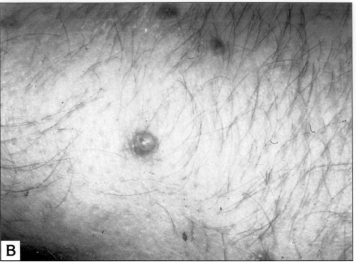

**FIGURE 11-36**
Multiple, painless skin lesions due to cryptococcosis. A man aged 50 years with Hodgkin's disease developed fever, shortness of breath, and multiple nontender skin lesions. **A**, Lesions on his face arose over the course of a week. **B**, Close-up view of the forearm shows several pustular lesions, which were shown to be caused by *Cryptococcus neoformans*.

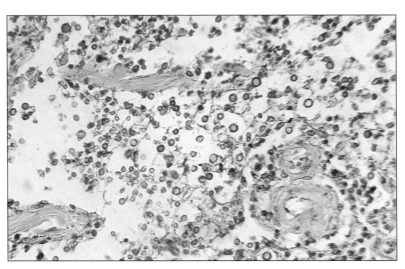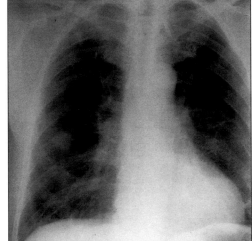

**FIGURE 11-38**
Chest radiograph in cryptococcosis showing multiple nodules. Biopsy of the nodules showed that they were due to *Cryptococcus neoformans*. The patient (*see* Fig. 11-36) also had cryptococcal meningitis.

**FIGURE 11-37** Mucicarmine staining of tissue biopsy in cryptococcosis. Biopsy revealed many mucicarmine-positive budding yeasts with large capsules. The mucicarmine stain is specific for the cell wall of *Cryptococcus neoformans* and can be very helpful in confirming a diagnosis of cryptococcosis. The capsule appears as a large clear area around the yeast cell.

# ASPERGILLOSIS

| Major disease manifestations of invasive aspergillosis |
| --- |
| Systemic |
|   Fever |
|   Chills |
|   "Toxic" appearance |
| Pulmonary |
|   Cough |
|   Dyspnea |
|   Hemoptysis |
|   Pleuritic pain |
| Other organ involvement |
|   Skin (pustules, necrosis) |
|   Central nervous system (confusion, seizures) |
|   Multisystem organ failure |

**FIGURE 11-39** Major disease manifestations of invasive aspergillosis.

| Risk factors for invasive aspergillosis | |
|---|---|
| **Predisposing conditions** | **Contributing factors** |
| Hematologic malignancy, especially leukemia | Neutropenia |
| Transplantation | Corticosteroids |
| AIDS | Cytotoxic chemotherapy |
| | Broad-spectrum antibiotics |

**FIGURE 11-40** Risk factors for invasive aspergillosis.

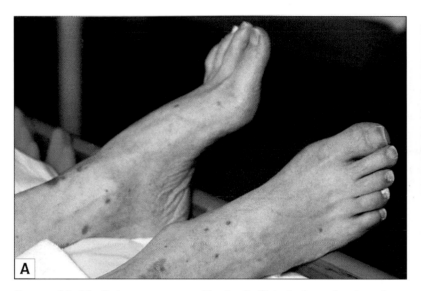

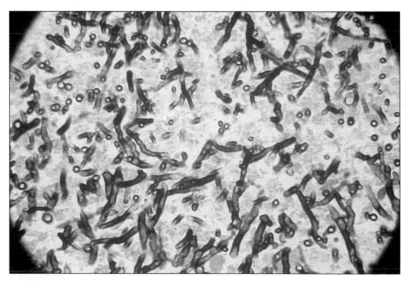

**FIGURE 11-41** Cutaneous aspergillosis. **A**, Skin lesions developed over the lower extremities of a man aged 65 years with polymyositis treated with high-dose corticosteroids for 3 months. The patient had bilateral nodular pulmonary infiltrates at the time these lesions developed, was febrile, and looked ill. **B**, Close-up view of pustular skin lesions. These lesions appeared over the course of 3 days. (*Courtesy of* D. Katz, MD.)

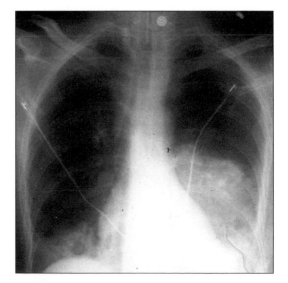

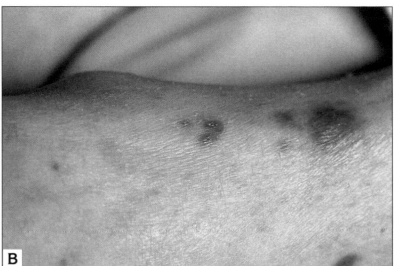

**FIGURE 11-42** Chest radiograph showing cavitary lesions in pulmonary aspergillosis. A patient with sarcoidosis on high-dose prednisone for 2 months came to the hospital with acute dyspnea, pleuritic chest pain, fever, and confusion. Cavitation is obvious in the lesion in the right lower lobe.

**FIGURE 11-43** Lung biopsy in pulmonary aspergillosis. A lung biopsy specimen from the patient (*see* Fig. 11-42), stained with methenamine silver, shows acutely branching, septate hyphae consistent with *Aspergillus* species. Culture yielded *Aspergillus fumigatus*.

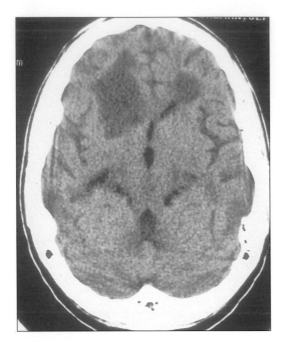

**FIGURE 11-44** Computed tomography scan showing multiple cerebral lesions in disseminated aspergillosis. The patient (*see* Fig. 11-42) developed seizures and became obtunded on day 3 of hospitalization and died on day 5.

# CANDIDIASIS

### Major disease manifestations of disseminated candidiasis

Systemic
 Fever
 Chills
 Septic shock (indistinguishable from bacterial infection)
Specific organ involvement
 Skin (pustules on erythematous base)
 Eye (blurring of vision, pain)
 Central nervous system (headache, confusion, obtundation,
  seizures)
 Osteomyelitis (pain, swelling)
 Multisystem organ failure

**FIGURE 11-45** Major disease manifestations of disseminated candidiasis.

### Risk factors for disseminated candidiasis

| Patient groups at risk | Contributing factors |
|---|---|
| Hematologic malignancies, especially leukemias | Neutropenia |
| | Corticosteroids |
| Transplant recipients | Cytotoxic chemotherapy |
| Burn patients | Broad-spectrum antibiotics |
| Premature infants | Intravenous catheters |
| Injectable drug users | Total parenteral nutrition |
| Surgery patients | Bowel perforation, surgery |

**FIGURE 11-46** Risk factors for disseminated candidiasis.

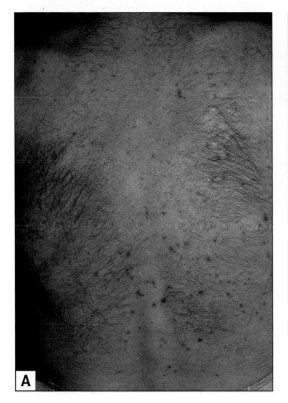

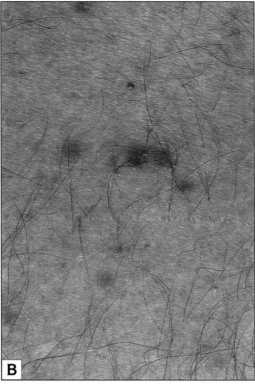

**FIGURE 11-47** Pustular cutaneous lesions of disseminated candidiasis. **A**, Diffuse erythematous pustular lesions arose over the course of 24 hours on the trunk of a man aged 67 years with chronic lymphocytic leukemia and neutropenia. He had been febrile and on broad-spectrum antibiotics for 8 days when these lesions occurred. **B**, Close-up view of the lesions shows small pustules on an erythematous base. The lesions were nontender.

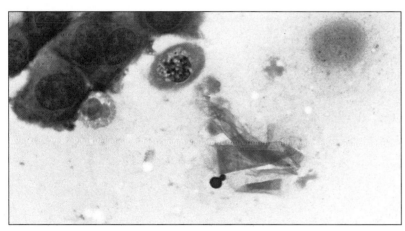

**FIGURE 11-48** Smear of pustular lesion. Wright's stain of tissue scraped from the base of a pustule in the patient in Figure 11-47 shows epithelial cells and budding yeast. The organism was later identified as *Candida albicans*.

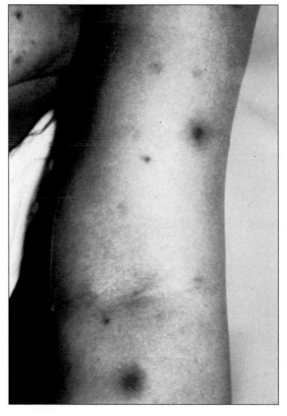

**FIGURE 11-49** Skin lesions of disseminated candidiasis in a young woman with acute leukemia who was neutropenic and on broad-spectrum antibiotics. These lesions have an erythematous base and necrotic center. Aspirate from one of the lesions grew *Candida albicans*, and biopsy showed budding yeast and pseudohyphae. (*Courtesy of* P.G. Jones, MD.)

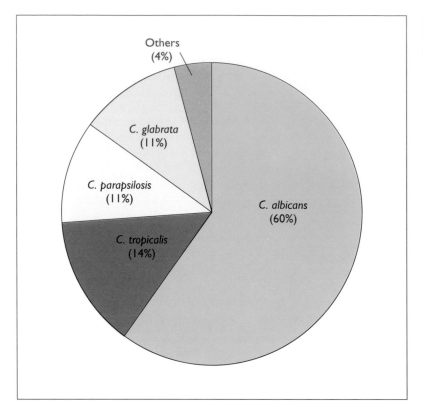

**FIGURE 11-50**  Major species of *Candida* causing fungemia in humans. Data are taken from a large multicenter treatment trial of candidemia between 1989 and 1993 [5].

# MUCORMYCOSIS (ZYGOMYCOSIS)

**Major disease manifestations of invasive mucormycosis**

Systemic
  Fever
  Chills
  "Toxic" appearance
Rhinocerebral
  Facial pain
  Necrosis (palate, sinuses, facial tissues)
  Sinus drainage
  Cavernous sinus thrombosis
  Stroke
  Obtundation

Pulmonary
  Cough
  Dyspnea
  Hemoptysis
  Pleuritic pain
Other organ involvement
  Skin (necrosis, cellulitis)
  Bowel (perforation, obstruction)
  Multisystem organ failure

**FIGURE 11-51**  Major disease manifestations of invasive mucormycosis (zygomycosis).

**Risk factors for invasive mucormycosis (zygomycosis)**

| Predisposing condition | Contributing factors |
| --- | --- |
| Diabetes mellitus | Ketoacidosis |
| Hematologic malignancy | Neutropenia |
| Aluminum or iron overload | Corticosteroids |
|   (hemodialysis, myelodysplastic | Cytotoxic chemotherapy |
|   syndromes, thalassemia, etc) | Deferoxamine therapy |

**FIGURE 11-52**  Risk factors for invasive mucormycosis (zygomycosis).

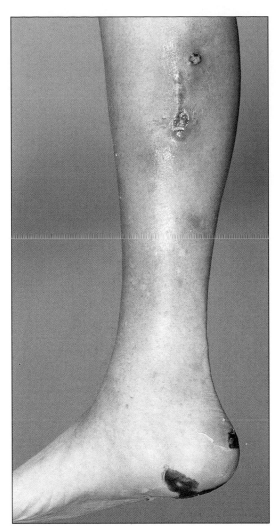

**FIGURE 11-53** Cutaneous mucormycosis affecting the lower leg. A man aged 72 years who had myelodysplastic syndrome received deferoxamine for iron overload related to repeated transfusions. He developed cellulitis that did not respond to antistaphylococcal antibiotics; the lesions became necrotic, very painful, and drained purulent material. Two weeks later, he developed painful nodules on the heel, and these progressed to necrosis. Biopsy of the calf lesion revealed broad nonseptate hyphae, and culture grew *Rhizopus* species.

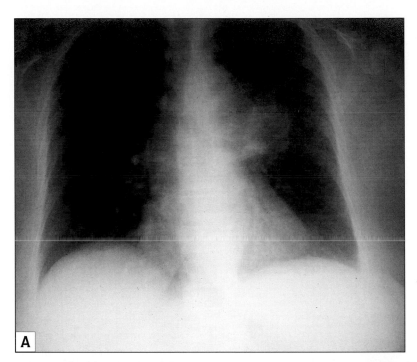

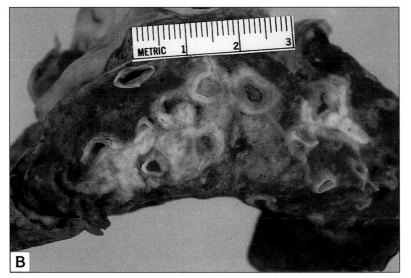

**FIGURE 11-54** Pulmonary mucormycosis. **A**, Chest radiograph from a woman aged 60 years with myelodysplastic syndrome who was receiving deferoxamine for iron overload. She presented to the hospital with fever and confusion, became hypotensive, and died within 4 days of hospitalization. A chest radiograph revealed a left hilar masslike infiltrate. **B**, Lung specimen obtained at necropsy showed multiple thrombi in major pulmonary arteries.

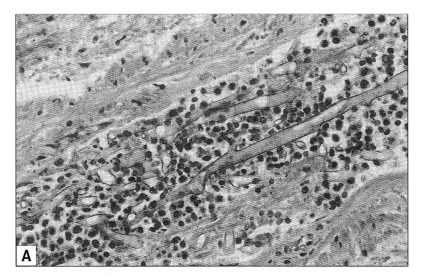

**FIGURE 11-55** Histopathologic examination in mucormycosis. **A**, Histopathologic section of lung from this patient (*see* Fig. 11-54) shows broad, nonseptate hyphae invading the pulmonary artery. (Hematoxylin-eosin stain.) Culture from this specimen yielded *Rhizopus* species. (*continued*)

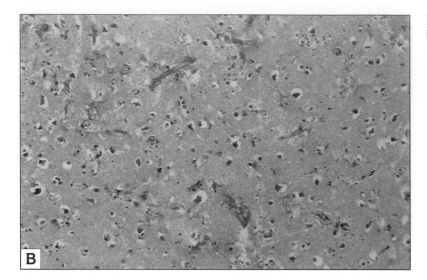

**FIGURE 11-55** (*continued*) **B,** Histopathologic preparation of the brain revealed large nonseptate hyphae invading the cerebrum. (Hematoxylin-eosin stain.)

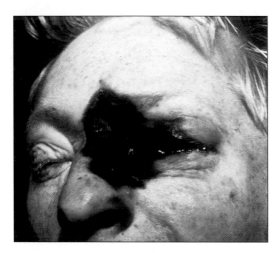

**FIGURE 11-56** Rapidly progressive rhinocerebral mucormycosis. A middle-aged man with insulin-dependent diabetes mellitus and recurrent ketoacidosis presented with rapidly progressive mucormycosis of the sinus, leading to cerebral infarction and death. (*Courtesy of* T. Walsh, MD; *from* Walsh *et al.* [6]; with permission.)

# REFERENCES

1. Kauffman CA: Non-resolving pneumonia: Is endemic mycosis to blame? *J Respir Dis* 1995, 16:1008–1024.

2. Kauffman CA: Fungal infections in the elderly. *Emerg Med* 1993, 25:24–32.

3. Kauffman CA: Fungal infections. *Clin Geriatr Med* 1992, 8:777–791.

4. Kauffman CA, Terpenning MS: Deep fungal infections in the elderly. *J Am Geriatr Soc* 1988, 36:548–557.

5. Rex JH, Bennett JE, Sugar AM, *et al.*: A randomized trial comparing fluconazole with amphotericin B for the treatment of candidemia in patients without neutropenia. *N Engl J Med* 1994, 331:1325–1330.

6. Walsh T, Rinaldi M, Pizzo PA: Zygomycosis of the respiratory tract. *In* Sarosi GA, Davies SF (eds.): *Fungal Diseases of the Lung.* New York: Raven Press; 1993.

# SELECTED BIBLIOGRAPHY

Galgiani JN: Coccidioidomycosis. *West J Med* 1993, 159:153–171.

Goodwin RA, Shapiro JL, Thurman GH, *et al.*: Disseminated histoplasmosis: Clinical and pathologic correlations. *Medicine* 1980, 59:1–33.

Kwon-Chung KJ, Bennett JE: *Medical Mycology.* Philadelphia: Lea & Febiger; 1992.

Odds FC: *Candida and Candidosis*, 2nd ed. London: Balliere Tindall; 1988.

Rippon JW: *Medical Mycology: The Pathogenic Fungi and the Pathogenic Actinomycetes*, 3rd ed. Philadelphia: W.B. Saunders; 1988.

# CHAPTER 12

# Manifestations of Protozoal and Helminthic Diseases in Latin America

Anastacio de Q. Sousa
Thomas G. Evans
Richard D. Pearson

## Major helminthic pathogens of humans in Latin America

| Group or class | Infection | Organism | Mode of transmission to humans |
| --- | --- | --- | --- |
| Nematodes (roundworms) | Trichuriasis | *Trichuris trichiura* | Ingestion of eggs |
| | Enterobiasis | *Enterobius vermicularis* | Ingestion of eggs |
| | Ascariasis | *Ascaris lumbricoides* | Ingestion of eggs |
| | Hookworm | *Ancylostoma duodenale, Necator americanus* | Skin penetration by larvae |
| | Strongyloidiasis | *Strongyloides stercoralis* | Larvae penetrate skin or colon |
| | Trichinosis | *Trichinella spiralis* | Ingestion of larvae in muscle |
| | Lymphatic filariasis | *Wuchereria bancrofti, Brugia malayi* | Transference of larvae during mosquito bite |
| | Onchocerciasis | *Onchocerca volvulus* | Transference of larvae during black fly bite |
| Trematodes (flukes) | Schistosomiasis | *Schistosoma mansoni* | Penetration of intact human skin by cercariae |
| | Fascioliasis | *Fasciola hepatica* | Ingestion of metacercariae on aquatic plants |
| | Paragonimiasis | *Paragonimus westermani* | Ingestion of metacercariae in crayfish or freshwater crabs |
| Cestodes (tapeworms) | Echinococcosis | *Echinococcus granulosus* | Ingestion of eggs |
| | Taeniasis saginata | *Taenia saginata* | Ingestion of cysticerci in beef |
| | Taeniasis solium | *Taenia solium* | Ingestion of cysticerci in pork |
| | Cysticercosis | *Taenia solium* | Ingestion of eggs |

**FIGURE 12-1** Major helminthic pathogens of humans in Latin America. Helminthic and protozoal infections are important causes of morbidity and mortality in Latin America. Helminths are multicellular organisms with complex organ systems and complicated life cycles. They can be subdivided into nematodes (roundworms), trematodes (flukes), and cestodes (tapeworms). Some helminthic genera are parasites of the gastrointestinal tract, whereas others produce systemic disease. Helminths do not multiply in their definite human hosts, although in a few instances, such as with the intestinal helminth *Strongyloides stercoralis*, they can produce autoinfection. The severity of helminthic disease generally correlates with the worm burden, but on occasion, a single adult worm may produce life-threatening damage, as is the case with an adult *Ascaris lumbricoides*, which can induce pancreatitis if it migrates into the common bile duct. Helminths frequently stimulate eosinophilia as they migrate through the body. (*Adapted from* Mahmoud [1].)

## Major protozoal pathogens of humans in Latin America

| Organism (infection) | Means of transmission | Major clinical syndrome |
| --- | --- | --- |
| *Acanthamoeba* spp | Contact lens, water, soil, air-borne (?) | Keratitis, granulomatous encephalitis in immunocompromised patients |
| *Balantidium coli* | Zoonosis (pigs) (?), water, human fecal-oral | Colitis |
| *Blastocystis hominis* | Fecal-oral, water | Diarrhea (?) |
| *Cryptosporidium* spp | Water, fecal-oral, zoonosis | Self-limited noninflammatory diarrhea; chronic severe diarrhea and cholangitis in AIDS patients |
| *Dientamoeba fragilis* | Water, fecal-oral | Diarrhea, eosinophilia |
| *Entamoeba histolytica* (amebiasis) | Water, fecal-oral, food-borne | Rectocolitis, liver abscess |
| *Giardia lamblia* | Water, fecal-oral, food-borne | Noninflammatory diarrhea with malabsorption |
| *Isospora* spp | Fecal-oral | Self-limited diarrhea; chronic severe diarrhea in AIDS patients |
| *Leishmania* spp  L. mexicana  L. amazonensis  L. chagasi  L. braziliensis | Sandfly | Cutaneous or mucosal ulceration; visceral disease with fever, cachexia, hepatosplenomegaly |
| *Naegleria* spp | Freshwater, intranasal exposure | Granulomatous amebic encephalitis |
| *Plasmodium* spp (malaria) | Female anopheline mosquitoes | Paroxysmal fever, chills, headache, hepatosplenomegaly |
| *Sarcocystis* spp | Food-borne | Myositis, fever, eosinophilia |
| *Toxoplasma gondii* | Zoonosis (cats), food-borne (meat), blood or organ transplantation, congenital | Fever, malaise, lymphadenopathy; chorioretinitis; congenital abnormalities; in immunocompromised host; encephalitis, myocarditis, pneumonitis |

(*continued*)

## Major protozoal pathogens of humans in Latin America  (*continued*)

| Organism (infection) | Means of transmission | Major clinical syndrome |
|---|---|---|
| *Trichomonas vaginalis* | Venereal, during birth, nonvenereal (?) | Vaginitis, urethritis |
| *Trypanosoma cruzi* (Chagas' disease) | Reduviid bugs | Acute disease: fever, lymphadenopathy, meningoencephalitis, myocarditis<br>Chronic disease: megaesophagus and megacolon, congestive cardiomyopathy |

**FIGURE 12-2**  Major protozoal pathogens of humans in Latin America. Protozoa are single-cell organisms that divide and multiply in their human hosts. Infection with even a single protozoan can result in overwhelming parasite numbers and life-threatening disease. Protozoal infections are not typically associated with eosinophilia, although there are exceptions. (*Adapted from* Ravdin [2].)

## A. Distribution of the major parasitic diseases in the Americas

| | Mainland Central America | Caribbean | Tropical South America | Temperate South America |
|---|:---:|:---:|:---:|:---:|
| Intestinal protozoa (*Entamoeba histolytica, Giardia lamblia*, etc) | X | X | X | X |
| Intestinal helminths (*Necator americanus, Ascaris lumbricoides*, etc) | X | X | X | X |
| Malaria (*Plasmodium falciparum, P. vivax, P. malariae*) | X | X | X | X |
| Chagas' disease (*Trypanosoma cruzi*) | X | — | X | X |
| Leishmaniasis (*Leishmania* spp) | | | | |
| Cutaneous | X | X | X | X |
| Mucosal | X | — | X | X |
| Visceral | X | — | X | — |
| Onchocerciasis (*Onchocerca volvulus*) | X | — | X | — |
| Bancroftian filariasis (*Wuchereria bancrofti*) | X | X | X | — |
| Schistosomiasis (*Schistosoma mansoni*) | — | X | X | — |
| Taeniasis/cysticercosis (*Taenia solium*) | X | X | X | X |
| Paragonimiasis (*Paragonimus westermani*) | X | — | X | — |
| Echinococcosis (*Echinococcus* spp) | — | — | X | X |
| Fascioliasis (*Fasciola hepatica*) | — | X | — | — |

**FIGURE 12-3**  Distribution of the major parasitic diseases in the Americas. **A,** The distribution of parasitic diseases in Latin America varies among four major geographic areas: mainland Central America, the Caribbean, tropical South America, and temperate South America. It is important to be aware of this distribution in developing prophylactic strategies for travelers and in evaluating returning travelers or immigrants with diseases. The risk of specific diseases also varies within these regions. (*continued*)

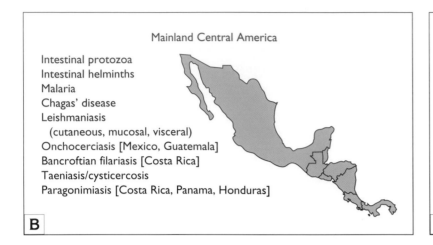

Mainland Central America

Intestinal protozoa
Intestinal helminths
Malaria
Chagas' disease
Leishmaniasis
   (cutaneous, mucosal, visceral)
Onchocerciasis [Mexico, Guatemala]
Bancroftian filariasis [Costa Rica]
Taeniasis/cysticercosis
Paragonimiasis [Costa Rica, Panama, Honduras]

**B**

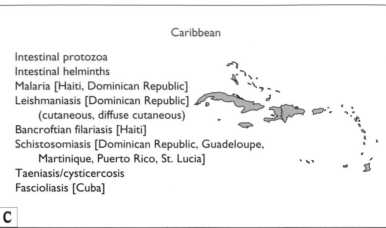

Caribbean

Intestinal protozoa
Intestinal helminths
Malaria [Haiti, Dominican Republic]
Leishmaniasis [Dominican Republic]
   (cutaneous, diffuse cutaneous)
Bancroftian filariasis [Haiti]
Schistosomiasis [Dominican Republic, Guadeloupe,
       Martinique, Puerto Rico, St. Lucia]
Taeniasis/cysticercosis
Fascioliasis [Cuba]

**C**

Tropical South America

Intestinal protozoa
Intestinal helminths
Malaria
Chagas' disease
Leishmaniasis
   (cutaneous, mucosal, visceral)
Onchocerciasis [Ecuador, Venezuela, northern Brazil]
Bancroftian filariasis [Brazil, Guyana, Suriname]
Schistosomiasis [Brazil, Suriname, Venezuela]
Taeniasis/cysticercosis
Paragonimiasis [Ecuador, Peru, Venezuela]
Echinococcosis

**D**

Temperate South America

Intestinal protozoa
Intestinal helminths
Malaria [northwestern Argentina]
Chagas' disease
Leishmaniasis
   (cutaneous)
Taeniasis/cysticercosis
Echinococcosis

**E**

**FIGURE 12-3** (*continued*) **B**, Mainland Central America: Belize, Costa Rica, El Salvador, Guatemala, Honduras, Mexico, Nicaragua, and Panama. **C**, Caribbean: Antigua and Barbuda, Aruba, Bahamas, Barbados, British Virgin Islands, Cayman Islands, Cuba, Dominica, Dominican Republic, Grenada, Guadeloupe, Haiti, Jamaica, Martinique, Montserrat, Netherlands Antilles, Puerto Rico, St. Christopher and Nevis, St. Lucia, St. Vincent and the Grenadines, Trinidad and Tobago, Turks and Caicos Islands, and the Virgin Islands (USA). **D**, Tropical South America: Bolivia, Brazil, Colombia, Ecuador, French Guiana, Guyana, Paraguay, Peru, Suriname, and Venezuela. **E**, Temperate South America: Argentina, Chile, Falkland Islands (Malvinas), and Uruguay. The risks of various parasitic diseases vary within each region. When a disease is restricted to one or a limited number of countries, the endemic location(s) is given in *brackets*. (Panel 3A *adapted from* Centers for Disease Control and Prevention [3].)

# VECTOR-BORNE SYSTEMIC PROTOZOAL INFECTIONS

**Major vector-borne protozoal diseases in Latin America**

Malaria
   (*Plasmodium falciparum, P. vivax, P. malariae*)
Leishmaniasis (*Leishmania* spp)
   Cutaneous
   Mucosal
   Visceral
Chagas' disease
   (*Trypanosoma cruzi*)

**FIGURE 12-4** Major vector-borne protozoal diseases in Latin America. There are three major vector-borne pathogenic protozoal genera in Latin America: *Plasmodium* species that produce malaria; *Leishmania* species that produce cutaneous, mucosal, and visceral leishmaniasis; and *Trypanosoma cruzi*, the cause of Chagas' disease.

# *Plasmodium* Species (Malaria)

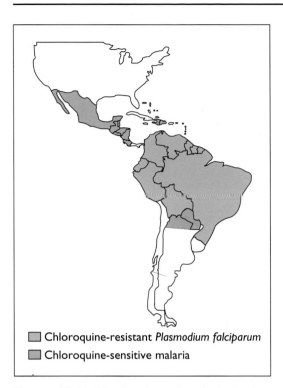

FIGURE 12-5 Distribution of malaria in the Americas, showing range of chloroquine-resistant *Plasmodium falciparum* in 1995. *Plasmodium* species are endemic throughout the Amazon basin and in other rural areas of Latin America. *P. falciparum*, which causes the most severe form of malaria, is found east and south of the Panama Canal Zone in Central America, in South America, and in Haii and adjacent areas of the Dominican Republic. The distributions of chloroquine-sensitive malaria and chloroquine-resistant *P. falciparum* malaria are reported yearly by the Centers for Disease Control and Prevention (CDC). Recommendations by country are available in the CDC's *Health Information for International Travel* and through its travelers' hotline ([404] 332-4559) [3].

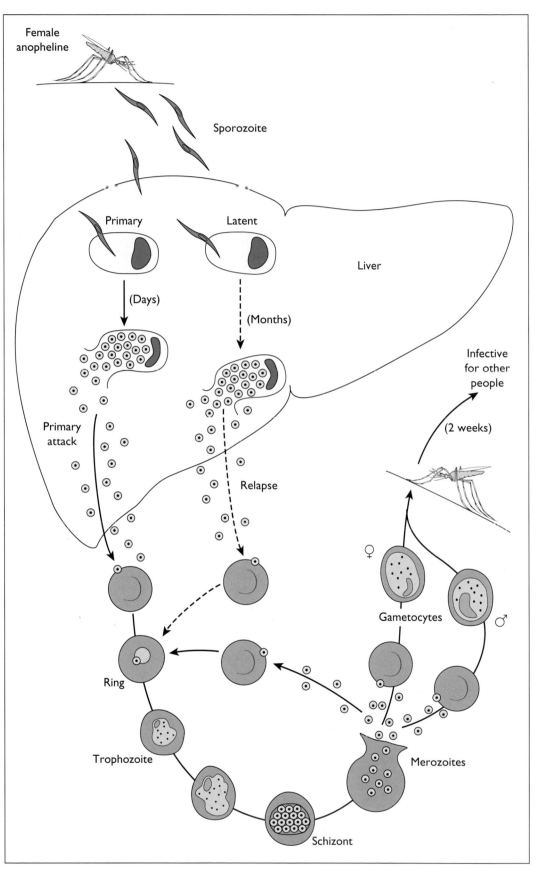

FIGURE 12-6 Life cycle of plasmodia. The life cycle of *Plasmodium* species involves development in *Anopheles* mosquitoes and sexual and asexual reproduction in humans. *P. vivax* and *P. ovale* have latent forms (hypnozoites) that persist in the liver and can result in relapses, whereas *P. falciparum* and *P. malariae* do not. (*Adapted from* Wyler [4].)

### Manifestations of severe falciparum malaria

| | |
|---|---|
| Unarousable coma/cerebral malaria | Failure to localize or respond appropriately to noxious stimuli; coma should persist for > 30 mins after generalized convulsion |
| Convulsions | > 2 generalized seizures in 24 hrs |
| Severe normochromic, normocytic anemia | Hematocrit < 15% or hemoglobin < 5 g/dL with parasitemia level > 10,000/mL |
| Hemoglobinuria | Macroscopic black, brown, or red urine; not associated with effects of oxidant drugs or red blood cell enzyme defects (such as G6PD deficiency) |
| Renal failure | Urine output < 400 mL/24 hrs in adults or 12 mL/kg/24 hrs in children; no improvement with rehydration; serum creatinine > 265 µmol/L (> 3.0 mg/dL) |
| Pulmonary edema/adult respiratory distress syndrome | |
| Hypoglycemia | Glucose < 2.2 mmol/L (< 40 mg/dL) |
| Hypotension/shock | Systolic blood pressure < 50 mm Hg in children 1–5 yrs or < 80 mm Hg in adults; core skin temperature difference > 10° C |
| Bleeding/DIC | Significant bleeding and hemorrhage from the gums, nose, gastrointestinal tract, and/or evidence of DIC |
| Acidemia/acidosis | Arterial pH < 7.25 or plasma bicarbonate < 15 mmol/L, venous lactate > 6 mmol/L |
| Jaundice | Serum bilirubin level > 50 mmol/L (> 3.0 mg/dL) |
| Hyperpyrexia | Rectal temperature > 40° C |

DIC—disseminated intravascular coagulation; G6PD—glucose-6-phosphate dehydrogenase.

**FIGURE 12-7** Manifestations of severe falciparum malaria. *Plasmodium falciparum* can produce severe, life-threatening disease. Nonimmune travelers, children, and pregnant women are at greatest risk. Patients with malaria typically present with fever, chills, headache, and other constitutional symptoms. Splenomegaly may be present, but there are no specific findings on physical examination. Malaria must be considered in the differential diagnosis of any febrile resident or traveler with exposure in an endemic region. The diagnosis is confirmed by identifying parasites in thick or thin blood smears. (*Adapted from* White et al. [5].)

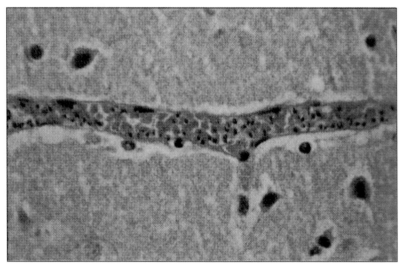

**FIGURE 12-8** Histologic section of brain tissue in cerebral malaria. Much of the damage done by *Plasmodium falciparum* comes from local anoxia, due to the cytoadherence of *P. falciparum*–parasitized erythrocytes in capillaries and venules and the release of cytokines. *P. falciparum* is shown lining venules in the brain of a patient who died of cerebral malaria. (*Courtesy of* M. Aikawa, MD; *from* Miller et al. [6]; with permission.)

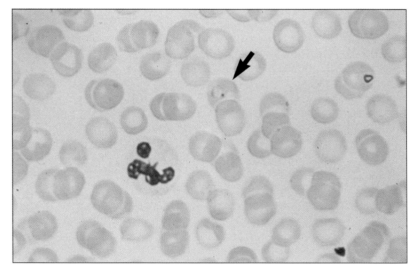

**FIGURE 12-9** *Plasmodium falciparum* ring-form. *P. falciparum* infection, which can be life threatening, is characterized by delicate ring-forms (*arrow*), high levels of parasitemia, multiple parasites within infected erythrocytes, and double chromatin bodies, but none of these findings allows for a species-specific diagnosis.

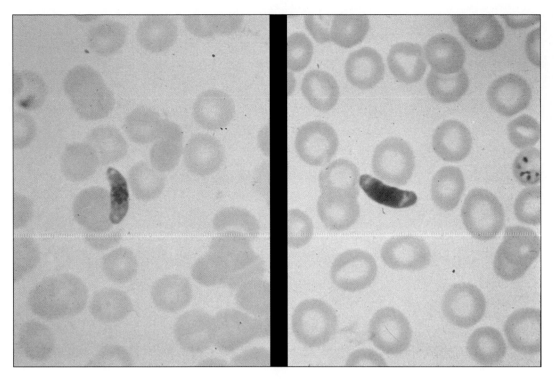

**FIGURE 12-10** *Plasmodium falciparum*, gametocytes. The gametocytes of *P. falciparum* are banana-shaped, in contrast to the gametocytes of *P. vivax*, *P. ovale*, and *P. malariae*, all of which are round. (*From* Smith *et al.* [7]; with permission.)

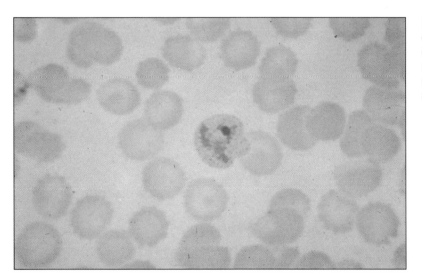

**FIGURE 12-11** *Plasmodium vivax*, amoeboid trophozoite. *P. vivax* is endemic in many rural areas of Central and South America. All stages of asexual development, including ring-forms, amoeboid tropho-zoites, and schizonts, may be seen in peripheral blood. Schuffner's dots, brown pigmented granules, are found in *P. vivax*–infected erythrocytes. (*From* Smith *et al.* [7]; with permission.)

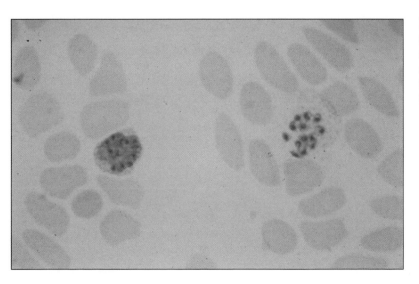

**FIGURE 12-12** *Plasmodium vivax*, schizont, and merozoites. After a period of growth in the erythrocyte, parasites undergo nuclear division followed by segmentation (*left*), a process known as *schizogony*. Individual merozoites are released when the infected erythrocyte ruptures (*right*). Merozoites subsequently invade uninfected erythrocytes. (*From* Smith *et al.* [7]; with permission.)

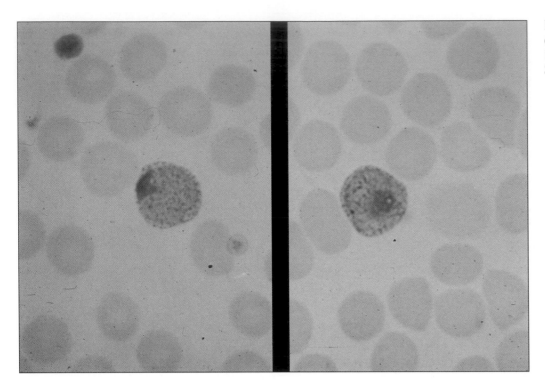

**FIGURE 12-13** *Plasmodium vivax*, gametocyte. The gametocytes of *P. vivax* are round, in contrast to those of *P. falciparum*. (*From* Smith *et al.* [7]; with permission.)

**A. Treatment of malaria: Chloroquine-resistant** *Plasmodium falciparum* **malaria**

| | | Adults | Children |
|---|---|---|---|
| **Oral** | | | |
| Drugs of choice | Quinine sulfate *plus* pyrimethamine-sulfadoxine | 650 mg every 8 hrs × 3–7 days | 25 mg/kg/day in 3 doses × 3–7 days |
| | | Three tablets at once on last day of quinine | < 1 yr: 1/4 tablet |
| | | | 1–3 yrs: 1/2 tablet |
| | | | 4–8 yrs: 1 tablet |
| | | | 9–14 yrs: 2 tablets |
| | *or plus* tetracycline* | 250 mg four times a day × 7 days | > 8 yrs: 20 mg/kg/day in 4 doses × 7 days* |
| | *or plus* clindamycin[†] | 900 mg three times a day × 3–5 days | 20–40 mg/kg/day in 3 doses × 3–5 days |
| Alternatives | Mefloquine | 750 mg, then 500 mg 6–8 hrs later | 25 mg/kg once (< 45 kg) |
| | Halofantrine[‡] | 500 mg every 6 hrs × 3 doses; repeat in 1 wk | 8 mg/kg every 6 hrs × 3 doses (< 40 kg); repeat in 1 wk |
| **Parenteral** | | | |
| Drug of choice | Quinidine gluconate[§] | 10 mg/kg loading dose (max 600 mg) in normal saline slowly over 1–2 hrs, followed by continuous infusion of 0.02 mg/kg/min until oral therapy can be started | Same as adult dose |
| | *or* | | |
| | Quinine dihydrochloride[§] | 20 mg/kg loading dose in 10 mg/kg 5% dextrose over 4 hrs, followed by 10 mg/kg over 2–4 hrs every 8 hrs (max 1800 mg/day) until oral therapy can be started | Same as adult dose |

*Not recommended for children < 8 yrs of age and pregnant women.

[†]In pregnancy.

[‡]Causes dose-related lengthening of *PR* and *QTc* intervals. Sudden deaths have been reported. Cardiac monitoring is recommended.

[§]Continuous electrocardiographic, blood pressure, and glucose monitoring recommended.

**FIGURE 12-14** Treatment of malaria. The optimal treatment of malaria depends on the infecting *Plasmodium* species and its sensitivity to chemotherapeutic agents, which varies among geographic areas. The treatment recommendations must be revised periodically because of increasing antimicrobial resistance around the world. **A,** Treatment of chloroquine-resistant *Plasmodium falciparum* malaria. (*continued*)

## B. Treatment of malaria: Chloroquine-sensitive *Plasmodium* malaria

| | Adults | Children |
|---|---|---|
| **Oral** | | |
| Chloroquine phosphate | 1 gm (600 mg base), then 500 mg (300 mg base) 6 hrs later, then 500 mg (300 mg base) at 24 and 48 hrs | 10 mg base/kg (max 600 mg base), then 5 mg base/kg 6 hrs later, then 5 mg base/kg at 24 and 48 hrs |
| **Parenteral** | | |
| Quinidine gluconate | Same as above | Same as above |
| *or* quinine dihydrochloride | Same as above | Same as above |

## C. Treatment of malaria: Prevention of relapses (*P. vivax* and *P. ovale* only)

| | Adults | Children |
|---|---|---|
| Primaquine phosphate*† | 26.3 mg (15 mg base)/day × 14 days *or* 79 mg (45 mg base)/wk × 8 wks | 0.3 mg base/kg/day × 14 days |

*Primaquine can cause hemolytic anemia in persons with glucose-6-phosphate dehydrogenase deficiency. It should not be used during pregnancy.

†Some relapses have been reported with this regimen; relapses should be treated with chloroquine plus primaquine, 22.5 to 30 mg base/day × 14 days.

**FIGURE 12-14** (*continued*) **B,** Treatment of chloroquine-sensitive *Plasmodium* malaria. **C,** Prevention of relapses (*P. vivax* and *P. ovale* only). (*Adapted from* [8].)

## Chemoprophylaxis regimens for malaria

| | Adults | Children |
|---|---|---|
| **Chloroquine-sensitive areas** | | |
| Drug of choice | | |
| Chloroquine phosphate | 500 mg (300 mg base), once/wk* | 5 mg/kg base once/wk, up to adult dose of 300 mg base |
| **Chloroquine-resistant areas** | | |
| Drug of choice | | |
| Mefloquine | 250 mg once/wk* | 15–19 kg: 1/4 tablet 20–30 kg: 1/2 tablet 31–45 kg: 3/4 tablet >45 kg: 1 tablet |
| *or* doxycycline† | 100 mg daily† | > 8 yrs: 2 mg/kg/d, up to 100 mg/day |
| Alternatives | | |
| Chloroquine phosphate *plus* pyrimethamine-sulfadoxine for presumptive treatment | Same as above Carry a single dose (3 tablets) for self-treatment of febrile illness when medical care is not immediately available | Same as above < 1 yr: 1/4 tablet 1–3 yrs: 1/2 tablet 4–8 yrs: 1 tablet 9–14 yrs: 2 tablets |
| *or plus* proguanil‡ (in Africa south of Sahara) | 200 mg daily | < 2 yrs: 50 mg daily 2–6 yrs: 100 mg daily 7–10 yrs: 150 mg daily > 10 yrs: 200 mg daily |

*Beginning 1 week before travel and continuing weekly for the duration of stay and for 4 weeks after leaving.

†Beginning 1 day before travel and continuing for the duration of stay and for 4 weeks after leaving. Use of tetracyclines is contraindicated in pregnancy and in children less than 8 years of age. Doxycycline can cause gastrointestinal disturbances, vaginal moniliasis, and photosensitivity reactions.

‡Proguanil (Paludrine–Ayerst, Canada; ICI, England), which is not available in the United States but is widely available overseas, is recommended mainly for use in Africa south of the Sahara. Prophylaxis is recommended during exposure and for 4 weeks afterward. Failures in prophylaxis with chloroquine and proguanil have been reported in travelers to Kenya.

**FIGURE 12-15** Chemoprophylaxis regimens for malaria. Malaria is transmitted by *Anopheles* mosquitoes. Measures that limit mosquito exposure can decrease the risk of transmission. These include remaining in well-screened areas or wearing long-sleeve shirts and long pants at peak anopheles feeding times (between dusk and dawn); sleeping under mosquito nets; and the judicious use of insect repellents on exposed skin (formulations with 30%–35% DEET) or clothing (permethrin). In addition, chemoprophylaxis is necessary. Recommendations by country are updated yearly in the Centers for Disease Control and Prevention's *Health Information for International Travel* [3]. (Adapted from [8].)

# *Leishmania* Species (Leishmaniasis)

## Clinical variants of leishmaniasis in Latin America

| Clinical syndromes | *Leishmania* spp | Location |
|---|---|---|
| Visceral leishmaniasis | | |
| Kala-azar: generalized involvement | *L. (L.) chagasi* | Latin America |
| of the reticuloendothelial system | *L. (L.) amazonesis* | Brazil (Bahia) |
| | | |
| New-world cutaneous leishmaniasis | | |
| Single or limited skin lesions | *L. (L.) mexicana* (chiclero ulcer) | Mexico, Central America, Texas |
| | *L. (L.) amazonensis* | Amazon basin, neighboring areas, Bahia and other states in Brazil |
| | *L. (L.) pifanoi* | Venezuela |
| | *L. (L.) garnhami* | Venezuela |
| | *L. (L.) venezuelensis* | Venezuela |
| | *L. (Viannia) braziliensis* | Multiple areas of Latin America |
| | *L. (V.) guyanensis* (Forest yaws) | Guyana, Suriname, northern Amazon basin |
| | *L. (V.) peruviana* (uta) | Peru (western Andes), Argentinian highlands |
| | *L. (V.) panamensis* | Panama, Costa Rica, Columbia |
| | *L. (L.) chagasi* | Latin America |
| Diffuse cutaneous leishmaniasis | *L. (L.) amazonensis* | Amazon basin, neighboring areas, Bahia and other states in Brazil |
| | *L. (L.) pifanoi* | Venezuela |
| | *L. (L.) mexicana* | Mexico, Central America, Texas |
| | *Leishmania (L.)* spp | Dominican Republic |
| Mucosal leishmaniasis | *L. (V.) braziliensis* | Multiple areas in Latin America |
| (Espundia) | Other *Leishmania* spp (rare) | Multiple areas in Latin America |

**FIGURE 12-16** Clinical variants of leishmaniasis in Latin America. *Leishmania* species are enzootic in scattered areas across Central and South America. *Lutzomyia* sandflies are responsible for transmission. In most instances, leishmaniasis is a zoonosis involving rodents in forested areas or, in the case of *L. chagasi*, domestic dogs, wild foxes, and possibly humans as reservoirs. The clinical manifestations depend on complex interactions between the virulence factors of the infecting *Leishmania* species and the immune responses of its human host. The clinical spectrum includes visceral, cutaneous, and mucosal leishmaniasis. Although individual *Leishmania* species tend to produce the same clinical syndrome, there are many exceptions. For example, *L. chagasi*, which usually causes visceral leishmaniasis, has been isolated from skin ulcers in patients with simple cutaneous leishmaniasis, and *L. amazonensis*, which usually causes cutaneous disease, has been isolated from patients with visceral leishmaniasis [9].

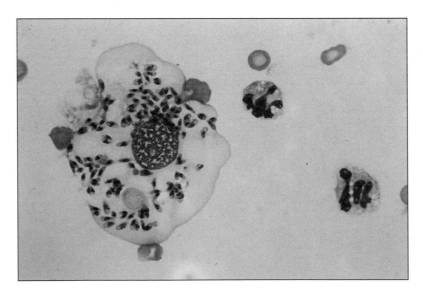

**FIGURE 12-17** *Leishmania* amastigotes in an infected macrophage (Wright-Giemsa stain), seen in a cytocentrifuged preparation of pleural fluid from a patient with visceral leishmaniasis and AIDS. *Leishmania* exist within mononuclear phagocytes as intracellular amastigotes. Although slight ultrastructural differences exist among amastigotes of different *Leishmania* species, they are not sufficient to allow for species-specific identification [10]. (*Courtesy of* D.M. Markovitz, MD, and R.F. Betts, MD.)

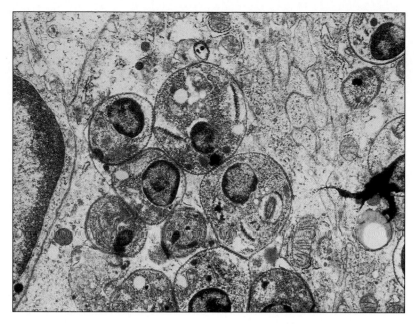

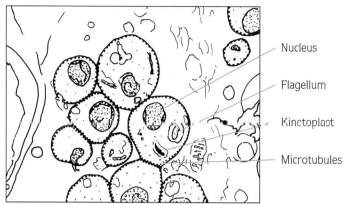

**FIGURE 12-18** Electron micrograph of *Leishmania* amastigotes in a human mononuclear phagocyte infected *in vitro*. Amastigotes are 2 × 3 μm in diameter and oval or round in shape. They have an eccentrically located nucleus, a bar-shaped specialized mitochondrial structure (kinetoplast), and a flagellum that lies within a flagellar pocket. A layer of microtubules is present under the plasma membrane. A dividing amastigote is seen in the center, lower half of the micrograph.

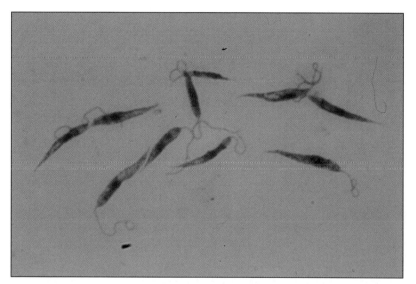

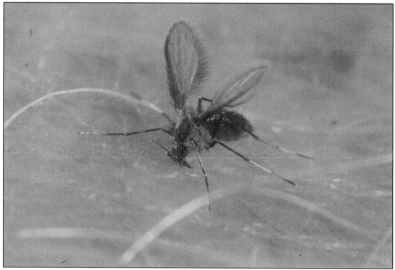

**FIGURE 12-19** *Leishmania* promastigotes (Wright-Giemsa stain). *Leishmania* exist as extracellular promastigotes in the gut of their sandfly vectors and in axenic cultures maintained at 24° to 26° C.

**FIGURE 12-20** Phlebotomine sandfly (*Lutzomyia longipalpus*). *Lutzomyia* species are responsible for transmitting *Leishmania* species in Latin America. Sandflies are modified pool-feeders and ingest amastigotes in macrophages. *Leishmania* convert to promastigotes in the sandfly gut and then go through a series of developmental stages before infective metacyclic promastigotes migrate to the proboscis. They are transmitted when infected phlebotomine sandflies attempt to take their next blood meal. (*Courtesy of* E.D. Rowton.)

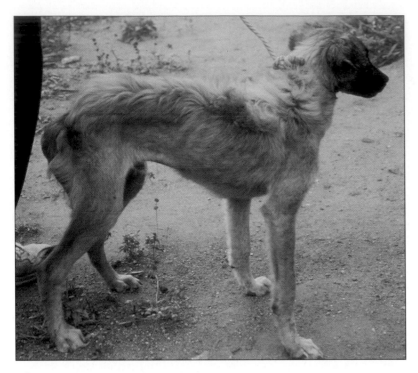

**FIGURE 12-21** *Leishmania (L.) chagasi*–infected domestic dog in northeastern Brazil. Leishmaniasis is a zoonosis in most geographic areas. The domestic dog, wild fox, and possibly infected humans serve as reservoirs of *L. (L.) chagasi* in northeastern Brazil. A number of rodent species are reservoirs of *L. (L.) mexicana* and *L. (Vianna) braziliensis*.

## *Cutaneous leishmaniasis*

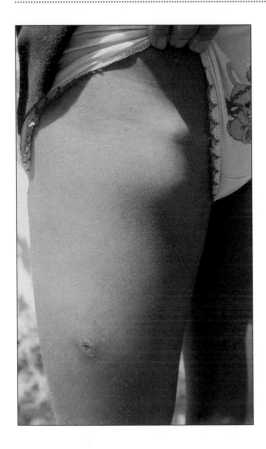

**FIGURE 12-22** Early American cutaneous leishmaniasis with associated regional lymphadenopathy due to *Leishmania (Vianna) braziliensis*. A number of *Leishmania* species can produce cutaneous leishmaniasis. The skin lesion develops weeks to months after promastigotes are inoculated by an infected sandfly. Some persons infected with *L. (V.) braziliensis*, such as this patient, develop regional lymphadenopathy, fever, malaise, and constitutional symptoms prior to the appearance of the skin lesion. The systemic findings resolve as the skin lesion develops.

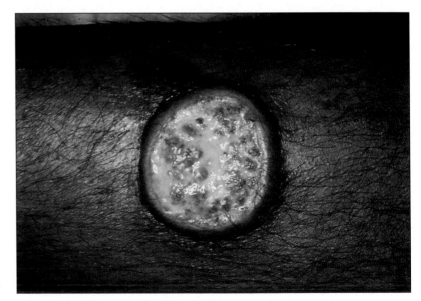

**FIGURE 12-23** Cutaneous leishmaniasis due to *Leishmania (Vianna) braziliensis*. The classic leishmanial lesion has a central area of ulceration, overlying exudate, and raised margin, with a "pizza-like" appearance.

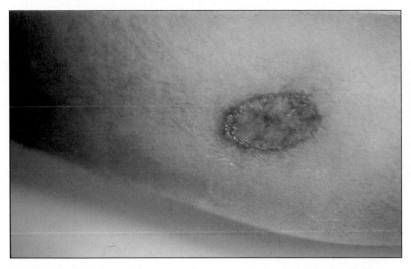

**FIGURE 12-24** Healing lesion of cutaneous leishmaniasis. Cutaneous leishmaniasis persists for several months (variable) before healing occurs.

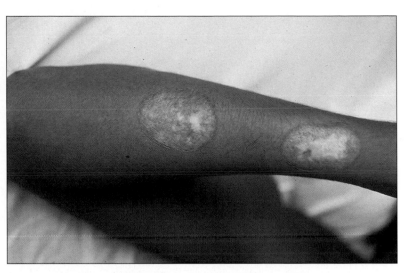

**FIGURE 12-25** Healed cutaneous leishmaniasis. Patients are left with nonspecific, flat, atrophic, burnlike scars as evidence of disease.

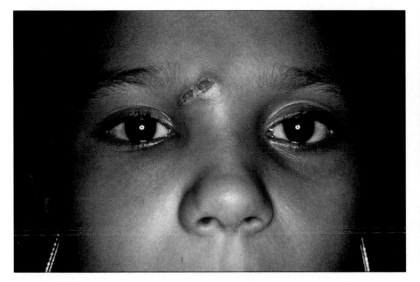

**FIGURE 12-26** American cutaneous leishmaniasis involving the face. The appearance of cutaneous leishmaniasis varies widely. The clinical manifestations depend on a complex interplay between the infecting *Leishmania* species and the cell-mediated immune responses of the host.

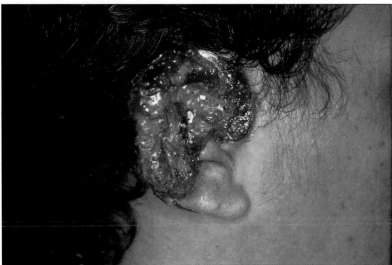

**FIGURE 12-27** American cutaneous leishmaniasis involving the ear. Such involvement is common in Mexico, where it is known as "chiclero ulcer."

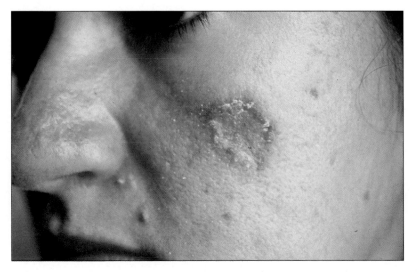

**FIGURE 12-28** American cutaneous leishmaniasis on a patient's cheek. Not all infections result in ulceration. Cutaneous leishmaniasis must be considered in the differential diagnosis of any chronic skin lesion in a person who has been exposed in an endemic area.

## *Mucosal leishmaniasis*

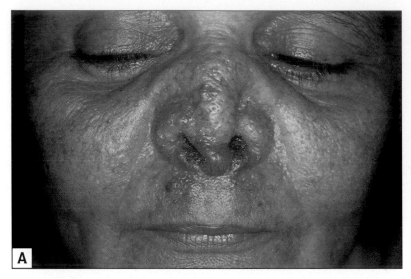

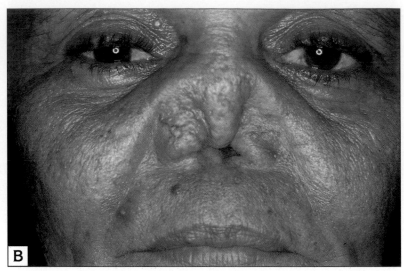

**FIGURE 12-29** American mucosal leishmaniasis due to *Leishmania (Vianna) braziliensis* with involvement of the nasal septum. **A,** A small subset of persons with skin lesions due to *L. (V.) braziliensis* manifest mucosal disease months to years after the initial cutaneous lesion(s) resolves. Those affected frequently present with chronic nasal stuffiness. **B,** The patient is seen after chemotherapy with meglumine antimoniate, a pentavalent antimonial. The nasal septum was destroyed during infection, and the bridge of the nose has collapsed.

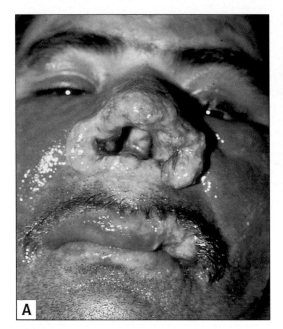

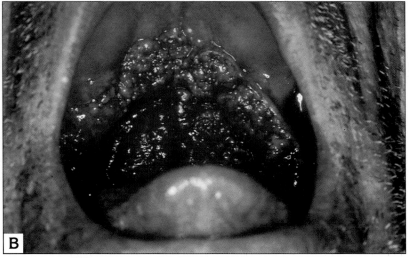

**FIGURE 12-30** American mucosal leishmaniasis involving the nose, lips, cheeks, and palate. **A** and **B,** Although deaths are rare with mucosal leishmaniasis, morbidity can be severe, as illustrated by these patients [11].

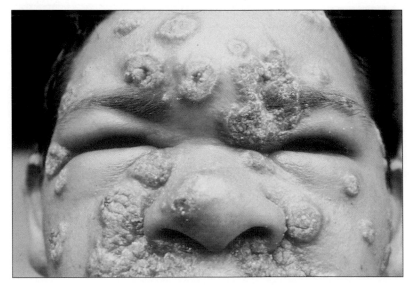

**FIGURE 12-31** Diffuse cutaneous leishmaniasis. A small percentage of patients infected with *Leishmania (L.) mexicana* develop diffuse cutaneous leishmaniasis, an anergic variant of cutaneous leishmaniasis. Skin lesions contain large numbers of amastigote-infected macrophages.

## *Visceral leishmaniasis*

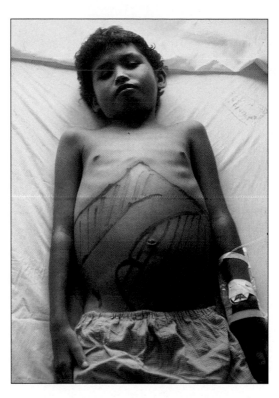

**FIGURE 12-32**
American visceral leishmaniasis with hepatosplenomegaly due to *Leishmania (L.) chagasi*. Amastigotes are found in macrophages throughout the reticuloendothelial system in persons with visceral leishmaniasis. The spleen is often massively enlarged.

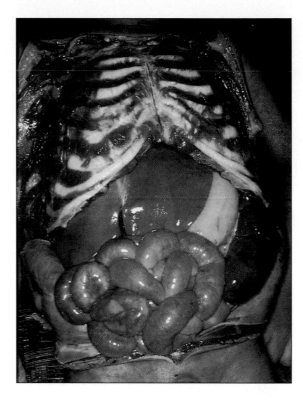

**FIGURE 12-33**
Autopsy of a child who died of visceral leishmaniasis due to *Leishmania (L.) chagasi*. Note the massive enlargement of the spleen and liver.

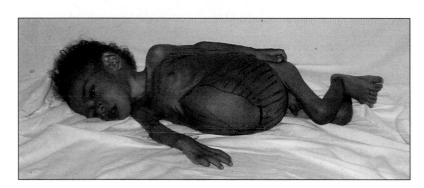

**FIGURE 12-34** Severe wasting associated with visceral leishmaniasis due to *Leishmania (L.) chagasi*. Evidence from animal models suggests that wasting is due to cytokines such as tumor necrosis factor/cachectin. (*From* [12]; with permission.)

# *Trypanosoma cruzi* (Chagas' Disease)

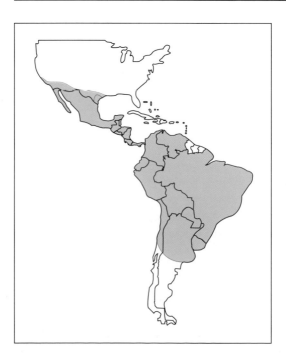

**FIGURE 12-35** Distribution of *Trypanosoma cruzi* (Chagas' disease). *T. cruzi*, the cause of Chagas' disease, is widely distributed in rural areas extending from the southern United States to central Argentina. Autochthonous transmission is rare in the United States. (*Adapted from* Kirchhoff [13].)

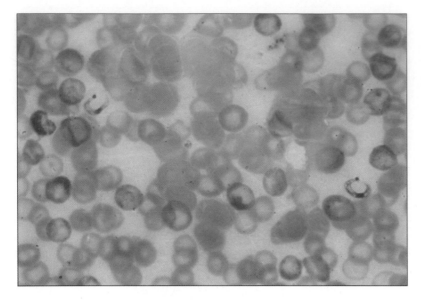

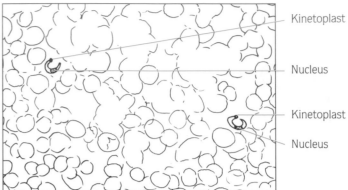

**FIGURE 12-36** *Trypanosoma cruzi* trypomastigotes in the peripheral blood of a person with Chagas' disease. *T. cruzi* is an important cause of morbidity and mortality in many impoverished rural areas of Latin America.

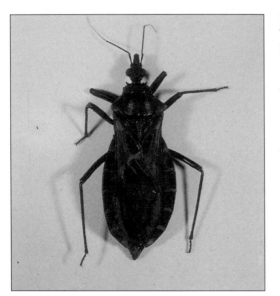

**FIGURE 12-37** Triatome (reduviid bug) vector of *Trypanosoma cruzi*. Members of the Triatominae subfamily of the family Reduviidae are responsible for transmitting *T. cruzi*.

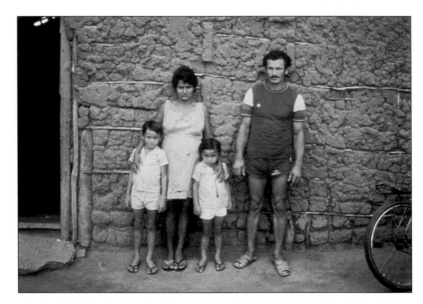

**FIGURE 12-38** Typical adobe house in an area endemic for *Trypanosoma cruzi* in northeastern Brazil. Thousands of reduviid bugs live in the walls of such adobe dwellings and feed on blood while the human hosts sleep. The bugs defecate as they take a blood meal. Metacyclic trypomastigotes in the feces are scratched into the bite site or enter through the conjunctivae.

**FIGURE 12-39** Romaña's sign. A woman shows unilateral swelling about the eye, a typical early finding in Chagas' disease, which results when metacyclic trypomastigotes enter the body via the conjunctiva. (*Courtesy of* E. Kuschnir, MD.)

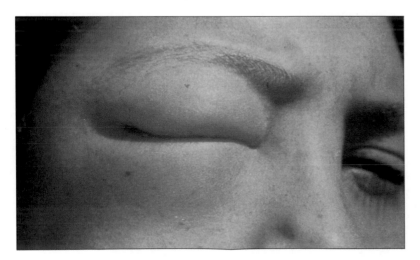

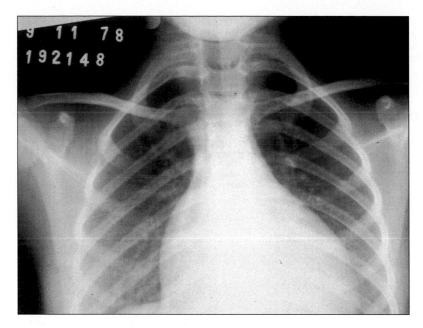

**FIGURE 12-40** Cardiomegaly in a patient with chronic Chagas' disease. Although acute *Trypanosoma cruzi* infections can be fatal, most are asymptomatic or mild and resolve spontaneously. However, parasitemia can persist for decades. A subset of infected persons develop chagasic cardiomyopathy with congestive heart failure, conduction abnormalities, arrhythmias, and thromboemboli.

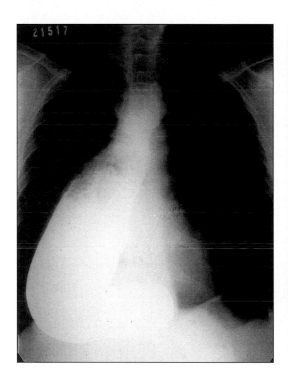

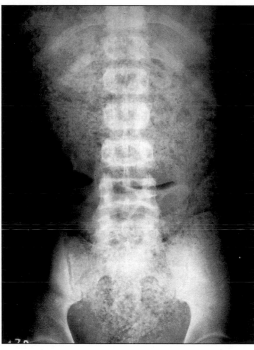

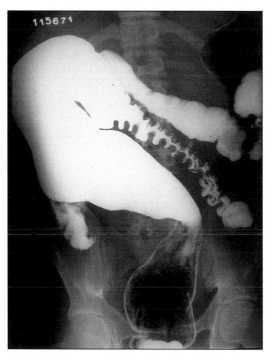

**FIGURE 12-41** Barium swallow demonstrating megaesophagus in chronic Chagas' disease. Progressive esophageal dilatation occurs as a result of autoimmune destruction of the myenteric plexus. Affected persons experience dysphagia, odynophagia, chest pain, and regurgitation. Aspiration pneumonia can complicate advanced disease.

**FIGURE 12-42** Abdominal radiograph showing retained feces in a patient with megacolon due to chronic Chagas' disease. Megacolon results from the destruction of the myenteric plexus. Constipation and abdominal pain are common symptoms.

**FIGURE 12-43** Barium enema demonstrating chagasic megacolon.

# SYSTEMIC MANIFESTATIONS OF INTESTINAL NEMATODES

## Important intestinal roundworm infections of humans

| Infection | Mode of transmission | Superfamily | Species infecting humans | Infective stage | Final habitat |
|---|---|---|---|---|---|
| Trichuriasis | Direct | Trichuroidea | *Trichuris trichiura* | Eggs | Large intestines |
| Enterobiasis | Direct | Oxyuroidea | *Enterobius vermicularis* | Eggs | Cecum |
| Ascariasis | Modified direct | Ascaroidea | *Ascaris lumbricoides* | Mature eggs | Small intestines |
| Hookworm | Skin penetration | Strongyloidea | *Ancylostoma duodenale* | Larvae | Small intestines |
| | | | *Necator americanus* | Larvae | Small intestines |
| Strongyloidiasis | Skin penetration | Rhabditoidea | *Strongyloides stercoralis* | Larvae | Small intestines |

**FIGURE 12-44** Important intestinal roundworm (nematode) infections of humans. A number of important intestinal nematodes (roundworms) are endemic in Latin America. *Ascaris lumbricoides*, *Necator americanus*, and *Trichuris trichiura* are prevalent where sanitation and hygiene are poor. The adult worms of these species typically reside in the human intestinal tract. Ova are excreted in the stool. (*Adapted from* Mahmoud [1].)

## *Ascaris lumbricoides* (Ascariasis)

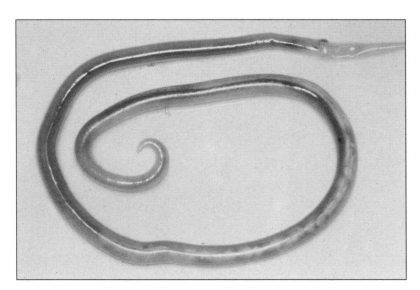

**FIGURE 12-45** Adult *Ascaris lumbricoides*. Adult *Ascaris* can migrate from the intestine to produce biliary tract obstruction or pancreatitis. On occasion, they emerge from the nose or are coughed up, much to the chagrin of the host. Adult *Ascaris* are white or pink. Males range from 10 to 31 cm in length and females from 22 to 35 cm. *Ascaris* is the only human pathogen that resembles an earthworm in size and shape. (*From* Pearson [14]; with permission.)

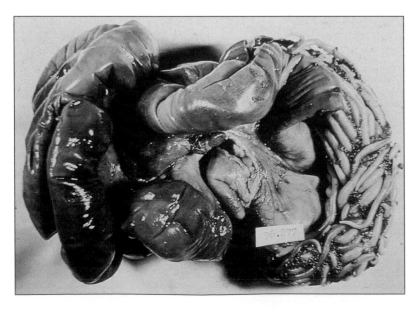

**FIGURE 12-46** Intestinal obstruction due to an entangled mass of *Ascaris lumbricoides*. Symptoms of intestinal obstruction with *Ascaris* include crampy abdominal pain, distension, and vomiting. (*From* Smith *et al.* [7]; with permission.)

## *Strongyloides* Species (Strongyloidiasis)

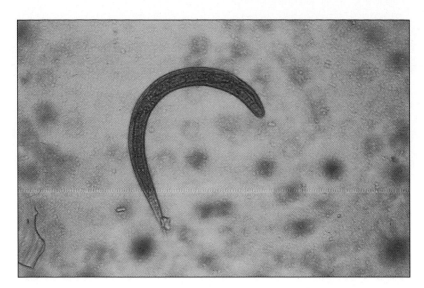

**FIGURE 12-47** Rhabditiform larva of *Strongyloides stercoralis* in stool. *S. stercoralis* can persist for decades in humans due to autoinfection. Persons who become immunocompromised, particularly following organ transplantation, may develop hyperinfection as rhabditiform convert to filariform larvae in the gastrointestinal tract. From there, they can invade in massive numbers through the intestinal wall, resulting in pneumonia, polymicrobial sepsis, or polymicrobial meningitis. (*Courtesy of* R.L. Guerrant, MD)

## *Trichinella spiralis* (Trichinosis)

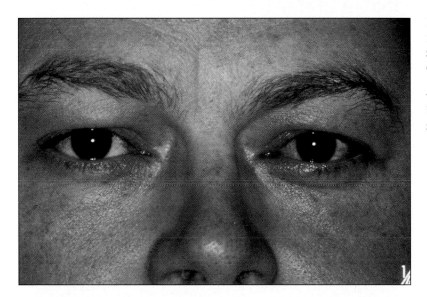

**FIGURE 12-48** Periorbital edema and conjunctival injection in a man with trichinosis. Trichinosis is characterized by the triad of severe myalgia, eosinophilia, and periorbital edema. Most cases develop following ingestion of inadequately cooked pork, but *Trichinella spiralis* is also found in bear, walrus, and other carnivores. The diagnosis of trichinosis can be confirmed by muscle biopsy, but that is seldom necessary, or by serology, but it takes several weeks for antibodies to develop [15]. (*Courtesy of* W.A. Petri, Jr, MD, PhD.)

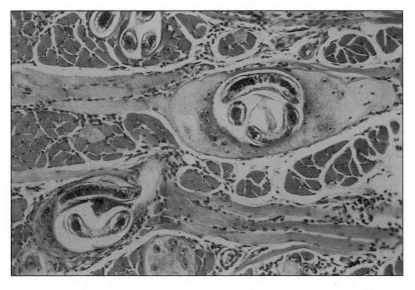

**FIGURE 12-49** Infective larvae of *Trichinella spiralis* in tissue section of tongue. Infective larvae are approximately 1 mm long and become adults within a few days after ingestion. (Hematoxylin-eosin stain). (*From* Smith *et al.* [7]; with permission.)

## *Ancylostoma* Species (Hookworm)

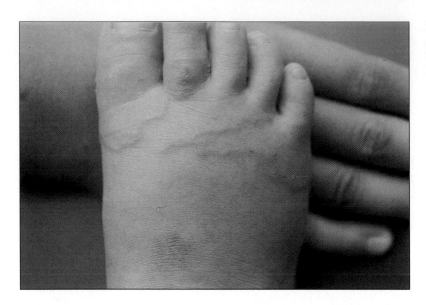

**FIGURE 12-50** Cutaneous larva migrans. *Ancylostoma braziliensis*, and other nematodes whose definitive hosts are animals, can invade human skin but wander beneath it, unable to complete their life cycle. They produce serpiginous, erythematous, pruritic tracts.

# MANIFESTATIONS OF TISSUE NEMATODES

## *Onchocerca volvulus* (Onchocerciasis)

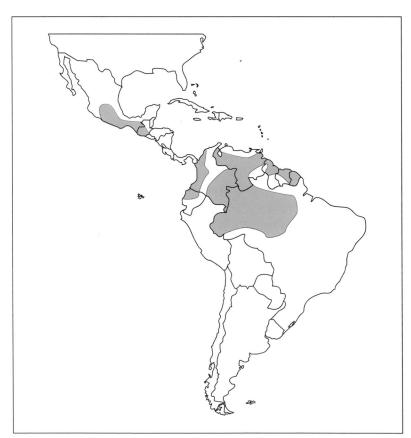

**FIGURE 12-51** Distribution of *Onchocerca volvulus* (onchocerciasis) in Latin America. Onchocerciasis is found in several areas of Central America and northern South America. *Simulium* blackflies, which breed in rapidly flowing water, are responsible for transmission.

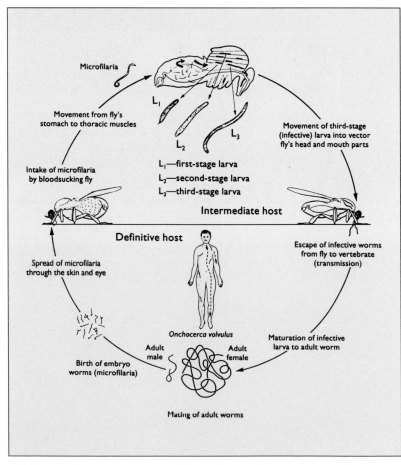

**FIGURE 12-52** Life cycle of *Onchocerca volvulus*. The life cycle of *Onchocerca volvulus* includes the blackfly *Simulium* species and humans. The adult worms can produce palpable subcutaneous nodules in humans, but the important manifestations of disease are caused by microfilariae in the skin and eye. (*Courtesy of* M. Trpis, MD.)

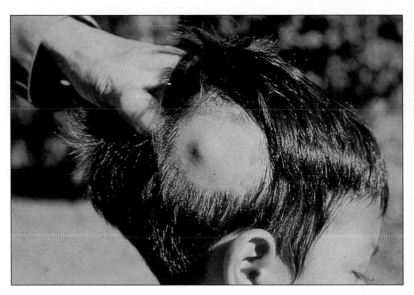

**FIGURE 12-53** Subcutaneous nodule due to *Onchocerca volvulus* infection. Onchocerciasis is endemic in several areas of Latin America. Adult worm pairs form nodules in the subcutaneous tissue. (*From* Smith *et al.* [7]; with permission.)

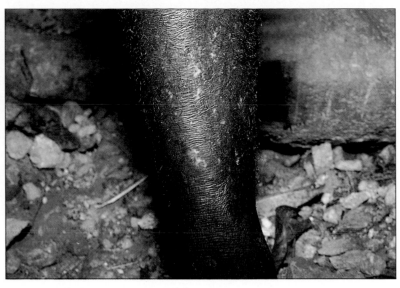

**FIGURE 12-54** Altered skin pigmentation and wrinkling due to onchocerciasis. Microfilariae of *Onchocerca volvulus* can produce substantial pruritus. Chronic skin changes include depigmentation (leopard skin), lichenification, wrinkling, and atrophy. (*Courtesy of* M. Trpis, MD.)

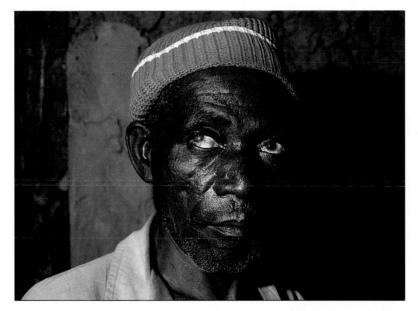

**FIGURE 12-55** Blindness due to onchocerciasis. The most important impact of onchocerciasis is on vision. This patient is blind in the right eye and has impaired vision in the left. The ocular damage of onchocerciasis is largely irreversible. (*Courtesy of* M. Trpis, MD.)

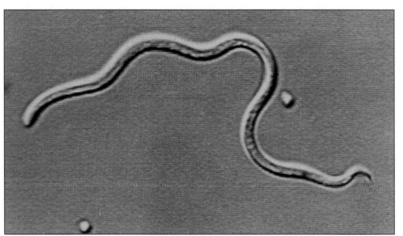

**FIGURE 12-56** Electron micrograph of microfilaria of *Onchocerca volvulus*. A Nomarski photomicrograph shows a microfilaria from the skin of a patient with onchocerciasis. Microfilariae, which range from 220 to 260 μm by 5 to 9 μm, are responsible for inflammation and damage in the skin and eye. (*From* Joyce and Pearson [16]; with permission.)

# *Wuchereria bancrofti* (Bancroftian Filariasis)

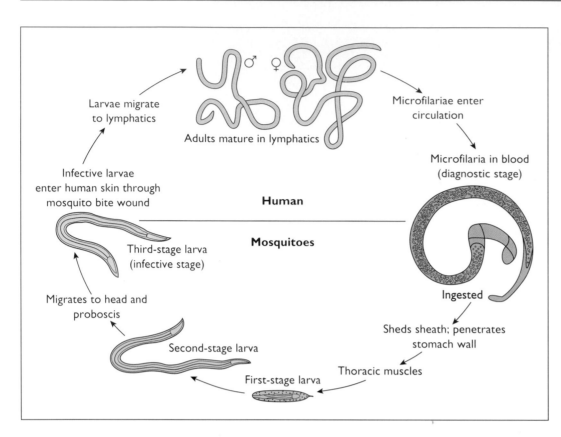

Larvae migrate to lymphatics

Adults mature in lymphatics

Microfilariae enter circulation

Infective larvae enter human skin through mosquito bite wound

Microfilaria in blood (diagnostic stage)

**Human**

**Mosquitoes**

Third-stage larva (infective stage)

Migrates to head and proboscis

Ingested

Sheds sheath; penetrates stomach wall

Second-stage larva

Thoracic muscles

First-stage larva

**FIGURE 12-57** Life cycle of *Wuchereria bancrofti*. Microfilariae enter the human host through a mosquito bite. Developing larvae migrate to the human lymphatics (where they produce clinical lymphadenopathy, often visible in the inguinal area) and, over the course of 1 year, mature, mate, and produce microfilariae. These microfilariae circulate in the bloodstream, where they are withdrawn by another mosquito. The larvae develop through three metamorphic stages in the thoracic musculature of the mosquito, over 6 to 20 days, before migrating to the mosquito's head and proboscis for transmission to another human. (*Adapted from* Muller [17].)

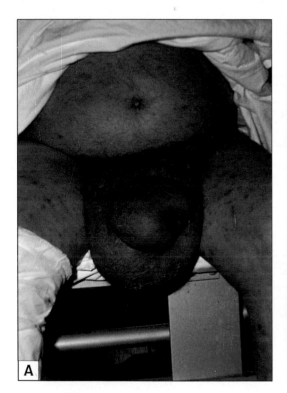

**A**

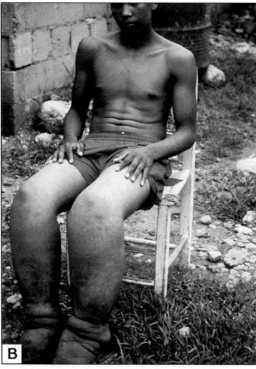

**B**

**FIGURE 12-58** Tissue enlargement in lymphatic filariasis. Chronic infection is associated with lymph stasis, fibrosis, and development of collateral circulation, with continued tissue growth; ultimately, massive growth and enlargement result. **A**, Scrotal edema with marked genital enlargement in filariasis. **B**, Lymphedema involving both lower extremities in a young man from the Dominican Republic. (Panel 58A *courtesy of* M. Wittner, MD, PhD; panel 58B *courtesy of* A.L. Vincent, PhD.)

# MANIFESTATIONS OF TREMATODES

## Important trematodes in Latin America

*Schistosoma mansoni* (schistosomiasis)
*Fasciola hepatica* (fascioliasis)
*Paragonimus westermani* (paragonimiasis)

**FIGURE 12-59** Important trematodes in Latin America. Of the trematodes, or flukes, *Schistosoma mansoni* is the most important cause of disease in Latin America. Cercariae invade through skin when persons swim or bath in infected water.

## *Schistosoma mansoni* (Schistosomiasis)

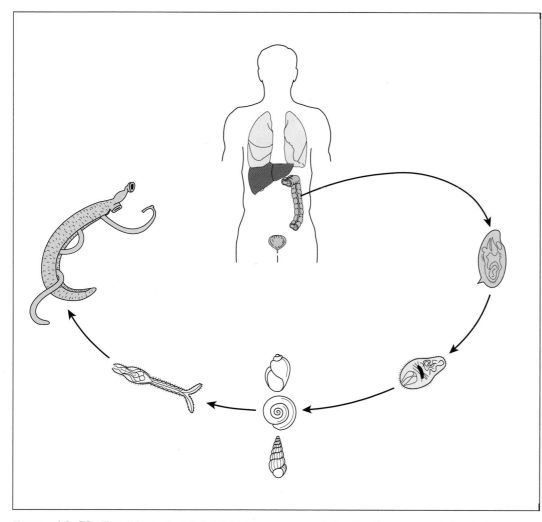

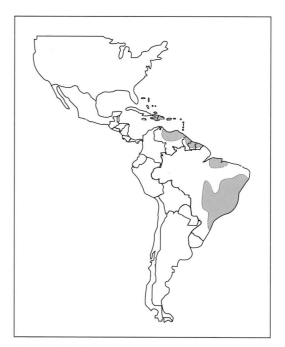

**FIGURE 12-61** Distribution of *Schistosoma mansoni* in the Americas. Schistosomiasis is endemic in some islands of the Caribbean and in multiple areas of northern and eastern South America. (*Adapted from* Laughlin [19]).

**FIGURE 12-60** The life cycle of *Schistosoma mansoni*. Snails, the reservoir host, become infected when ova in human feces reach freshwater and hatch, releasing miracidia, which invade snails. Forked-tailed cercariae invade humans when they come in contact with freshwater during agricultural or recreational activities. (*Adapted from* Mahmoud [18].)

## Clinical manifestations of *Schistosoma mansoni* infection

Schistosome dermatitis
    Onset within 24 hrs of invasion by cercariae
    Pruritic papular eruption on exposed skin (swimmer's itch)
Acute schistosomiasis (Katayama fever)
    Onset 4–8 wks after infection
    Fever, chills, headache, malaise, fatigue, other constitutional symptoms
    Lymphadenopathy and mild hepatosplenomegaly
    Eosinophilia
    Symptoms usually resolve spontaneously within a few weeks
Chronic schistosomiasis
    Asymptomatic (common in persons with low parasite burdens)
    Intestinal—fatigue, abdominal pain, intermittent diarrhea, anemia, granulomatous
      lesions in bowel, colonic polyps
    Hepatic—hepatomegaly, portal hypertension with splenomegaly, abdominal pain,
      portosystemic collateral circulation, esophageal varices, hematemesis
    Pulmonary—cor pulmonale due to inflammatory response to eggs shunted to the
      lungs through portosystemic collaterals
    Central nervous system (rare)—transverse myelitis due to eggs in spinal cord

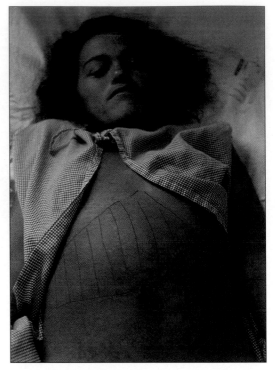

**FIGURE 12-62** Clinical manifestations of *Schistosoma mansoni* infection. *S. mansoni* can produce schistosome dermatitis (swimmer's itch), which occurs within 24 hours of penetration by cercariae. Acute schistosomiasis (Katayama fever) is a serum sickness–like syndrome that develops 4 to 8 weeks after invasion and is associated with the onset of ova production. Chronic schistosomiasis may be asymptomatic, particularly in patients with low parasite burdens. Heavy infections can result in abdominal pain and intermittent diarrhea due to involvement of the intestines; hepatomegaly resulting from the granulomatous response to eggs that reach the liver; portal hypertension and accompanying findings such as splenomegaly and esophageal varices; cor pulmonale; and rarely, involvement of the spinal cord resulting in transverse myelitis.

**FIGURE 12-63** Hepatosplenic schistosomiasis due to *Schistosoma mansoni* infection. Adult schistosomes live and produce eggs in mesenteric vessels. Infection is perpetuated when the eggs, which secrete lytic enzymes, gain entrance to the lumen of the bowel and are excreted in feces. However, many eggs are swept back to the liver through the portal circulation, where they can elicit an inflammatory reaction and fibrosis that result in hepatomegaly.

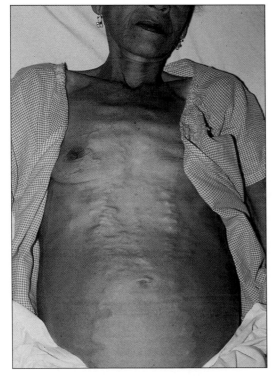

**FIGURE 12-64** Advanced hepatosplenic schistosomiasis due to *Schistosoma mansoni*, with portal-systemic shunting through abdominal veins. Progressive periportal fibrosis results in portal hypertension and shunting through superficial abdominal veins as well as esophageal varices.

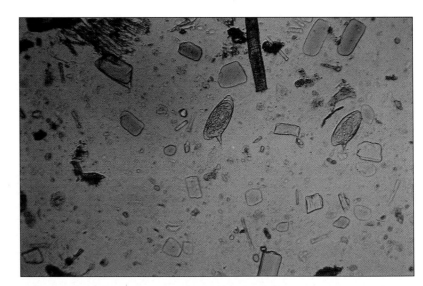

**FIGURE 12-65** Ova of *Schistosoma mansoni* in stool (iodine stain). Note the relatively thin, yellowish, transparent shell with the prominent, sharply pointed lateral spine. A miracidium is within the egg. In wet mounts, tapping the coverslip to reorient eggs so that the lateral spine lies to the side may facilitate identification. Eggs measure 114 to 180 μm by 45 to 73 μm. (*From* Smith *et al.* [7]; with permission.)

# MANIFESTATIONS OF CESTODES

| Important cestodes (tapeworms) in Latin America |
| --- |
| *Echinococcus granulosus* (echinococcosis)<br>*Taenia saginata* (taeniasis)<br>*Taenia solium* (taeniasis, cysticercosis) |

**FIGURE 12-66** Important cestodes (tapeworms) in Latin America. Humans are the definitive host for several species of tapeworms. Adult tapeworms reside in the gastrointestinal tract and release proglottides and ova into the feces. *Taenia solium*, the pork tapeworm, is important because humans also serve as an intermediate host when they ingest ova in fecally contaminated water or food. The resulting condition, cysticercosis, is responsible for substantial morbidity and mortality in Latin America.

## *Taenia solium* (Taeniasis)

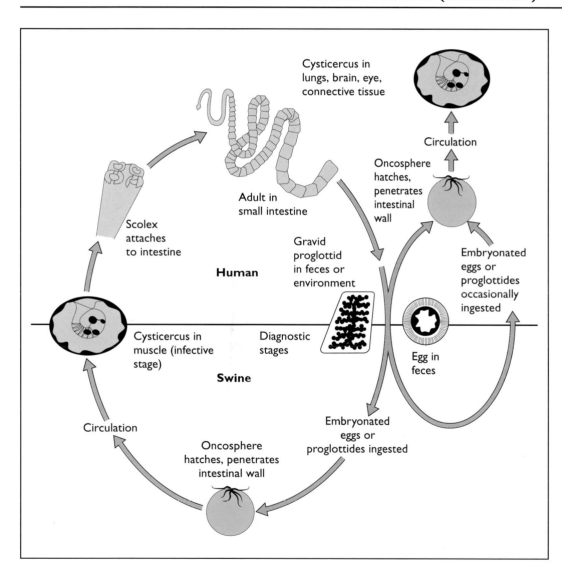

**FIGURE 12-67** Life cycle of *Taenia solium*. The ingestion of pork infected with cysticerci, the tissue larval stage, results in infestation of the human small intestine (definitive host) by the adult tapeworm. The terminal gravid proglottides of the adult tapeworm that develop in the intestine are excreted in the feces. The eggs released from these proglottides contaminate the environment and can be ingested by pigs or man. The eggs mature into true larvae in the small intestine and migrate through the intestinal mucosa into blood vessels, migrating to various tissues including muscle (intermediate host). (*Adapted from* Melvin *et al.* [20].)

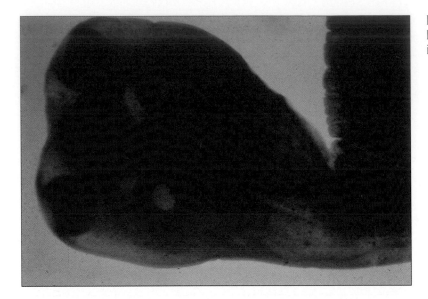

**FIGURE 12-68**    *Taenia solium* scolex. Humans are the definitive host for *T. solium*. The adult worm resides in the human small intestine. (*From* Smith *et al.* [7]; with permission.)

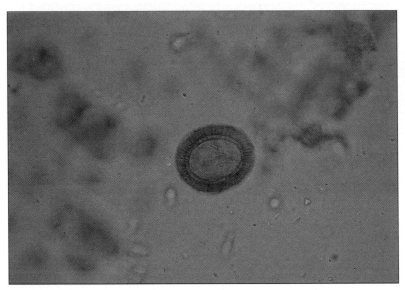

**FIGURE 12-69**    *Taenia* species, ova. Ova and proglottides of *Taenia solium* are excreted in the stool. Humans become an intermediate host when they ingest the ova. This ovum demonstrates the thick, bile-stained, radially striated shell enclosing a six-hooked embryo. The ova may stain so darkly with iodine that the egg resembles a pollen grain. Confirmation of the diagnosis depends on visualization of the six hooks of the embryo. Ova measure 31 by 43 μm in diameter. The ova of *T. solium* and *T. saginata*, the beef tapeworm, are morphologically indistinguishable. (*From* Smith *et al.* [7]; with permission.)

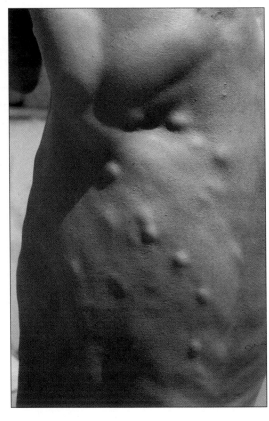

**FIGURE 12-70**    Cysticerci in subcutaneous tissue.

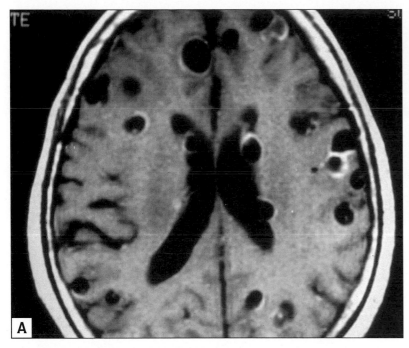

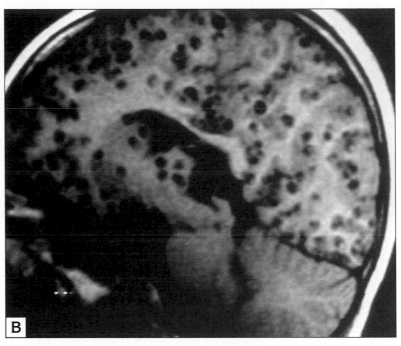

**FIGURE 12-71** Neurocysticercosis due to *Taenia solium* seen on magnetic resonance scans. **A**, Some cysts are surrounded by edema and inflammation resulting from the release of cysticercal antigens. Neurocysticercosis is a common cause of seizures and focal neurologic abnormalities in Latin America. **B**, Severe neuro-cyticercosis seen on a sagittal view in a magnetic resonance image.

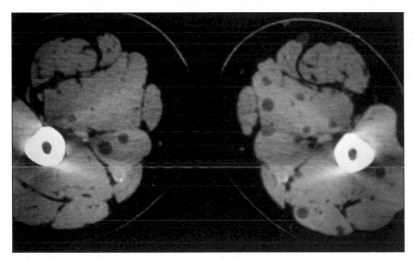

**FIGURE 12-72** *Taenia solium*, cysticerci in muscle seen on magnetic resonance imaging.

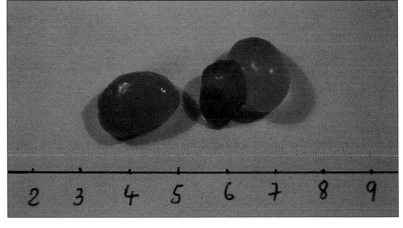

**FIGURE 12-73** *Taenia solium*, cysticerci dissected from tissue. Each larval cyst, formerly known as *Cysticercus cellulosae*, contains a single scolex inverted in a fluid-filled bladder. The cysticercus develops into an adult tapeworm in the gut of the definitive human host.

**FIGURE 12-74** *Taenia solium* cysticercus seen in a tissue section of brain. The scolex region of the cysticercus is in the center. The typical hooks are evident within the inverted scolex. (Hematoxylin-eosin stain, low power). (*From* Smith *et al.* [7]; with permission.)

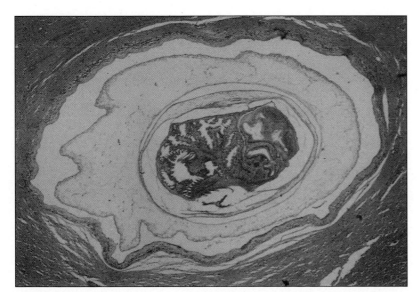

# REFERENCES

1. Mahmoud AAF: Diseases due to helminths: Introduction. *In* Mandell GL, Bennett JE, Dolin R (eds.): *Principles and Practice of Infectious Diseases*, 4th ed. New York: Churchill Livingstone; 1995:2525–2526.

2. Ravdin JI: Protozoal diseases: Introduction. *In* Mandell GL, Bennett JE, Dolin R (eds.): *Principles and Practice of Infectious Diseases*, 4th ed. New York: Churchill Livingstone; 1995:2393–2395.

3. *CDC Health Information for International Travel 1995*. Atlanta: Centers for Disease Control and Prevention; 1995:163–165. (HHS publ. no. [CDC] 95-8280.)

4. Wyler DJ: *Plasmodium* species (malaria). *In* Mandell GL, Douglas RG Jr, Bennett JE (eds.): *Principles and Practice of Infectious Diseases*, 3rd ed. New York: Churchill Livingstone; 1990:2057.

5. White NJ, Breman JG: Malaria and babesiosis. *In* Isselbacher KJ, Braunwald E, Wilson JD, *et al.* (eds.): *Harrison's Principles of Internal Medicine*, 13th ed. New York: McGraw-Hill; 1994:889.

6. Miller LH, Good MF, Milon G: Malaria pathogenesis. *Science* 1994, 264:1880.

7. Smith WJ, *et al.*: Blood and tissue parasites [revised reprint]. *In Atlas of Diagnostic Medical Parasitology Series*. Chicago: American Society of Clinical Pathology, 1976 [revised 1984].

8. Drugs for parasitic infections. *Med Lett Drugs Ther* 1995, 37:102–104.

9. Pearson RD, Sousa AQ: *Leishmania* species: Visceral (kala-azar), cutaneous and mucosal leishmaniasis. *In* Mandell GL, Bennett JE, Dolin R (eds.): *Principles and Practice of Infectious Diseases*, 4th ed. New York: Churchill Livingstone; 1995:2428.

10. Chenoweth CE, Singal S, Pearson RD, *et al.*: AIDS-related visceral leishmaniasis presenting in a pleural effusion. *Chest* 1993, 103:648–649.

11. Pearson RD, Wheeler DA, Harrison LH, *et al.*: The immunobiology of leishmaniasis. *Rev Infect Dis* 1983, 5:907–927.

12. *Curr Opinion Infect Dis* 1989, 2:631–638.

13. Kirchhoff LV: Trypanosoma species (American trypanosomiasis, Chagas' disease): Biology of trypanosomes. *In* Mandell GL, Bennett JE, Dolin R (eds.): *Principles and Practice of Infectious Diseases*, 4th ed. New York: Churchill Livingstone; 1995:2443.

14. Pearson RD: Parasitic diseases: Helminths. *In* Yamada T, *et al.* (eds.): *Atlas of Gastroenterology*. Philadelphia: J.B. Lippincott Co; 1991:394–399.

15. Petri WA Jr, Holsinger JR, Pearson RD: Common-source outbreak of trichinosis associated with eating raw home-butchered pork. *South Med J* 1988, 81:1056–1058.

16. Joyce MP, Pearson RD: Upper extremity swelling and hyperpigmentation due to onchocerciasis in an American. *South Med J* 1987, 81:1452–1454.

17. Muller R: Helminths. *In* Warren KS (ed.): *Immunology and Molecular Biology of Parasitic Infections*, 3d ed. Boston: Blackwell; 1993:567–598.

18. Mahmoud AAF: Trematodes (schistosomiasis) and other flukes. *In* Mandell GL, Bennett JE, Dolin R (eds.): *Principles and Practice of Infectious Diseases*, 4th ed. New York: Churchill Livingstone; 1995:2539.

19. Laughlin LW: Schistosomiasis. *In* Strickland GT (ed.): *Hunter's Tropical Medicine*, 6th ed. Philadelphia: W.B. Saunders, 1984:714.

20. Melvin DM, Brooke MM, Sadun EH: *Common Intestinal Helminths of Man*. Atlanta: Centers for Disease Control and Prevention; 1964. (DHEW publ. no. [CDC] 72-8286.)

# SELECTED BIBLIOGRAPHY

Guerrant RL, Sousa MA, Nations MK (eds.): *At the Edge of Development: Health Crisis in a Transitional Society*. Chapel Hill, NC: North Carolina University Press; 1996 (in press).

Mandell GL, Bennett JE, Dolin R (eds.): *Principles and Practice of Infectious Diseases*, 4th ed. New York: Churchill Livingstone; 1995.

Neva FA, Brown HW: *Basic Clinical Parasitology*, 8th ed. Norwalk, CT: Appleton & Lange; 1994.

Strickland GT (ed.): *Hunter's Tropical Medicine*, 7th ed. Philadelphia: W.B. Saunders Co.; 1991.

# CHAPTER 13

## Cutaneous Manifestations of Infection in the Immunocompromised Host

Donald Armstrong

## A. Epidemiologic considerations in opportunistic infections: Geographic factors

| Types of organisms | Comments |
|---|---|
| **Bacteria** | |
| *Mycobacterium tuberculosis* | More common in developing countries, inner cities in the United States |
| **Fungi** | |
| *Histoplasma capsulatum* | More common in Mississippi and Ohio River valleys in North America and in Central and South America; latent infection |
| *Coccidioides immitis* | |
| **Parasites** | |
| *Strongyloides stercoralis* | More common in tropics and subtropics |
| *Babesia* spp | Distribution nationally and internationally |
| *Plasmodium* spp | May be latent infection |
| **Viruses** | |
| Measles | Still endemic in developing countries; reappearing in United States |

## B. Epidemiologic considerations in opportunistic infections: Household exposures

| Types of organisms | Comments |
|---|---|
| **Bacteria** | |
| *Mycobacterium tuberculosis* | Household contacts at high risk |
| **Fungi** | |
| *Aspergillus* spp | Flourish in moist environments, including air conditioners and humidifiers |
| **Parasites** | |
| Scabies (*Sarcoptes scabiei*) | Children may bring home |
| **Viruses** | |
| Varicella-zoster | Home contacts a regular source |
| Cytomegalovirus | |
| Respiratory syncytial virus | |
| Influenza | |

**FIGURE 13-1** Epidemiologic considerations in opportunistic infections. Infections in the immunocompromised host depend on two main variables—the epidemiologic background of the patient and the specific area of the immune defense that is most compromised. Almost everyone of these organisms can cause skin lesions. Infections in immunocompromised hosts can reflect the different sources of infection, varying with geographic region as well as by occupational and avocational exposures. Hospitalization is a major contributing factor to infection in the immunocompromised patient. **A,** Geographic factors. **B,** Household exposures. (*continued*)

**C. Epidemiologic considerations in opportunistic infection: Work, habits, and hobbies**

**FIGURE 13-1** (*continued*) **C**, Work, habits, and hobbies. **D**, Hospital exposures. (*Adapted from* Armstrong [1].)

| Types of organisms | Comments |
| --- | --- |
| Bacteria | |
| *Capnocytophaga canimosis* | Dogs |
| *Campylobacter* spp | Pets |
| *Listeria monocytogenes* | Farm animals, pets; ingestion of various foods |
| *Rhodococcus equi* | Farm animals |
| *Aeromonas hydrophila* | Freshwater (wading) |
| Fungi | |
| *Cryptococcus neoformans* | Pigeons |
| *Histoplasma capsulatum* | Chicken coops, pigeons, birding, spelunking |
| Parasites | |
| *Toxoplasma gondii* | Cats, raw meat consumption |
| *Strongyloides stercoralis* | Walking barefooted |
| Scabies | Nursery schools; crowded, poor environments |
| *Giardia lamblia* | Outbreaks in ski resorts and certain countries |
| *Plasmodium* | Outdoor recreation increases risk |
| *Babesia* | |
| Viruses | |
| Cytomegalovirus | STD especially among promiscuous persons |
| Herpes simplex | STD |

STD—sexually transmitted disease.

**D. Epidemiologic considerations in opportunistic infections: Hospital exposures**

| Types of organisms | Comments |
| --- | --- |
| Bacteria | |
| *Streptococcus viridans* | Organisms vary among hospitals; some are associated |
| *Enterococcus faecium* | with colonization, such as Enterobacteriaceae and |
| *Staphylococcus* spp | *P. aeruginosa*, and others with procedures, such as |
| *Pseudomonas aeruginosa* | *S. marcescens* and *Pseudomonas* |
| *Klebsiella pneumoniae* | |
| *Serratia marcescens* | |
| *Pseudomonas* | |
| *Corynebacterium* CDC-JK | |
| *Salmonella* spp | |
| *Legionella* spp | |
| *Mycobacterium tuberculosis* | |
| Fungi | |
| *Candida albicans* | All associated with neutropenia |
| *Candida tropicalis* | Associated with administration of total parenteral |
| *Candida parapsilosis* | nutrition |
| *Candida krusei* | |
| *Aspergillus* spp | *A. flavus* associated with construction |
| Mucoraceae | |
| Parasites | |
| *Pneumocystis carinii* | Can be prevented by early diagnosis and isolation |
| Scabies (*Sarcoptes scabiei*) | techniques |
| Viruses | |
| Influenza | Spread by aerosolization and contact with |
| Varicella-zoster | secretions/excretions |
| Cytomegalovirus | |
| Respiratory syncytial virus | |

## A. Immune defects and anticipated infecting organisms in immunocompromised hosts: Surgical and invasive procedures

| Immune defect | Bacteria | Fungi | Parasites | Viruses |
|---|---|---|---|---|
| Interrupted integument<br> IV needles and catheters<br> Chemotherapy-induced GI ulcers<br> Finger or bone marrow puncture<br> Bladder catheters | Streptococci<br>Staphylococci<br>Enterobacteriaceae<br>*Pseudomonas aeruginosa*<br>*Corynebacterium* spp<br>Water-borne organisms<br> (*eg, Serratia marcescens,*<br> *Pseudomonas*) | *Candida*<br>Mucoraceae<br>*Aspergillus*<br>*Fusarium*<br>*Rhodotorula* | — | — |
| Infusion infection<br> Blood products<br> IV fluids | *Salmonella* spp<br>*Enterobacter* spp | *Candida* | *Plasmodium* spp<br>*Toxoplasma gondii*<br>*Babesia* spp<br>*Trypanosoma cruzi* | Hepatitis B, C virus<br>Cytomegalovirus<br>Epstein-Barr virus<br>HIV-1<br>Human T-cell lymphotropic<br> virus I, II |
| Surgical procedure<br> Tracheostomy<br> Respiratory assistance endoscopies<br> GI or gynecologic surgery | Streptococci<br>Staphylococci<br>Enterobacteriaceae<br>*Pseudomonas aeruginosa*<br>*Bacteroides fragilis* | *Candida* | — | Herpes simplex virus |

GI—gastrointestinal; IV—intravenous.

## B. Immune defects and anticipated infecting organisms in immunocompromised hosts: Neutrophil and T-lymphocyte dysfunction

| Immune defect | Bacteria | Fungi | Parasites | Viruses |
|---|---|---|---|---|
| Neutrophil dysfunction<br> Acute leukemia<br> Chemotherapy | *Streptococcus* spp<br>*Staphylococcus aureus*<br>Enterobacteriaceae<br>*Pseudomonas aeruginosa*<br>Enterococci | *Candida*<br>*Aspergillus*<br>Mucoraceae<br>*Trichosporon*<br>*Fusarium*<br>*Pseudallescheria boydii* | — | — |
| T-lymphocyte dysfunction<br> Hodgkin's disease<br> Transplantation<br> HIV infection | *Listeria monocytogenes*<br>*Salmonella* spp<br>*Nocardia asteroides*<br>*Mycobacterium* spp<br>*Legionella* spp<br>*Rhodococcus equi* | *Cryptococcus neoformans*<br>*Candida* spp<br>*Histoplasma capsulatum*<br>*Coccidioides immitis*<br>*Penicillin marnefii* | *Pneumocystis carinii*<br>*Toxoplasma gondii*<br>*Strongyloides stercoralis*<br>*Cryptosporidium*<br>*Isospora belli*<br>*Microsporidium* | Measles<br>Varicella-zoster virus<br>Cytomegalovirus<br>Adenovirus<br>Respiratory syncytial<br> virus |

**FIGURE 13-2** Immune defects and anticipated infecting organisms in immunocompromised hosts. The specific immune defects that characterize each patient's case help to direct evaluation and management. Patients may have a neutrophil defect, splenic or B-cell defect, T-cell dysfunction, dysfunction of gamma globulin or complement, and/or an interrupted integument or other invasive in-hospital procedure. Each of these disorders is likely to be associated with its own spectrum of potential pathogens. Of these predisposing factors to infection, neutrophil and splenic defects are the most serious. Most of the organisms listed in these tables can cause skin lesions. **A**, Surgical and invasive procedures. **B**, Neutrophil and T-lymphocyte dysfunction. (*continued*)

**C. Immune defects and anticipated infecting organisms in immunocompromised hosts: Globulin, complement, and splenic dysfunction**

| Immune defect | Bacteria | Fungi | Parasites | Viruses |
|---|---|---|---|---|
| **Globulin dysfunction** | | | | |
| Multiple myeloma | *Streptococcus pneumoniae* | — | *Pneumocystis carinii* | Echovirus |
| Chronic lymphocytic leukemia | *Haemophilus influenza* | | *Giardia lamblia* | |
| | *Neisseria meningitidis* | | | |
| **Complement dysfunction** | | | | |
| Congenital defects | *Neisseria* spp | — | — | — |
| **Splenic dysfunction** | | | | |
| Staging laporatomy for | *Haemophilus influenzae* | — | *Plasmodium* spp | — |
| Hodgkin's disease | *Streptococcus pneumoniae* | | *Babesia* spp | |
| Posttraumatic | *Neisseria meningitidis* | | | |

**FIGURE 13-2** (*continued*) **C**, Globulin, complement, and splenic dysfunction. (*Adapted from* Armstrong [1].)

**A. Microorganisms most often associated with skin lesions in opportunistic infections, by type of immune defect: Neutrophil defects**

| Bacteria | Fungi | Parasites | Viruses |
|---|---|---|---|
| Streptococci | *Candida* | — | — |
| S. pyogenes | | | |
| Viridans | | | |
| *Staphylococcus aureus* | *Aspergillus* | | |
| *Clostridium perfringens* | Mucoraceae | | |
| *Pseudomonas aeruginosa* | Fusarium | | |
| *Aeromonas hydrophila* | *Pseudallescheria boydii* | | |
| Enterobacteriaceae | *Trichosporon bigellei* | | |

**B. Microorganisms most often associated with skin lesions in opportunistic infection, by type of immune defect: T-lymphocyte defects**

| Bacteria | Fungi | Parasites | Viruses |
|---|---|---|---|
| *Listeria monocytogenes* | *Cryptococcus neoformans* | *Toxoplasma gondii* | Measles |
| *Salmonella* spp | | | |
| *Nocardia asteroides* | *Candida* spp | *Strongyloides stercoralis* | Varicella-zoster virus |
| *Legionella* spp | | | |
| *Rhodococcus equi* | *Histoplasma capsulatum* | | Cytomegalovirus |
| *Mycobacterium* *haemophilum* | *Coccidioides immitis* | | Herpes simplex virus |
| *Mycobacterium* spp | *Penicillium marnefei* | | Adenovirus |

**FIGURE 13-3** Microorganisms most often associated with skin lesions in opportunistic infections, by type of immune defect. Skin lesions usually are not diagnostic on history and physical examination, with a few exceptions, such as herpes zoster. Even these lesions may be atypical in the immunocompromised patient. It is essential to try to make a specific microbial diagnosis in such patients because the appearance of a skin lesion often represents late, hematogenous spread of the infection, and because the identification plus susceptibility studies, when available, can direct therapy. Testing almost always requires an aspirate, if not a biopsy of the lesion, and the sooner the better. If the aspirate is not revealing on direct smear and the patient's condition requires rapid action, a biopsy should be done immediately, including appropriate cultures and histopathologic studies. The more common causes of skin lesions according to the immune defect are listed: **A**, Neutrophil defect. **B**, T-lymphocyte defect. (*continued*)

**C. Microorganisms most often associated with skin lesions in opportunistic infections, by type of immune defect: Globulin, complement, and splenic defects**

| | Bacteria | Fungi | Parasites | Viruses |
|---|---|---|---|---|
| Globulin defect | *Neisseria meningitidis* | — | — | Echovirus |
| | *Streptococcus pneumoniae* | | | |
| Complement defect | *Neisseria* spp | — | — | — |
| Splenic defect | *Neisseria meningitidis* | — | — | — |
| | *Streptococcus pneumoniae* | | | |

**Figure 13-3** (*continued*) **C,** Globulin, complement, and splenic defects.

# NEUTROPHIL DEFECTS

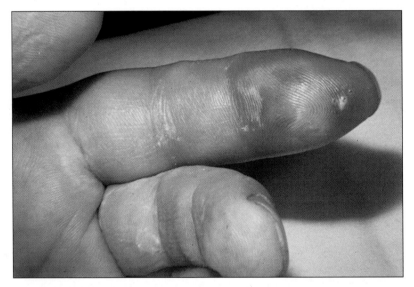

**Figure 13-4** Skin lesion on a finger due to *Staphylococcus aureus*. Skin lesions due to *S. aureus* in the immunocompromised host can take many forms, ranging from papules to pustules to ulcers or blebs. Cellulitis also may be seen. The bleb on this patient's finger was at the site of a skin puncture for a complete blood count. On aspiration, the bleb yielded gram-positive cocci on staining and *S. aureus* in culture. Sensitivity studies showed it to be sensitive to methicillin. The patient responded to intravenous therapy with oxacillin. We have isolated mixed cultures of *S. aureus* and *Clostridium perfringens* from such lesions and have added high-dose penicillin to the oxacillin. Mixed infections with *Streptococcus pyogenes* and *S. aureus* also may be seen. Viridans streptococci can cause acute septic syndromes with a maculopapular skin rash and rapid progression to septic shock. The organisms may be resistant to β-lactam antibiotics and require vancomycin. Smears, cultures, and susceptibility studies are all important studies in the patient's evaluation.

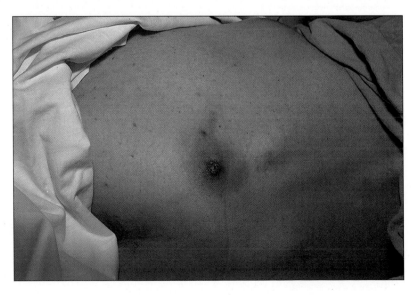

**Figure 13-5** Lesion due to mixed infection on a patient's lower back. This lesion, in a neutropenic patient, was due to a mixture of *Staphylococcus aureus* and *Pseudomonas aeruginosa*. Patients may become septic due to more than one organism when they are profoundly neutropenic or when intravenous catheters become contaminated and result in polymicrobial sepsis.

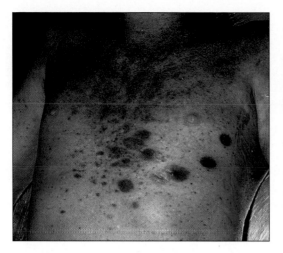

**FIGURE 13-6** Classic ecthyma gangrenosum secondary to *Pseudomonas aeruginosa* infection. The black centers set on a red raised papule result from invasion of blood vessels, with clotting and subsequent infarction and necrosis of tissue. *P. aeruginosa* also can produce vesicles, blebs, and cellulitis.

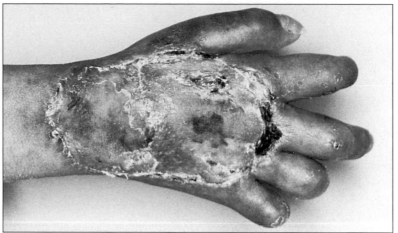

**FIGURE 13-7** Ecthyma gangrenosum due to *Pseudomonas aeruginosa* with sloughing of the skin of the hand down to the muscle. The lesion occurred at the site of an intravenous line in a patient with leukemia. The patient went into remission following cytotoxic chemotherapy and produced neutrophils, which then appeared as pus in the lesion. The black infarcted tissue then sloughed, and skin grafting was required to fill the defect.

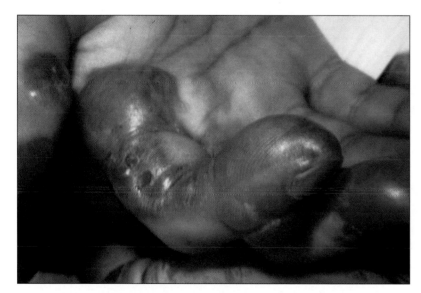

**FIGURE 13-8** Cellulitis of the hand due to *Proteus* species. *Escherichia coli* or *Klebsiella pneumoniae* also may cause papular lesions after hematogenous spread to the skin, and if there is hemorrhage into the center of the lesion, they can look like ecthyma gangrenosum due to *Pseudomonas aeruginosa* or *Aeromonas hydrophila*. Rarely, a cellulitis may appear due to the Enterobacteriaceae, including *Proteus* species or *Enterobacter* species as well as *P. aeruginosa* or *A. hydrophilia*. If aspiration of one of these lesions is unproductive, then injection and aspiration of 0.5 to 1 mL of sterile saline into the lesion may yield organisms. If not, the lesion should undergo biopsy for smear, culture, and histopathology. A methenamine silver stain should be done on the histopathologic section as well as a Gram stain. Fungi are more readily detectable on silver stain. These lesions of the hand started as cellulitis, developed into blebs, and were due to *Proteus rettgeri*.

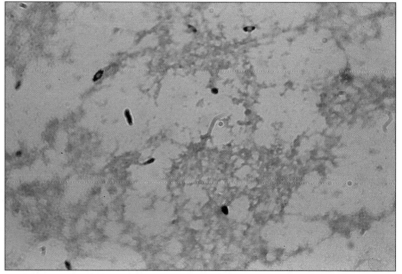

**FIGURE 13-9** Gram-positive rods of *Clostridium perfringens* seen on an aspirate of cellulitis with *C. perfringens* sepsis. The organisms are large, box-shaped rods and suggest the diagnosis by their appearance. An anaerobic culture also is necessary. After the cellulitis appears in both flanks, it rapidly, within hours, spreads toward the midline. The cellulitis darkens as hemorrhage occurs, and crepitation then becomes evident. By this time, the prognosis is grave. Alertness, despite hypotension, and a pulse more rapid than expected with the degree of fever are hallmarks of this syndrome. Because of hemolysis, pulses of 150 bpm may be seen with temperatures of 102° F. Because these infections arise in necrotic tumors of lymphoma or leukemic infiltrates of the bowel, Enterobacteriaceae or other bowel flora may accompany the *C. perfringens* and should be anticipated in empiric treatment. With this approach, the mortality rate has fallen from 90% to 50%.

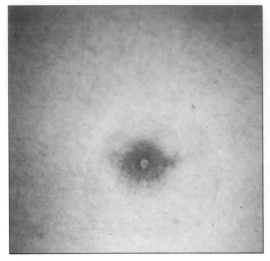

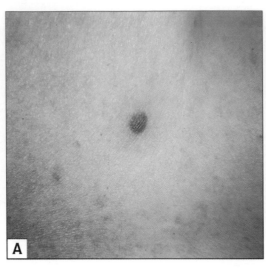

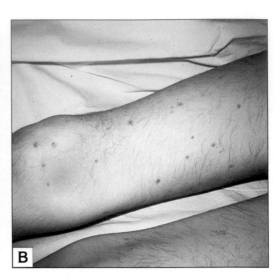

**FIGURE 13-10** Skin lesion in disseminated candidiasis. Fungi may produce a variety of skin lesions, but they are usually papular with or without a necrotic or pustular center. This lesion was due to *Candida albicans*; the source was probably the gastrointestinal tract, with the skin being infected by hematogenous spread. The patient also had hematogenous spread of infection to the lungs. Another route of entry for *Candida* species is an indwelling intravenous catheter.

**FIGURE 13-11** Skin lesions in disseminated candidiasis. Candidiasis may result in few or many lesions, and the lesions can be expected to contain the organisms. If a Gram stain of an aspirate is negative, a biopsy should be done immediately. **A**, A patient with a few isolated lesions due to *Candida*. **B**, A patient with many scattered lesions over the legs due to *Candida*. These lesions have a purplish hue due to hemorrhage into them.

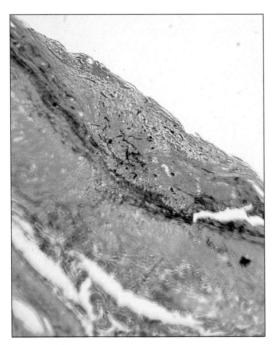

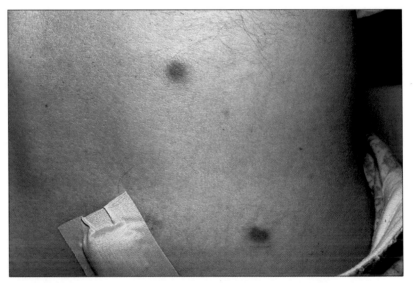

**FIGURE 13-12** Gomori methenamine silver stain showing pseudohyphae of *Candida tropicalis*. Smears of a skin lesion of a febrile, neutropenic patient proved to be negative, so a biopsy was done. Yeasts with pseudohyphae can be readily seen. The culture yielded *C. tropicalis*. The blood cultures were positive, but the source was not clear and thus was assumed to be the gastrointestinal tract. Quantitative blood cultures often reveal higher counts from an intravenous catheter than from a peripheral vein, a finding which is diagnostic for a catheter-induced infection if the catheter count is 10 times higher than the peripheral vein count.

**FIGURE 13-13** Skin lesions of trichosporosis. This febrile neutropenic patient developed skin lesions while receiving broad-spectrum antibacterial therapy. He also had a hemorrhagic pharyngitis. Biopsy of a skin lesion and the hemorrhagic material from the throat yielded *Trichosporon beigelii*. It is important to isolate the organism, because *T. beigelii* may be resistant to amphotericin B and most azoles except miconazole.

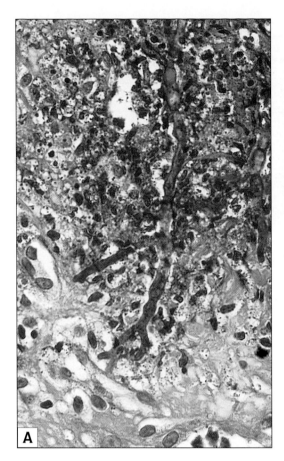

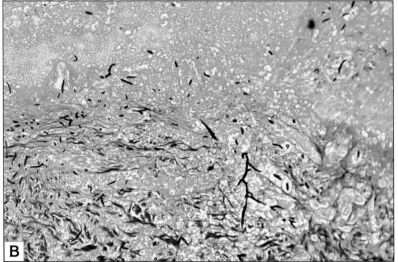

**FIGURE 13-14** Tissue stains in disseminated aspergillosis. A skin lesion that was indistinguishable from those caused by bacteria, *Candida, Mucoraceae, Trichosporon,* or other fungi yielded a few organisms or *Aspergillus flavus* when cultured. The source in a case of *A. flavus* infection may be the sinuses, as in this case, but more often it will be the lungs, where *A. flavus* causes pneumonia. **A,** The organism is seen on hematoxylin-eosin stain. **B,** The same biopsy specimen, at lower power on methamine silver stain. Acutely branching septate hyphae typical of an *Aspergillus* species can be seen. We usually use higher doses of amphotericin B (*eg,* in the 1.25-mg/g range) to treat *Aspergillus* infection, because of relative resistance.

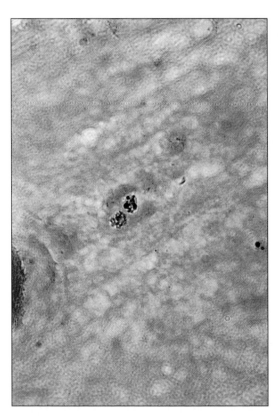

**FIGURE 13-15** Gram stain of tissue showing atypical organisms of *Candida albicans* from a cold abscess. The patient had leukemia and cytotoxic chemotherapy-induced neutropenia and went into remission. At the same time, a swelling, which was not hot or erythematous and only slightly tender, appeared below her mandible. On biopsy, organisms were seen, isolated, and identified as *C. albicans.* They are atypical in appearance—stippled rather than solidly gram-positive—and resemble those organisms (often difficult to grow) found in the livers and spleens of patients with hepatosplenic candidiasis following remission of leukemia. They presumably have been affected by the host's immune response.

# T-CELL DEFECTS

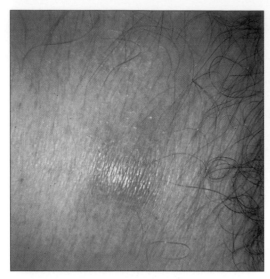

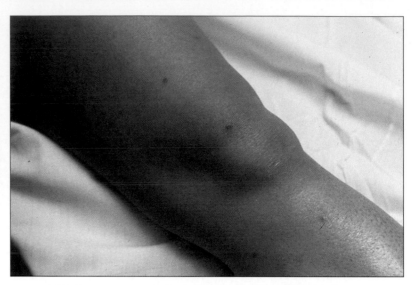

**FIGURE 13-16** Nodular lesion of nocardiasis in the groin of a patient with Hodgkin's disease. The lesion was not tender or warm and only slightly red. It presented as a cold abscess along with a pneumonia. Aspiration with a #21 needle did not yield any organisms, but a #18 needle yielded thick, purulent material that contained *Nocardia asteroides*. Some *Nocardia* skin lesions present as cold abscesses, and others may be typically warm, red, and tender. It may require a #15 needle to aspirate the thick pus. Because sputum specimens may be repeatedly negative, a skin lesion can offer an early diagnosis of *N. asteroides* infection.

**FIGURE 13-17** Vesicular skin lesions and joint disease due to *Mycobacterium haemophilum* in a bone marrow transplant recipient. The patient developed papular, vesicular, and pustular lesions along with an arthritis of the knee. Aspirate of a vesicular skin lesion revealed numerous acid-fast bacilli but no growth on routine mycobacterial cultures. The specimen was, however, grown at room temperature with hemosiderin to encourage the growth of *M. haemophilum*. The laboratory must be alerted to the need for special culture requirements when *M. haemophilum* is suspected. The disease is seen in patients with AIDS, lymphomas, multiple myeloma, and bone marrow or solid organ transplants and should be anticipated in anyone with a T-cell defect and skin and joint disease. In severe cases, pneumonia may result.

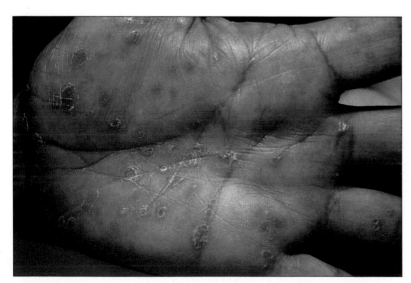

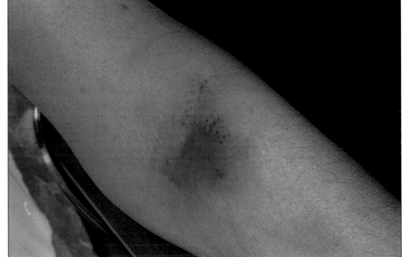

**FIGURE 13-18** Palmar skin lesions of secondary syphilis in a patient with suspected lymphoma. Speculation as to the cause of these lesions was far-reaching. A Venereal Disease Research Laboratories test lead to the diagnosis of the great imitator, syphilis, in its secondary stage. The lymph nodes, which were markedly enlarged, disappeared after treatment with penicillin. The biopsy showed spirochetes in an inflamed lymph node. (*Courtesy of* M.J. Chiu, MD.)

**FIGURE 13-19** Cryptococcal cellulitis at a venipuncture site in the forearm of a patient with chronic lymphocytic leukemia. A patient with chronic lymphocyte leukemia but normal neutrophils on chemotherapy developed fever and an area of cellulitis at the site of a venipuncture. An aspirate of this area of cellulitis yielded *Cryptococcus neoformans*, and a subsequent blood culture was positive. Cryptococcosis is the leading life-threatening fungal infection in AIDS patients and is seen in other patients with T-helper lymphocyte defects. It can cause a variety of skin lesions, ranging from papules to ulcers to cellulitis, as seen in this patient.

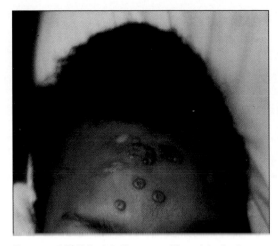

**FIGURE 13-20** Molluscum-like skin lesions due to disseminated cryptococcosis. Skin lesions due to *C. neoformans* in AIDS patients frequently take the form of umbilicated, raised, molluscum-like lesions. Biopsies reveal large numbers of cryptococci, and the antigen test is strongly positive. In these patients, serum antigens usually are strongly positive, and a lumber puncture should be done to look for evidence of central nervous system infection.

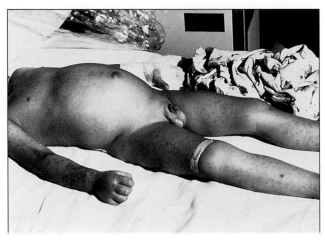

**FIGURE 13-21** Rash of disseminated histoplasmosis on the abdomen and legs of a child with leukemia. Histoplasmosis takes advantage of T-cell defects, often reactivating and disseminating years after the patient has left the endemic area. This diffuse rash appeared on the abdomen of a child aged 6 years after treatment for acute lymphoblastic leukemia, which included adenocorticosteroids, had induced remission. The lesions yielded *Histoplasma capsulatum* (small budding yeasts on smear), as did a blood culture of a bone marrow. The quickest method to establish the diagnosis is by biopsy of a skin lesion; the next is by aspiration and/or biopsy of the bone marrow.

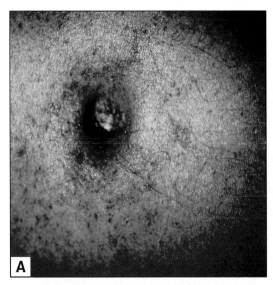

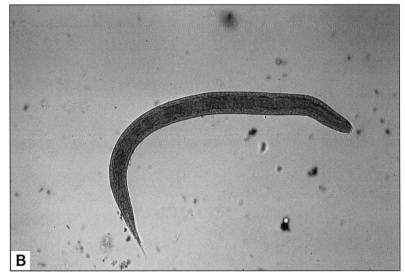

**FIGURE 13-22** Disseminated strongyloidiasis. This bone marrow transplant recipient developed abdominal signs and a pneumonia. **A,** A "thumbprint" rash developed around his umbilicus due to distended venules in that area secondary to a disseminated (hyperinfection syndrome) *Strongyloides stercoralis* infection. **B,** The organisms seen on a bronchoalveolar lavage specimen. (Panel 22A *from* Raffalli *et al.* [2]; with permission.)

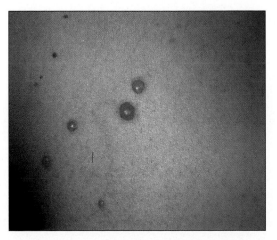

**FIGURE 13-23** Lesions of herpes zoster. Herpes zoster may disseminate in patients with T-cell defects and is easy to diagnose clinically if the sensory nerve distribution is obvious. Lesions can be atypical, particularly with acyclovir-resistant varicella-zoster virus, which may cause hemorrhagic lesions. In the immunocompromised patient, it is prudent to provide intravenous therapy until the disease is under control and then switch to oral therapy. Involvement of the central nervous system (CNS) can occur weeks to months after the skin lesions resolve, and this possibility should be considered in patients who develop CNS disease. CNS involvement may even resemble a brain abscess on computed tomography or magnetic resonance imaging scan. When the suspicion is high and toxoplasmosis or other causes of CNS disease such as lymphoma are unlikely, empiric therapy with acyclovir might be considered; however, a needle aspirate with direct fluorescent antibody studies for antigen and culture should be done when possible.

# REFERENCES

1.  Armstrong D: Management of fever and sepsis in the immunocompromised host. *Hosp Formul* 1994, 29(suppl 3):8–22.

2.  Raffalli J, Friedman C, Reid D, *et al.*: Diagnosis: Disseminated *Strongyloides stercoralis* infection. *Clin Infect Dis* 1995, 21:1459.

# SELECTED BIBLIOGRAPHY

Armstrong D: Empiric therapy for the immunocompromised host. *Rev Infect Dis* 1991, 13(suppl 9):S763–S769.

Armstrong D: Management of fever and sepsis in the immunocompromised host. *Hosp Formul* 1994, 29(suppl 3):8–22.

Brown AE, White MH: Controversies in the management of infections in immunocompromised patients. *Clin Infect Dis* 1992, 17(suppl 2):317–551.

Hughes WT, Armstrong D, Bodey GP, *et al.*: Guidelines for the use of antimicrobial agents in neutropenic patients with unexplained fever. *J Infect Dis* 1990, 161:381–396.

# INDEX